# NEURAL TUBE DEFECTS – ROLE OF FOLATE, PREVENTION STRATEGIES AND GENETICS

Edited by **Kannan Laksmi Narasimhan**

**Neural Tube Defects – Role of Folate, Prevention Strategies and Genetics**
Edited by Kannan Laksmi Narasimhan

**Published by InTech**
Janeza Trdine 9, 51000 Rijeka, Croatia



**Publishing Process Manager** Petra Nenadic

**Technical Editor** Teodora Smiljanic

**Cover Designe**r InTech Design Team

Additional hard copies can be obtained from orders@intechopen.com

Neural Tube Defects – Role of Folate, Prevention Strategies and Genetics,
Edited by Kannan Laksmi Narasimhan
p. cm.
ISBN 978-953-51-0317-2

For EU product safety concerns:
IN TECH d.o.o., Prolaz Marije Krucifikse Kozulić 3, 51000 Rijeka, Croatia,
info@intechopen.com or visit our website at intechopen.com.

# Meet the editor

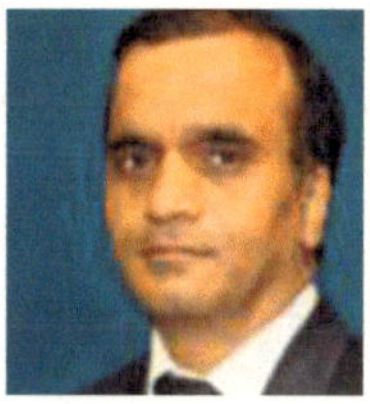

Professor K.L. Narasimhan completed his training in Pediatric Surgery in 1987 and has been interested in Pediatric Urology. He has been working on spina bifida from 1990. He has over 110 scientific publications in peer reviewed journals. He has special interest in prevention of neural tube defects. He also has several publications related to myelomeningoceles, neurogenic bladder, posterior urethral valves and obstructive uropathy.

# Contents

# Preface

The book Neural Tube Defects - Role of Folate, Prevention Strategies and Genetics has several eminent international authors and the book is a resource for anybody who is interested in this very important subject. The book has been divided into 3 sections; The role of Folic acid and prevention of Neural Tube disease which has seven chapters. Genetics of Neural Tube Defects having 3 chapters and a Surgical Treatment of Large Thoraco-lumbar Neural Tube Defects which includes a chapter on surgical treatment of large lumbo - sacral defects. The authors are distinguished and the chapters are a product of their extensive research.

I am glad that Intech took the initiative to publish this book for online free access.

**Dr. Kannan Laksmi Narasimhan**
Consultant in Ped Surgery,
KK women's and children's hospital,
Bukit Timah Road,
Singapore

# Part 1

# The Role of Folic Acid and Prevention of Neural Tube Disease

# 1

# The Role of Folic Acid in the Prevention of Neural Tube Defects

Lourdes García-Fragoso[1], Inés García-García[1] and Carmen L. Cadilla[2]
[1]*University of Puerto Rico, School of Medicine, Department of Pediatrics, Neonatology Section*
[2]*Department of Biochemistry*
*Puerto Rico*

## 1. Introduction

### 1.1 What is folic acid?

Folate is a water-soluble B vitamin that occurs naturally in food. Folic acid is the synthetic form of folate that is found in supplements and added to fortified foods. Folate gets its name from the Latin word "folium" for leaf. A key observation of researcher Lucy Wills nearly 70 years ago led to the identification of folate as the nutrient needed to prevent the anemia of pregnancy. Dr. Wills demonstrated that the anemia could be corrected by a yeast extract. Folate was identified as the corrective substance in yeast extract in the late 1930s, and was extracted from spinach leaves in 1941. Folate helps produce and maintain new cells. This is especially important during periods of rapid cell division and growth such as infancy and pregnancy. Folate is needed to make DNA and RNA, the building blocks of cells. It also helps prevent changes to DNA that may lead to cancer. Both adults and children need folate to make normal red blood cells and prevent anemia. Folate is also essential for the metabolism of homocysteine, and helps maintain normal levels of this amino acid (NIH, n.d).

Folic acid (pteroylmonoglutamic acid), which is the most oxidized and stable form of folate, occurs rarely in food but is the form used in vitamin supplements and in fortified food products. Folic acid consists of a *p*-aminobenzoic acid molecule linked at one end to a pteridine ring and at the other end to one glutamic acid molecule. Most naturally occurring folates, called *food folate* in some reports, are pteroylpolyglutamates, which contain one to six additional glutamate molecules joined in a peptide linkage to the γ-carboxyl of glutamate (IOM, 1998). Mammals are able to synthesize the pteridine ring but are unable to couple it to other compounds and are thus dependent on either dietary intake or bacterial synthesis within the intestine (Birn, 2006).

Dietary folates are a complex mixture of pteroylglutamates of various chain lengths and with a variety of substitutions on the pteridine ring. More than 90% of dietary folates exist as pteroylpolyglutamates, while the remaining is pteroymonoglutamate. The process of folate absorption requires a process involving hydrolysis to convert it to the monoglutamate form in the gut before absorption. An intestinal brush border pteroylpolyglutamate hydrolase (BB-PPH) has been identified in human and pig jejunum (Halsted, 1989). The pteroylmonoglutamyl folate form is absorbed along the entire length of the small intestine, although the jejunum is the primary site for its absorption. Pteroylglutamic acid is rapidly absorbed from the duodenum and jejunum by an active carrier-mediated transport mechanism involving the reduced folate carrier, and also by passive diffusion (Matherly & Goldman, 2003). Folate is not absorbed from the large intestine (otherwise, folate-producing colonic bacteria would be able to supply the body with considerable amounts of the vitamin). Enterohepatic circulation of folate occurs. A rise in blood folate level occurs as soon as 15 minutes after an oral dose (Butterworth, 1968; Olinger et al., 1973). The dominant folate form in serum is 5-methyl-tetrahydrofolate (5-MTHF) present either free, bound to high-affinity folate-binding protein (FBP), or loosely associated with other serum proteins including albumin (Matherly & Goldman, 2003).

Folates are widely distributed in tissues, most of them as polyglutamate derivatives. The main storage organ is the liver, which contains about half of the body's stores and represents 5 to 15 mg/kg of liver weight (Higdon, 2003). Total body content of folate has been estimated to be 38–96 mg (86–165 micromol) (Birn, 2006). A small amount is excreted in the feces and urine but the additional amounts are presumed to be metabolized and also lost by cells coming off in scales from body surfaces. Folate can be found in human milk. Folate is mainly required by organs or systems involved on the rapid proliferation of new cells. Folates are essential for normal cell division and growth. There are three stages of folic acid deficiency and high index of suspicion is needed because at the beginning may be subtle. After four to five months of continuing deficient intake of folates the clinical stage of folic megaloblastic acid anemia can be established. Aside of the bone marrow tissue, the immune system, mucous membranes, hair and fingernails may be affected as well (Shills, et al., 2006). Folate deficiency manifest primarily as anemia and physical symptoms that are considered to be classic include anemia, pallor, generalized weakness, mouth ulcers, an inflamed and sore tongue, peptic ulcers, a general numbness or tingling sensation in the hands and the feet, problems like indigestion and diarrhea, persistent depression, constant irritability and neurologic syndromes. In infants and children folate deficiency can be associated with slow overall growth rate. Folate deficiency during pregnancy increases the risk of prematurity and low birth weight (Herbert, 1999).

The folates cannot be significantly stored in the body and its replacement then requires a constant supply of the vitamin for preventing deficiency.The most common cause of folate deficiency is a low daily intake due to lack of ingestion of folate containing food, chronic alcoholism or total parenteral nutrition. Other causes can be related to impaired absorption, inadequate utilization, increased demand, and or increased excretion, or a combination of them. Impaired absorption includes Celiac disease (Sprue), gastric diseases that cause low stomach acid, congenital or acquired folate malabsorption and certain medications such as phenytoin, primidone and barbiturates. Numerous drugs are also known to inhibit the body's ability to utilize folate, including aspirin, cholesterol lowering drugs, oral birth control pills, antacids, and methotrexate when used for rheumatoid arthritis. Other nutrient deficiencies (zinc, riboflavin, niacin and vitamin $B_{12}$) may affect folates absorption and metabolism. Inadequate utilization may be seen in congenital or acquired enzyme deficiency and alcoholism. Alcohol interferes with folate metabolism and increases folate breakdown. Deficiency may be seen in the presence of an increased demand during pregnancy, lactation, infancy, increased metabolism as seen in paraneoplastic syndrome and in hemolytic anemia. Increased excretion can be secondary to renal dialysis (Johnson LE et al., 2007; Shills et al., 2006).

The primary indicator selected to determine folate adequacy is erythrocyte folate. Because folate is taken up only by the developing erythrocyte in the bone marrow and not by the circulating mature erythrocyte during its 120-day lifespan, erythrocyte folate concentration is an indicator of long-term status (IOM, 1998). If serum folate is < 3 ng/mL (< 7 nmol/L), deficiency is likely. Serum folate reflects folate status unless intake has recently increased or decreased. If intake has changed, erythrocyte (RBC) folate level better reflects tissue stores. A level of < 140 ng/mL (< 305 nmol/L) indicates inadequate status (Johnson LE et al., 2007).

### 1.2 Folate metabolism

Folate coenzymes play an important role in the metabolism of several amino acids, which are the building blocks of proteins. Tetrahydrofolic acid is involved in the formation of purines (adenine and guanine) and pyrimidines (thymidine) which are essential for the synthesis of the nucleic acids (DNA and RNA), responsible to carry the genetic instructions used in the development and functioning of all known living organisms. The 5-methyl THFA participates as a folate cofactor with vitamin $B_{12}$ in the methylation cycle where the methyl group is transferred to homocysteine to produce the aminoacid methionine. Methionine reacts with adenosine-5'-triphosphate (ATP) to produce S-adenosylmethionine which is the key methyl group donor. The methylation cycle is then essential to regulate deoxyribonucleic acid (DNA) gene expression, post-translational modification in proteins formation and synthesis of lipid synthesis. Methylation is also important step in the metabolism of neurotransmitters and detoxification of xenobiotics. Deficiency of 5-MeTHF causes accumulation of possible toxic metabolites such as homocysteine and, consequently, the inhibition of methyltransferases affecting gene expression, protein function and lipid and neurotransmitter metabolism (Blom et al., 2006; Gentili et al., 2009).

Folate in the 5-methyl THFA form is a cosubstrate required by methionine synthase when it converts homocysteine to methionine. As a result, in the scenario of folate deficiency, homocysteine accumulates (Gentili et al., 2009). High homocysteine levels are associated with an increased risk for atherosclerotic diseases, which has been linked with the risk of arterial disease, dementia and Alzheimer's disease. Accumulation of possibly toxic levels of homocysteine and impairment of methylation reactions involved in the regulation of gene expression also increase the neoplastic risks. Homocysteine and cysteine are associated with oxidative damage and metabolic disorders, which may lead to carcinogenesis (Eikelboom et al., 1999; Lin et al., 2010; Ray, 1998; Sedhadri et al., 2002).

### 1.3 Sources of folic acid in food

Natural foods like leafy green vegetables, spinach, brussel sprouts, turnip greens, potatoes, wheat germ, yeast, dried beans, legumes, fruits (such as citrus fruits and juices), and organ foods such as liver are rich sources of folate. Most dietary folates exist as polyglutamates, which are converted to the monoglutamate form and absorbed in the proximal small intestine. However, the body absorbs only about 50% of food folate. This problem is compounded by cooking practices such as prolonged stewing, processing, and storage, which can destroy some of the folate in natural foods (Talaulikar & Arulkumaran, 2011).

Red blood cell folate, plasma homocysteine and folate levels are used to determine the Recommended Dietary Allowance (RDA) of folate which reflects how much of this vitamin should be consumed daily. This recommended value can vary depending on age, gender, health status and other metabolic conditions. The synthetic folic acid has a greater bioavailability and the absorption is approximately 1.7 times higher from supplements and fortified foods compared with natural sources of folate. The USA Food and Nutrition Board of the Institute of Medicine recommended intakes for individuals as Daily Reference Intakes (DRI). The World Health Organization and several countries have their own set of DRIs recommendations. The 1998 USA Dietary Reference Intakes express the new Recommended Dietary Allowances for folate in dietary folate equivalents, which adjust for the nearly 50 percent of differences in the absorption of naturally occurring food folate and the more bioavailable synthetic folic acid: 1 μg of dietary folate equivalent = 0.6 μg of folic acid from fortified food or as a supplement taken with meals = 1 μg of food folate = 0.5 μg of a supplement taken on an empty stomach. (de Bree, 1997; IOM, 1998; Suitor & Bailey, 2000).

### 1.4 Relation of folic acid and neural tube defects

During the last decades, major interest has been devoted to preventable causes of central nervous system malformations such as neural tube defects (NTD). This term is applied to a variety of malformations resulting from incomplete to total absence of closure of the neural tube between 17 and 30 postconceptional days (Siebert et al., 1990; Volpe, 1994). The neural tube defects may present with different phenotypes depending on the affected region. The most vulnerable areas of the neural tube are the anterior and posterior neuropores because they are the last to close. Failure to close the anterior neural tube region results in anencephaly. Anencephaly is the most severe form of neural tube defect and is considered a lethal malformation (AAP & AHA, 2010).

Neural tube defects are a major cause of mortality in newborns and have been estimated to affect 0.5 to 8 per 1000 live births. Anencephaly and spina bifida are the most common manifestations of the spectrum (Gilbert, 2000; Siebert et al., 1990). Neural tube defects are considered multifactorial in origin with a combination of genetic and environmental influences predisposing its occurrence. It can be seen along with chromosomal abnormalities (trisomies 13 and 18), and other rare syndromes, and is associated to uncertain modes of inheritance (Hoyme, 1990; Saitoh et al., 2005; Volpe, 1994). Medications such as phenytoin, valproic acid, cotrimazole, aminopterin, thalidomide, carbamazepine, acetyl salicylic acid and efavirenz have been associated with an increased risk of NTD (Gilbert, 2000; Holmes et al., 1976; Hoyme, 1990; Volpe, 1994). Other factors such as maternal hyperthermia, maternal health status and metabolic disorders, ethnic variations, genetic predisposition, plasma vitamin levels, plasma folate levels, smoking, alcohol consumption and differences in folate metabolism have been implicated (Holmes ,1976; Larroche & Encha-Razavi, 1991; Saitoh et al., 2005; Sandford et al., 1992; Volpe, 1994).

In 1952, Thiersch reported the association of neural tube defects with the use of 4-aminopteroglutamic acid (Aminopterin), a folic acid antagonist, during early pregnancy. Edwards (1958) and Stein & Susser (1976) reported the association between dietary deficiencies and neural tube defects. The teratogenic effect of compromised nutrient intakes was confirmed in animal models (Miller, 1963; Seller, 1983). Folic acid deficiency was identified as cause of NTD and other birth defects in 1965 by Hibbard & Smithells, other studies by the later suggested that its supplementation could greatly reduce the incidence of these central nervous system malformations (Smithells, 1959, 1983). Since then, multiple research investigations have validated the role of folic acid in preventing neural tube defects (Watkins, 1998). Folate metabolism evaluation revealed that it is an important co-factor necessary in the conversion of homocysteine to methionine. Steegers-Theunissen et al. (1994) and Mills et al . (1995) reported elevated homocysteine levels in mothers of children with neural tube defects. Homocysteine is a sulfur amino acid formed by the demethylation of methionine and remethylated to conserve methionine. The methylation hypothesis points that the reason for failure of neural tube closure may be a relative shortage of methionine (methylation capacity) at a crucial stage of fetal development (Mills et al., 1995). Methionine is required for neural tube closure.

## 2. Mutations in folate-related enzymes

### 2.1 Methylenetetrahydrofolatereductase (MTHFR)

MTHFR catalyzes the conversion of of 5,10-methylenetetrahydrofolate to 5-methyltetrahydrofolate (Figure 1).This reaction is required for conversion of homocysteine to methionine by the enzyme methionine synthase. This conversion of homocysteine to methionine can also be catalyzed by the folate-independent enzyme betaine-homocysteinemethyltransferase (BHMT). 5,10-methylenetetrahydrofolate is used to convert dUMP to dTMP for *de novo* thymidine synthesis.MTHFR contains a bound flavin cofactor and uses NAD(P)H as the reducing agent. Because of the genetic complexity of folate metabolism, MTHFR alleles may be expected to interact with other folate-related genes and with folate consumption (van der Linden et al., 2006a).

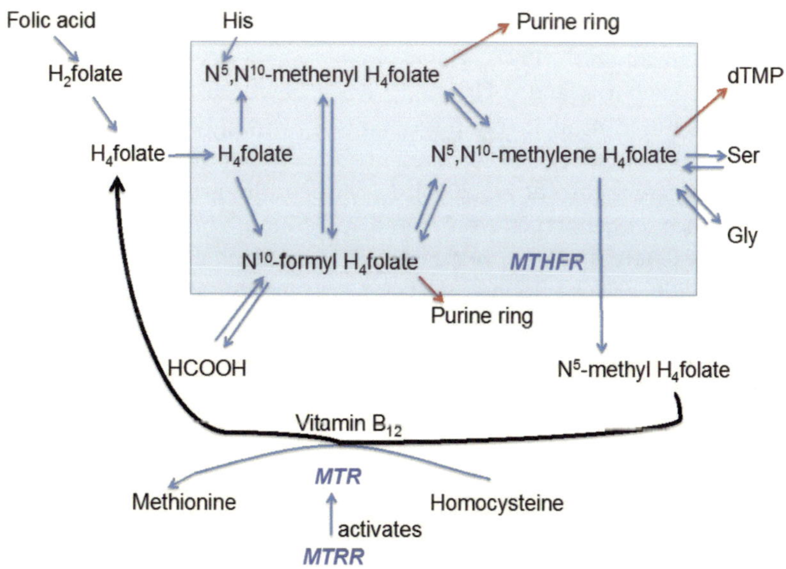


Fig. 1. One carbon metabolism. Interconversions of folic acid and its derivatives are indicated by blue arrows. Red arrows indicate pathways which depend exclusively on folate. A black arrow indicates the important B12-dependent reaction converting $N^5$-methyl tetrahydrofolate ($H_4$folate) back to $H_4$folate. The various one carbon derivatives of $H_4$folate are enclosed in the blue box overlay.

### 2.1.1 C677T

Among folate-related genes, the gene coding for 5,10-methylenetetrahydrofolate reductase (MTHFR) has been the principal focus of attention (Greene et al., 2009). A common polymorphism (677C-T, Ala222Val, rs1801133) was first identified as an important genetic risk factor in vascular disease (Frosst et al., 1995).This mutation creates a Hinf I site, which allows for easy screening of this missense mutation by PCR-RFLP. When lymphocyte extracts from individuals heterozygous or homozygous for this mutation were evaluated, reduced enzyme activity and increased thermolability was observed. In vitro expression of a cDNA bearing this missense mutation confirmed the thermolability of the mutant MTHFR. Thethermolabile enzyme with the 677C-T mutation is stabilized by folate (Frosst et al., 1995). When serum folate levels are greater than 15.4 nM, the effects of 677C-T mutations are neutralized (Jacques et al., 1996). In addition, individuals who are homozygous for the mutation have significantly elevated plasma homocysteine levels (Frosst et al., 1995). The first report that the 677C-T polymorphism was associated with increased risk of spina bifida (van der Put et al., 1995) was published shortly after, followed quickly by similar studies that included other NTDs (Botto & Yang, 2000a; Narasimhamurthy et al. 2010; Naushad et al, 2010; Possey et al., 1996; Shaw et al., 2009; van der Put et al., 1997; Whitehead et al., 1995). Homozygosity for 677C-T was associated with a 7.2 fold increased risk for NTDs (95% confidence interval: 1.8-30.3; p value: 0.001) (Ou, etal., 1996). Many subsequent studies had similar findings (García-Fragoso et al., 2002; Martínez de Villareal et al., 2001; Richter et al., 2001).

The 677C-T mutation was early on reported to be found more frequently among Caucasians than in African Americans (McAndrew, 1996). Among 151 consecutively born white infants in South Carolina, 20 were homozygous and 65 were heterozygous for the 677 T allele; among consecutive black newborns, none of 146 were homozygous, and 31 were heterozygous (Stevenson et al., 1997). The estimated allele frequency of the mutation was 0.35 among white newborns and 0.11 among black newborns. Subsequently, the 677C-T polymorphism was found in relatively high frequency throughout the world (for example, Schneider et al., 1998; Relton et al., 2004), even in admixed populations like that in the island of Puerto Rico (García-Fragoso et al., 2010). In Mexico, the proportion of CC (17.6%), CT (47.6%), and TT (34. 8%) genotypes were found to be high, with gene frequencies of 0.414 and 0.586% for the C and T alleles, respectively (Mutchinick et al., 1999). The 677T allele was, associated with one haplotype, G-T-A-C, in white and Japanese homozygotes (Rosenberg et al., 2002). Among the African individuals, analysis of maximum likelihood disclosed an association with the G-T-A-C haplotype, although none of the 174 subjects examined was homozygous for the 677C-T polymorphism. These results suggested that the 677C-T alteration occurred on a founder haplotype that may have had a selective advantage.

In contrast, other studies have found either no association of 677C-T with increased risk of NTD (for example, Boyles et al., 2006; Dávalos et al., 2000; Erdogan et al., 2010; Johnson WE et al., 1999; Stegmann et al., 1999,) or even a protective effect (Doudney et al., 2009 and Relton et al., 2003) of the 677C-T polymorphism. Yet, other studies suggested that additional candidate genes other than MTHFR may be responsible for an increased risk to NTD in some American Caucasian families (Rampersaud et al., 2003). A meta-analysis that included results from 27 studies concluded that the 677TT genotype confers an overall 1.9 times increase in risk of NTD (Blom et al., 2006). A more recent study included 37 different European populations from 32 studies and a total of 3,530 cases and 6,296 controls, where data was stratified according to geographical region and ethnicity, produced two separated meta-analyses for non-Latin European and Latin European descent populations (Amorim et al., 2007). No association was demonstrated for the 677TT genotype in Latin European populations (1.16; 0.95-1.43), while the non-Latin European meta-analyses (1.62; 1.38-1.90) indicated an association of the TT genotype and NTDs. The examination of non-Latin European studies revealed that the association of TT genotype with NTD has only been proven for Irish populations, both by case-control studies, and by family-based tests, such as the allele transmission disequilibrium test (TDT) (Amorim et al, 2007).

Genomic DNA methylation directly correlates with folate status and inversely with plasma homocysteine (tHcy) levels ($P < 0.01$) (Friso et al., 2002). The 677TT genotypes had a diminished levelof DNA methylation compared with those with the 677CC wild-type (32.23 vs.62.24 ng 5-methylcytosine/µg DNA, $P < 0.0001$). When analyzed according to folate status, however, only the 677TT subjects with low levels of folate accounted for the diminished DNA methylation ($P < 0.0001$). Moreover, in 677TT subjects, DNA methylationstatus correlated with the methylated proportion of red blood cell folate and was inversely related to the formylated proportion of red blood cell folates ($P < 0.03$), that is known to be solely represented in those individuals (Friso et al., 2002). These results indicate that the MTHFR C677T polymorphism influences DNA methylation status through an interaction with folate status.

It is clear from the many studies that have evaluated the MTHFR gene 677C-T polymorphism that it may elevate the risk of NTD in many populations, that the magnitude of the risk conferred by this mutation depends on nutritional factors and may range from close to 2-fold and possibly higher, depending on the ethnic group examined. Of all the folate gene polymorphisms, the 677C-T appears to be the most consistently present genetic factor conferring risk for NTDs.

### 2.1.2 A1298C

A second common mutation in the methylenetetrahydrofolatereductase gene (1298 A→C, glu429-to-ala (E429A, rs1801131) was reported in 1998 by van der Put et al. 1998 and Weisberg et al., 1998). The mutation destroys an MboII recognition site and had an allele frequency of 0.33 in Canadian subjects tested (van der Put, et al., 1998). This polymorphism was associated with decreased enzyme activity; homozygotes had approximately 60% of control activity in lymphocytes. Heterozygotes for both the C677T and the A1298C mutation, which accounted for approximately 15% of individuals in the Canadian study (Weisberg et al., 1998), had 50-60% of control activity, a value that was lower than that seen in single heterozygotes for the C677T variant. These results suggested that a combined heterozygosity for the two *MTHFR* common mutations may account for a proportion of folate-related neural tube defects. While the 677C-T transition occurs within the predicted catalytic domain of the MTHFR enzyme, the 1298A-C polymorphism is located in the presumed regulatory domain. Van der Put, et al., (1998) found that combined heterozygosity at the 2 polymorphic sites was associated with reduced MTHFR-specific activity, higher Hcy, and decreased plasma folate levels. This combined heterozygosity was observed in 28% of the neural tube defect (NTD) patients compared with 20% among controls, resulting in an odds ratio of 2.04. In NTD families in Italy and Turkey, the *MTHFR*A1298C polymorphism was found to be a genetic determinant for NTD risk

(Boduroğlu et al., 2005; De Marco et al., 2002) but there are conflicting studies in spina bifida occulta patients in Turkey (Eser et al., 2010). Other studies have failed to find an association between the 1298A-C polymorphism and risk of NTDs (Parle-McDermott et al., 2003).

Most 677T and 1298C alleles appear to be associated with 1298A and 677C alleles, respectively. There may be an increased frequency of the very rare cis 677T/1298C haplotype in some parts of the United Kingdom and Canada, possibly due to a founder effect (Ogino & Wilson, 2003). A Canadian study demonstrated that 677T and 1298C alleles could occur in both cis and trans configurations (Isotalo et al., 2000). Combined 677CT/1298CC and 677TT/1298CC genotypes, which contain three and four mutant alleles, respectively, were not observed in the neonatal group (P=.0402). This suggests decreased viability among fetuses carrying these mutations and a possible selection disadvantage among fetuses with increased numbers of mutant MTHFR alleles. Vaughn et al (2004) determined in 362 women 20–30 yrs of age that plasma homocysteine was inversely ($P < 0.0001$) associated with serum folate and plasma vitamin B-12 regardless of genotype. Plasma homocysteine was higher ($P < 0.05$) for women with the MTHFR 677 TT/1298 AA genotype combination compared with the CC/AA, CC/AC, and CT/AA genotypes.

### 2.2 Methionine synthase (MTR)

5-methyltetrahydrofolate-homocysteine S-methyltransferase (MTR), also known as methionine synthase, catalyzes the remethylation of homocysteine to form methionine. This remethylation reaction takes place in all cells, except erythrocytes. The MTR enzyme requires vitamin $B_{12}$ as a cofactor, and the MTR-cobalamin(I) complex then binds the methyl group of 5-methyl $H_4$folate to form methyl-cobalamin(III)MTR. When the methyl group is transferred to homocysteine, the cobalamin(I)MTR complex is reformed and available for another methyl donation step by 5-methyl $H_4$folate. Loss of function mutations in the *MTR* gene cause increased levels of plasma homocysteine. In liver and kidneys, homocysteine remethylation is carried out by another enzyme system, the betaine-homocysteinemethyltransferase enzyme, which is responsible for 50% of the homocysteine remethylation.

#### 2.2.1 A2756G

In 1996 Leclerc et al. identified a missense mutation and a 3 bp deletion in patients of the cobalamin (cblG) complementation group of inherited homocysteine/folate disorders by SSCP and DNA sequence analysis, as well as an amino acid substitution present in high frequency in the general population (2756A-G), which changes an aspartic acid residue to a glycine. This mutation is associated with relatively elevated homocysteine and relatively low vitamin B12 and red blood cell folate levels. In a study of 56 patients with spina bifida, 62 mothers of patients, 97 children without NTDs (controls), and 90 mothers of controls, the 2756A-G MTR polymorphism was associated with a decreased O.R. (O.R.); none of the cases and only 10% of controls were homozygous for this variant (Christensen et al., 1999). Doolin et al., (2002) studied the genetics of spina bifida in families (n = 209) that included at least one affected (i.e., with meningocele, meningomyelocele, or myelocele) member who were ascertained through several sources. Samples were obtained from the family member(s) affected with spina bifida (i.e., the proband) and his or her (their) parents, sibs, and maternal grandparents. Doolin et al (2002) assessed associations between maternal and offspring MTR and MTRR genotypes and spina bifida using the two-step TDT and using a log-linear approach. They determined that the risk of having a child with spina bifida appears to increase with the number of high-risk alleles in the maternal genotype for MTR (R1=2.16, 95% CI 0.92-5.06; R2=6.58, 95% CI 0.87-49.67). In contrast, Al Farra (2010) tested for both the 2756A-G and the 2758C-G and found no association between the two examined polymorphisms and the increase in maternal risk for giving birth to NTD children.

### 2.3 Methionine synthase reductase (MTRR)

The product of the methionine synthase reductase (MTRR) gene is required for the regeneration of functional methionine synthase by reductive methylation through a reaction catalyzed by MTRR gene in which the methyl donor used is S-adenosyltmethionine. Methionine synthase uses cobalamin(I) cofactor, which becomes oxidized to cobalamin (II), thus rendering the MTR enzyme inactive (Leclerc et al., 1998). Patients who are defective in the reductive activation of methionine synthase exhibit megaloblastic anemia, developmental delay, hyperhomocysteinemia and hypomethioninemia (Wilson et al., 1999a).

#### 2.3.1 A66G

A common MTRR polymorphism, i.e. a 66A-G substitution that results in an isoleucine to methionine substitution (I22M), was identified in a Canadian study, where this mutation has an allele frequency of 0.51 and increases NTD risk when cobalamin status is low or when the *MTHFR* mutant genotype is present (Wilson et al., 1999b). When a study population of 601 Northern-Irish men, aged 30-49, for which biochemical and genetic data relevant to folate/homocysteine metabolism had already been acquired, the 66AA genotype had a frequency of 29%.There was a significant influence of MTRR genotype on total Homocysteine ranking(tHcy)(P=0.004) and the 66AA genotype contributes to a moderate increase in tHcy levels across the distribution [OR 1.59 (95% CI: 1.10--2.25) for the 66AA genotype to be in the upper half of the tHcy distribution, P=0.03] (Gaughan et al., 2001). Doolin et al., (2002) also assessed the 66A-G mutation in their spina bifida study and determined that for the risk of having a child with spina bifida appears to increase with the number of high-risk alleles in the maternal MTR genotype as well as the MTRR genotype mentioned above (R1 p 2.16, 95% CI 0.92–5.06; R2 p 6.58, 95% CI 0.87–49.67) and MTRR (R1 p 2.05, 95% CI 1.05–3.99; R2 p 3.15, 95% CI 0.92–10.85). These findings highlight the importance of considering both the maternal and embryonic genotype when evaluating putative spina bifida susceptibility loci.

Vaughn and colleagues (2004) concluded from assaying for common genetic variants (MTHFR 677C3T, MTHFR 1298A3C, and MTRR 66A3G), folate, and vitamin B-12 status on plasma homocysteine in women (20–30 yrs old; n = 362) that coexistence of the MTHFR 677 TT genotype with the MTRR 66A3G polymorphism may exacerbate the effect of the MTHFR variant alone and that the potential negative effect of combined polymorphisms of the MTHFR and MTRR genes on plasma homocysteine in at-risk population groups with low folate and/or vitamin B-12 status, such as women of reproductive potential, deserves further investigation. Furthermore, women with the MTHFR 677 TT/MTRR 66 AG genotype had higher ($P < 0.05$) plasma homocysteine than all other genotype combinations except the TT/AA and TT/GG genotypes (Vaughn et al., 2004).Conflicting results were obtained in a case-control study by van der Linden and colleagues (2006b), where they studied the association between the MTRR 66A-Gpolymorphism and spina bifida risk in 121 mothers, 109 spina bifida patients, 292 control women, and 234 pediatric controls and found that the MTRR66A-G polymorphism had no influence on spina bifida risk.

Since the MTR and MTRR genes have been much less studied as genes conferring risk to NTD, the conflictive evidence still needs to be clarified with further studies that evaluate the metabolic as well as genetic factors that contribute to these developmental defects.

## 3. Folic acid supplementation

Epidemiological studies that associate folate supplementation with a decreased risk of NTDs date back to the 1960s. The most definitive research addressing the benefits of folic acid supplementation in decreasing the risk of NTDs was the multicentre, randomized, double-blind trial by the Medical Research Council in the United Kingdom (MRC Vitamin Study Research Group, 1991). The aim of this trial was to evaluate the efficacy of 4-mg doses of folic acid in preventing recurrent NTDs in women who had previously delivered children with NTDs. The trial showed that women randomized to take folic acid supplementation had a 1.0% chance of having children with NTDs (relative risk [RR] 0.28, 95% confidence interval [CI] 0.12 to 0.71), but women in the unsupplemented group did not show a decrease in the risk of NTDs (3.49%) (RR 0.8, 95% CI 0.37 to 1.72) (Czeizel & Dudas, 1992; MRC Vitamin Study Research Group, 1991). Overall, supplementation with folic acid reduced the rate of recurrence of NTDs by 72% (MRC Vitamin Study Research Group, 1991).

A second key trial evaluating folic acid–fortified multivitamin supplementation during pregnancy was a double-blind, randomized controlled trial, in which women were randomized to take a multivitamin supplement containing 0.8 mg of folic acid or a multivitamin containing trace-element supplementation (Czeizel & Dudas 1992). Five thousand women were randomized in each group; no NTDs were observed in babies from the folic acid–fortified group, whereas 6 NTDs were found in those from the trace-element group. A recent meta-analysis observed that use of multivitamin supplements provided consistent protection against neural tube defects with an odds ratio (OR) of 0.67 (95% CI 0.58 to 0.77) in case-control studies and an OR 0.52 (95% CI 0.39 to 0.69) in cohort and randomized controlled studies. An OR of 0.67 means 0.33 (or 33%) protective effect; an OR of 0.52 means 0.48 (or 48%) protective effect (Goh et al., 2006). A study investigating the relationship between serum and red blood folate concentrations and the risk of NTDs found an inverse relationship between maternal red blood cell folate and the risk of NTD (Daly LE et al., 1995). Daly et al showed that women receiving less than 150 μg and more than 400 μg of folic acid had a 6.6/1000 and 0.8/1000 chance of having children with NTDs, respectively. Supplementation at doses of 100 μg, 200 μg, and 400 μg of folic acid resulted in a 22%, 41%, and 47% decreased risk of NTDs, respectively (Daly S et al., 1997).

### 3.1 Recommendations for women without a previous pregnancy affected by NTD

In 1991, the British Medical Research Council Vitamin Study reported that folic acid supplements reduced the recurrence neural tube defects (spina bifida or anencephaly) by 71% (MRC Vitamin Study Research Group, 1991). Preliminary results from the Hungarian randomized controlled trial of multivitamin/mineral supplementation (including 0.8 mg of folic acid) among women who had not had a prior NTD-affected pregnancy were reported in 1989. This trial was stopped in May 1992 on the advice of an ad hoc scientific advisory committee because of evidence of an NTD-protective effect of the multivitamin/mineral preparation relative to the study placebo preparation (CDC, 1992). In September 1992, the United States Department of Health and Human Services Public Health Service Centers for Disease Control recommended that all women of childbearing age in the United States who are capable of becoming pregnant and without a previous pregnancy affected by NTD should consume 0.4 mg of folic acid per day for the purpose of reducing their risk of having a pregnancy affected with spina bifida or anencephaly (CDC, 1992).

### 3.2 Recommendations for women with a previous pregnancy affected by NTD

Among US couples who have had a child with an NTD, the recurrence risk is 2% to 3% in subsequent pregnancies. The Medical Research Council (MRC) Vitamin Study Group reported the results of a trial of folic acid supplementation for the prevention of NTDs in pregnancies of women who had a previous child with an NTD and the CDC published its recommendations (CDC, 1991; MRC Vitamin Study Research Group, 1991). The guideline called for the consumption of a 4.0- mg daily dose of folic acid, from at least 1 month before conception through the first 3 months of pregnancy. The guideline did not specifically address the issue of folic acid consumption among these women during the times when they are not planning to become pregnant. Women who have had an NTD-affected pregnancy should consume 0.4 mg of folic acid per day, unless they are planning a pregnancy. When these women are planning to become pregnant, they can follow the guideline and consult their physicians about the desirability of using 4.0 mg of folic acid per day. Because 4.0 mg of folic acid per day is a very high dose, there may be risks associated with these levels. Although it appears that a lower dose, such as 0.4 mg, may have as great a beneficial effect as 4.0 mg, women who are at very high risk of having an NTD-affected pregnancy may choose to follow the guideline because it is based on data from the most rigorous study directly pertinent to their risk of NTDs, and because their risk of having an NTD-affected pregnancy may outweigh any risk that may occur as the result of the use of 4.0 mg of folic acid (CDC, 1991). The South Carolina NTD prevention program has reported great success in preventing the recurrence of isolated NTDs by providing counseling and vitamins to women who have had a previous NTD-affected pregnancy. Over the 6 years of surveillance (1992-1998) there were no NTD recurrences in 113 subsequent pregnancies to mothers of infants with isolated NTDs who took periconceptional folic acid (Stevenson et al., 2000).

### 3.3 Folic acid campaigns

Despite folic acid's clear link with NTD prevention, folic acid education campaigns worldwide have had mixed results in terms of knowledge about the benefits and sources of folic acid, and especially in terms of understanding the correct, periconceptional timing of folic acid intake. Official health education initiatives have promoted folic acid supplementation and a diet rich in folates. Campaigns range from media communications and information kits, to free product samples and discount vouchers, to improved labeling and in-store displays promoting dietary sources of folic acid. A review of 38 scientific publications about folic acid campaigns showed that awareness of folic acid improved post-campaign, with the percentage improvement between pre- and post-campaigns ranging from 6 to 41%. Although knowledge regarding appropriate sources of folic acid (foods or supplements) improved post-campaign, in most studies <50% of women were able to provide details about supplements that contained folic acid. In general, folic acid consumption rose between 12.4 % and 25.3% after public health campaigns. Nevertheless, the percentage of women taking periconceptional folic acid as prescribed ranged from 13 to 57%. This suggests >43% of women were not taking folic acid as prescribed after campaigns ceased (Rofail, 2011).

Folate unawareness not only exists among general population but also among nurses, pharmacists and health professionals. A survey conducted among student pharmacists concluded that 94% knew folic acid supplements prevent birth defects, 74% knew supplementation should begin before pregnancy but only 55% knew the recommended levels or good folate sources (50%). A telephone survey among obstetricians in Delhi, India reported that although all of them were aware of folic acid, only 63% knew that it prevents birth defects and 30% knew that it should be given before pregnancy. None of them prescribed periconceptional folic acid or folate rich diet through child-bearing age. Interestingly, 80% of those surveyed were not aware of the preventive dose of folic acid (Gupta & Gupta, 2004).

Increased periconceptional consumption of dietary folates or supplements have had limited impact on decreasing the incidence of neural tube defects. In addition to unplanned pregnancy, factors such as adolescent pregnancies, ethnicity, low socio-economic status, maternal education, and access to preventive healthcare influence the consumption of folic acid supplements. Sustained educational health campaigns should continue but also they should address barriers and limitations for adequate preconceptional and reproductive health. These campaigns are needed to reassess the message sent and the ability people have to change their behaviors according to their own circumstances. Due to limited success of the folic acid campaigns in increasing the supplementation of folic acid, the primary prevention of these birth defects then relies on folic acid fortification (Gupta & Gupta, 2004; Ray et al., 2004; Rofail et al., 2011; Eichholzer et al., 2006).

## 4. Fortification of food with folic acid

### 4.1 Recommendations

In March 1996, the US Food and Drug Administration (FDA) mandated that enriched cereal-grain products be fortified with folic acid. The FDA determined that fortification of cereal-grain products with folic acid, along with fortification of ready-to-eat breakfast cereals and dietary supplements, would provide increased intakes of folate for women in their childbearing years, while keeping daily intakes for the non-target population within the recommended safe limit. Food fortification had the advantage of reaching a great number of women in the target population before conception and during early pregnancy. It also had the advantage of providing folic acid in a continuous and passive manner and, thus, represented a potentially effective means for improving the folate nutriture of women throughout their childbearing years (FDA, 1996). Many countries have not chosen mandatory folic acid fortification, in part because expected additional health benefits are not yet scientifically proven in clinical trials, in part because of feared health risks, and because of the issue of freedom of choice. In these countries, additional creative public-health approaches need to be developed to prevent neural tube defects and improve the folate status of the general population (Eichholzer et al., 2006).

### 4.2 Fortification results

The mandatory fortification of cereal grain products in the US resulted in a substantial increase in blood folate concentrations and a concomitant decrease in NTD prevalence (CDC, 2010). The prevalence estimates of low serum and RBC folate concentrations declined in women of childbearing age from 21% before to <1% after fortification. For RBC folate concentrations there was a decline from 38% to 5% (Pfeiffer et al., 2007). NTD prevalence decreased by 36% after fortification, from 10.8 per 10,000 population during 1995--1996 to 6.9 at the end of 2006 (CDC, 2010).

A similar trend has been seen in other countries. In Chile, mandatory wheat flour fortification started in 2000. A study was designed to measure the effect of such policy in a group of women of childbearing age in Santiago. Folate levels, as well as RBC folate concentrations, increased significantly, 2.8 and 1.4-fold, respectively. It is important to notice that none of the participants took folic acid supplements since there was no public health policy regarding their use in Chile (Hertrampt et al., 2003). During 2001-2002 the NTD rate in Chile was significantly reduced by 43% from 17.1/10,000 to 9.7/10,000 births (Hertrampt et al., 2008). In Argentina, fortification started in 2003. Hospital discharge statistics showed a decrease of 54% for anencephaly, 33% for encephalocele, and 45% for spina bifida between 2000 and 2005 (Calvo & Biglieri, 2008). Canada has also seen a 50% reduction in spina bifida (Godwin et al., 2008). Another fortification strategy was studied in New Zealand, where daily consumption of folic acid fortified milk in women of childbearing age for 12 weeks resulted in an increase in plasma folate and RBC folate concentrations (Green et al., 2005).

Improved survival of children with NTD has also been reported after fortification. A retrospective cohort study was conducted and included 2841 infants with spina bifida and 638 infants with encephalocele who were born between 1995 and 2001 and were registered in any of 16 participating birth defects monitoring programs in the United States. First-year survival rates for both spina bifida and encephalocele cohorts were measured and factors associated with improved chances of first-year survival, including birth before or during folic acid fortification, were measured with regression analysis. Infants with spina bifida experienced a significantly improved first-year survival rate of 92.1% (adjusted hazard ratio: 0.68; 95% confidence interval: 0.50-0.91) during the period of mandatory folic acid fortification, compared with a 90.3% survival rate for those born before fortification. Infants with encephalocele had a statistically nonsignificant increase in survival rates, ie, 79.1% (adjusted hazard ratio: 0.76; 95% confidence interval: 0.51-1.13) with folic acid fortification, compared with 75.7% for earlier births. It is possible that folic acid plays a role not only in preventing NTDs but also in ameliorating the severity of spina bifida among live-born infants. One possible mechanism for reduction of the severity of spina bifida is that folic acid may move the location of the lesion caudally along the developing spine (Bol et al., 2006). A study in Atlanta demonstrated lower survival rates for infants with high lesions (cervical or thoracic), compared with infants with low lesions (lumbar or sacral). In multivariable analysis, factors associated with increased mortality were low birthweight (<2500 g) and high lesions (Bol et al., 2006, Wong & Paulozzi, 2001).

### 4.3 Concerns

Before the mandatory fortification of grains, the average consumption of folic acid was estimated to be 0.25mg/day and the fortification is estimated to add 0.1 mg/day, leaving many women of childbearing age under the recommended levels (Chacko et al., 2003). A study by Boushey and colleagues (2001) showed that 61% of women in childbearing age after fortification had intakes of folic acid below the recommended levels and those who achieved the guidelines were those who consumed supplements. Brent and Oakley (2005) have suggested that there is a need to increase the amount of folic acid in the fortification of grains. The Food and Drug Administration disagreed since fortification is nonspecific and must be safe for all groups (Rader & Schneeman, 2006). With fortification, the possibility remains that certain segments of the population may benefit less and may even experience some adverse effects from increased folic acid intakes.

The main concern has been the potential masking of vitamin $B_{12}$ deficiency, a condition that affects 10–15% of the population over age 60 years. Increased folic acid intake may correct the hematologic signs of vitamin $B_{12}$ deficiency, thus delaying diagnosis and treatment of the condition while its neurologic manifestations progress The Public Health Service fortification recommendation cautioned against daily intakes of folate above 1 mg (Liu et al., 2004). The agency noted that even with supplement use, 95th percentile intakes by adults 51+ years of age could reach 0.84 to 0.86 mg/day if enriched cereal-grain products are fortified. . While the agency recognized that this level approached the recommended safe upper limit and did not take into account likely underreporting biases regarding food intakes and underestimation of folate content of foods, it tentatively concluded that fortification of cereal-grain products with 140 g folic acid /100 g was the most appropriate fortification level of three levels analyzed (FDA, 1996). A study in Canada showed that the average dietary intake of folic acid due to fortification was 0.7 mg/day in women aged 19–44 years and 0.74 mg/day in seniors. Among seniors, there were no significant changes in indices typical of vitamin $B_{12}$ deficiencies, and no evidence of improved folate status masking hematological manifestations of vitamin $B_{12}$ deficiency (Liu et al, 2004).

Another concern related to folic acid supplementation is an increase in the rate of twins. The United Services Preventive Services Task Force (USPSTF) found no clear, consistent evidence that preconceptional folic acid use results in an increased rate of twinning. Many studies with methodological problems posit an association between folic acid and twinning; however, most of these studies did not appropriately adjust for fertility interventions, an important confounder. A study examined the association between risk for twinning in 176,042 women and exposure to a multivitamin or folic acid supplementation before or during pregnancy. After adjustment for age and parity, the authors reported an OR of 1.59 (CI, 1.41 to 1.78) for twin delivery after preconceptional folic acid supplementation. After accounting for the underreporting of folic acid use and in vitro fertilization, the OR for twin delivery after preconceptional supplementation decreased to 1.02 (CI, 0.85 to 1.24) and was no longer statistically significantly greater than the risk for women who did not take folic acid (USPSTF, 2009).

### 4.4 Health disparities

After mandatory fortification, prevalence of NTD in the US declined 30%--40% among the three largest racial and ethnic groups. Nevertheless, Hispanic women continue to be at significantly greater risk for having a baby affected by an NTD than non-Hispanic white women. Non-Hispanic black women have consistently had lower NTD prevalence than Hispanic women and non-Hispanic white women, despite having the lowest folate levels before and after mandatory fortification. Factors suggested to be contributing to the inconsistency include genetic differences in folate metabolism, maternal diabetes, and obesity, which are known to vary by race and ethnicity; and intake of nutrients other than folic acid, such as Vitamin B12 (CDC, 2010).

Canfield and colleagues (1996) studied a group of women in Texas with the primary etiologic question of whether increased NTD risk in Hispanics is explained by maternal diabetes or by other factors (e.g., maternal birthplace, prenatal care, reproductive history, age, socioeconomic status). They found that having a Hispanic mother was a risk factor for anencephaly among infants born to women with early prenatal care but not for those born to latecomers. Earlier prenatal care seemed "protective" for non-Hispanics but not for Hispanics. After adjustment in multivariate analysis, having a Hispanic (versus non-Hispanic) mother remained a strong risk factor for both anencephaly and spina bifida. Hispanic mother was the only study variable significantly associated with spina bifida in multivariate analysis. An increased risk of NTDs among Hispanics remained after controlling for other factors. For anencephaly, this risk might be partially explained by economic and cultural differences between Hispanics and non-Hispanics, and the effect of these factors on rates of prenatal diagnosis and elective pregnancy termination (Canfield et al., 1996). They suggested that cultural differences between Hispanic and non-Hispanic groups, including access to and use of folic acid-fortified food products, may contribute to the increased prevalence of NTDs. These factors may in turn affect rates of prenatal diagnosis and elective pregnancy termination, yielding births with more severe NTDs and poorer prognoses (Bol et al., 2006; Canfield et al., 1996).

Data from the US National Birth Defects Prevention Study for expected delivery dates from October 1997 through 2003 was used to determine whether the increased risk in anencephaly and spina bifida in Hispanics was explained by selected sociodemographic, acculturation, and other maternal characteristics. Hispanic mothers who reported the highest level of income were 80% less likely to deliver babies with spina bifida. In addition, highly educated Hispanic and white mothers had 76 and 35% lower risk, respectively. Other factors showing differing effects for spina bifida in Hispanics included maternal age, parity, and gestational diabetes. For spina bifida there was no significant elevated risk for U.S.-born Hispanics, relative to whites, but for anencephaly, corresponding ORs ranged from 1.9 to 2.3. The highest risk for spina bifida was observed for recent Hispanic immigrant parents from Mexico or Central America residing in the United States <5 years (Canfield et al., 2009).

In 2008 we did a study in Puerto Rico and found consumption of folic acid supplements to be 30% with 21% reporting use at least 4 times per week, and only 14% consuming it the day before the survey. Knowledge about the recommendation for women to consume folic acid was reported by 97% of the participants. Knowledge about the role of folic acid in preventing birth defects was reported by 90% of the participants. Awareness did not translate into practice. The use of folic acid was lower among women of lower education and lower social class. Women with higher education were 8.3 times more likely to consume folic acid (Garcia-Fragoso et al., 2008).

In 2009, the results of a study to evaluate the associations between neural tube defects and maternal folic acid intake among pregnancies conceived after fortification were published. This was a multicenter, case-control study using data from the National Birth Defects Prevention Study, 1998-2003. Among controls, 35.6% of non-Hispanic white women compared with 63.3% of non-Hispanic black women and 71.3% of Hispanic women reported no use of supplement from 3 months before pregnancy through the first month of pregnancy. Only 7.2% of Hispanic controls and 14.9% of non-Hispanic black controls reported use of a supplement compared with 36.3% for non-Hispanic white controls. Case women were more likely than controls to be Hispanic, less likely to report educational levels beyond high school, and less likely to report household incomes at or above $50,000 (Mosley et al., 2009). Consideration of ways to enhance the intake of folic acid among Hispanics is a high priority (CDC, 2010). These include educational strategies as well as consideration of expanding the foods currently fortified. Prue and coworkers (2010) conducted Hispanics targeted folic acid promotion efforts in several major cities in the US. Efforts included paid and unpaid placements of Spanish language public service announcements and community-level education. Women who reported awareness of folic acid had greater folic acid knowledge and use of vitamins containing folic acid. Pregnancy waiters were most likely to use vitamins containing folic acid daily. For this group, however, awareness did not play as large a role in whether they reported consuming a vitamin containing folic acid or not, as it did for pregnancy waiters and avoiders (Prue et al., 2010). The possibility of selectively fortifying foods not included in the current fortification regulation that are staples in Hispanic communities, such as corn tortillas or other products made from corn masa flour, is being considered (CDC, 2010). Hamner et al. (2009) analyzed this possibility and found that with corn masa flour fortification, Mexican American women aged 15-44 y could increase their total usual daily folic acid intake by 19.9% and non-Hispanic white women by 4.2%.

## 5. Can folic acid reduce other births defects?

### 5.1 Down syndrome

Down syndrome (DS) is a complex genetic disease resulting from the presence and expression of 3 copies of the genes located on chromosome 21. In most cases, the extra chromosome stems from the failure of normal chromosomal segregation during meiosis (meiotic nondisjunction). Studies have shown that genomic DNA hypomethylation is associated with chromosomal instability and abnormal segregation. MTHFR acts at a critical metabolic juncture in the regulation of cellular methylation reactions (James et al., 1999). James and colleagues showed that a polymorphism of the MTHFR gene may be a direct genetic risk factor for meiotic non-disjunction such as Down's syndrome. A significant increase in plasma homocysteine concentrations and lymphocyte methotrexate cytotoxicity was observed in the mothers of children with Down syndrome, consistent with abnormal folate and methyl metabolism. Mothers with the 677CT polymorphism had a 2.6-fold higher risk of having a child with DS than did mothers without the T substitution. That study stimulated considerable investigation into the possible role of folate/homocysteine metabolism in the risk of having a DS child and several studies have been performed to better address this issue. Studies indicate that an impaired folate/homocysteine metabolism can result in chromosome 21 nondisjunction; however, the birth of a DS child seems to be the result of the interplay of several factors making it difficult to discriminate the single contribution of each of them (Coppedè, 2009).

If elevated homocysteine levels are associated with an increase risk of DS and folate can lower homocysteine levels, folic acid supplementation might be expected to decrease the incidence of DS. It has been possible to examine the incidence of births of children with DS both prior to and after supplementation was initiated, and to evaluate its effectiveness by measuring folate levels in individuals pre- and post initiation of supplementation. An elevation of serum and red blood cell folate is observed post supplementation. However, there is no evidence of a decreased incidence of births of children with Down syndrome and some studies actually provided evidence for a slight increase in the incidence (Patterson, 2008). In Puerto Rico, we have seen an increase in the 2001-2007 DS incidence despite folate fortification of cereal-grain products and an active folic acid campaign (Puerto Rico Health Department, 2010).

### 5.2 Congenital heart disease

In 1995, Shaw and colleagues (1995) reported that women who take multivitamins from one month before until two months after conception have 30% to 35% lower risk of delivering offspring with conotruncal defects. Botto and coworkers (2000b) suggested that approximately one in four major cardiac defects could be prevented by periconceptional multivitamins use. Junker and colleagues (2001) showed that the embryonal MTHFR 677TT genotype was significantly associated with the development of structural congenital heart malformations during early pregnancy. Another study in the Netherlands reported that the maternal MTHFR 677CT and TT genotypes in combination with no use of periconceptional folate supplements were associated with a three-fold and six-fold increased risk for conotruncal heart defects in offspring (van Beynum et al., 2006). A study performed in a Hispanic population in Puerto Rico by these authors (Garcia-Fragoso et al., 2010) showed the prevalence of the TT polymorphism to be higher in mothers of children with congenital heart disease (CHD) than in controls. Compound heterozygosity for the 677TT and 1298AC polymorphisms was 3.7 times more common in children with CHD than in the newborn controls. Mothers of children with CHD were more likely to be compound heterozygotes. The higher prevalence of C677T polymorphism in mothers of children with CHD and of compound heterozygozity for both polymorphisms suggested the possible role of folic acid in the prevention of CHD. The American Academy of Pediatrics endorsed a statement by the American Heart Association Council on Cardiovascular Disease in the Young emphasizing that periconceptional intake of multivitamin supplements that contain folic acid may reduce the risk of congenital cardiovascular defects in offspring, similar to the known risk reduction for neural tube defects that is seen with folic acid intake (AAP, 2007). In 2009, investigators from Canada reported a 6% decrease per year in the rates of severe congenital heart defects after folic acid fortification of grain products (Lonescu-lttu et al., 2009).

### 5.3 Cleft lip and palate (CL/P)

Epidemiologic and family studies suggest that nonsyndromic cleft lip with or without cleft palate is a complex disorder caused by both genetic and environmental factors. The neural tube and the craniofacial regions both arise from neural crest cells, leading to the hypothesis that folic acid deficiency may also contribute to nonsyndromic clefting Perturbation of any part of the interacting folate metabolism pathways could result in folate deficiency with the effect of disrupting important biologic processes, such as craniofacial development. High levels of homocysteine may also affect developmental activities such as neural crest cell motility and migration, which are important in early development (Blanton et al., 2011). A study by Hernández and co-workers (2000) evaluated data on exposure to folic acid antagonists, finding a correlation with cardiovascular defects and oral clefts. A national population-based study showed that folic acid supplementation during early pregnancy was associated with a reduced risk of isolated cleft lip with or without cleft palate. Independent of supplements, diets rich in fruits, vegetables, and other high folate containing foods reduced the risk somewhat. The lowest risk of cleft lip was among women with folate rich diets who also took folic acid supplements and multivitamins. Folic acid provided no protection against cleft palate alone (Wilcox et al., 2007).

In 2001, Martinelli and coworkers reported a significantly higher MTHFR C677T mutation frequency detected in mothers of patients with CL/P compared to controls supporting the involvement of the folate pathway in the etiology of CL/P, and indicating an effect of the maternal genotype, rather than influence of the embryo's genotype. In 2008, Boyles and coworkers analyzed multiple genes involved in folate and vitamin A metabolisms. Despite strong evidence for genetic causes of oral facial clefts and the protective effects of maternal vitamins, they found no convincing indication that polymorphisms in these vitamin metabolism genes play an etiologic role.

## 6. Summary

There is strong evidence that consumption of folic acid by women in childbearing age can prevent the occurrence of NTD in their children. Recommendations for supplementation and fortification of food products have been established in many countries. Mutations in folic related enzymes continue to be studied in an effort to explain the role of folic acid in the occurrence of NTD and other congenital anomalies.

## 7. References

Al Farra H.Y. (2010). Methionine synthase polymorphisms (MTR 2756 A>G and MTR 2758 C>G) frequencies and distribution in the Jordanian population and their correlation with neural tube defects in the population of the northern part of Jordan. *Indian J Hum Genet,* Vol. 16, No. 3, pp.138-43.

American Academy of Pediatrics (AAP)., & American Heart Association. (2010). *Neonatal Resuscitation,* American Academy of Pediatrics, Elk Grove Village, Illinois.

American Academy of Pediatrics (AAP). (2207). Noninherited risk factors and congenital cardiovascular defects: current knowledge. *Pediatrics,* Vol. 120, No.2, pp. 445-446.

Amorim, M.R., Lima, M.A., Castilla, E.E., & Orioli, I.M. (2006) Non-Latin European descent could be a requirement for association of NTDs and MTHFR variant 677C > T: a meta-analysis. *Am J Med Genet A,* Vol. 143A, No. 15, pp. 1726-1732.

Birn H. (2006). The kidney in vitamin B12 and folate homeostasis: characterization of receptors for tubular uptake of vitamins and carrier proteins. *Am J Physiol Renal Physiol,* Vol.291, No.1, pp.F22-36.

Blanton, S.H., Henry, R.R., Yuan, Q., Mulliken, J.B., Stal, S., Finnell, R.H., & Hecht, J.T. (2011). Folate pathway and nonsyndromic cleft lip and palate. *Birth Defects Res A Clin Mol Teratol,* Vol.91, No.1, pp. 50-60.

Blom, H.J., Shaw, G.M., den Heijer, M., & Finnell, R.H. (2006). Neural tube defects and folate: case far from closed. *Nat Rev Neurosci,* Vol.7, No.9. pp. 724-731.

Boduroğlu, K., Alanay, Y., Alikaşifoğlu, M., Aktaş, D., & Tunçbilek, E. (2005). Analysis of MTHFR 1298A>C in addition to MTHFR 677C>T polymorphism as a risk factor for neural tube defects in the Turkish population. *Turk J Pediatr,* Vol. 47, No. 4, pp. 327-333.

Bol, K.A., Collins, J.S., & Kirby, R.S. (2006). National Birth Defects Prevention Network. Survival of infants with neural tube defects in the presence of folic acid fortification. *Pediatrics,* Vol.117, No.3, pp. 803-813.

Botto, L.D., & Yang, Q. (2000a). 5,10-Methylenetetrahydrofolate reductase gene variants and congenital anomalies: a HuGE review. *Am J Epidemiol,* Vol. 151, No. 9, pp. 862-877.

Botto, L.D., Mulinare, J., & Erickson, J.D. (2000b). Occurrence of Congenital Heart Defects in Relation to Maternal Multivitamin Use. *Am J Epidemiol,* Vol.151, No.9, pp. 878-884.

Boushley, C.J., Edmons, J.W., & Welshimer, K.J. (2001). Estimates of the effects of folic acid fortification and folic acid bioavailability for women. *Nutrition,* Vol.17, No.10, pp. 873-879.

Boyles, A.L., Billups, A.V., Deak, L.L., Siegel, D.G., Mehltretter, L., Slifer, S.H., Bassuk, A.G., Kessler, J.A., & Nijhout, H.F. (2006). Neural tube defects and folate pathway genes: family-based association tests of gene-gene and gene-environment interactions. *Environ Health Perspect,* Vol. 144, pp. 1547-1552.

Boyles, A.L., Wilcox, A.J., Taylor, J.A., Shi, M., Weinberg, C.R., Meyer, K., Fredriksen, A., Ueland, P.M., Johansen, A.M., Drevon, C.A., Jugessur, A., Trung, T.N., Gjessing, H.K., Vollset, S.E., Murray, J.C., Christensen, K., & Lie, R.T. (2009). Oral facial clefts and gene polymorphisms in metabolism of folate/one-carbon and vitamin A: a pathway-wide association study. *Genet Epidemiol,* Vol.33, No.3, pp. 247-255.

Brent, R.L., & Oakley, G.P. (2005). The Food and Drug administration must require the addition of more folic acid in "enriched" flour and other grains. *Pediatrics,* Vol.116, No.3, pp. 753-755.

Butherworth, C.E. (1968). Absorption and Malabsorption of Dietary Folates. *Am J Clin Nutr,* Vol.21, No.9, pp. 1121-1127.

Calvo, E.B., & Biglieri, A. (2008). Impact of folic acid fortification on women's nutritional status and on the prevalence of neural tube defects. *Arch Argent Pediatr,* Vol.106, No.6, pp. 492-498.

Canfield, M.A., Annegers, J.F., Brender, J.D., Cooper, S.P., & Greenberg, F. (1996). Hispanic origin and neural tube defects in Houston/Harris County, Texas, II: risk factors. *Am J Epidemiol,* Vol. 143, No.1, pp. 12- 24.

Canfield, M.A., Ramadhani, T.A., Shaw, G.M., Carmichael, S.L., Waller, D.K., Mosley, B.S., Royle, M.H., & Olney, R.S. (2009). National Birth Defects Prevention Study. Anencephaly and spina bifida among Hispanics: maternal, sociodemographic, and acculturation factors in the National Birth Defects Prevention Study. *Birth Defects Res A Clin Mol Teratol,* Vol.85, No.7, pp. 637-646.

Centers for Disease Control (CDC). (1991). Use of folic acid for prevention of spina bifida and other neural tube defects -- 1983-1991. *MMWR Morb Mortal Wkly Rep,* Vol.40, No.30, pp. 513-516.

Centers for Disease Control (CDC). (1992). Recommendations for the use of folic acid to reduce the number of cases of spina bifida and other neural tube defects. *MMWR Morb Mortal Wkly Rep,* Vol.41, RR-14, pp. 1–7.

Centers for Disease Control and Prevention (CDC). (2010). CDC Grand Rounds: additional opportunities to prevent neural tube defects with folic acid fortification. *MMWR Morb Mortal Wkly Rep*, Vol.59, No.31, pp. 980-984.

Chacko, M.R., Anding, R., Kozinetz, C.A., Grover, J.L., & Smith, P.B. (2003). Neural tube defects: knowledge and preconceptional prevention practices in minority young women. *Pediatrics*, Vol. 112, No.3, pp. 536-542.

Christensen, B., Arbour, L., Tran, P., Leclerc, D., Sabbaghian, N., Platt, R., Gilfix, B.M., Rosenblatt, D. S., Gravel, R.A., Forbes, P., & Rozen, R. (1999). Genetic polymorphisms in methylenetetrahydrofolate reductase and methionine synthase, folate levels in red blood cells, and risk of neural tube defects. *Am J Med Genet*, Vol. 84, No.2, pp. 151-157.

Coppedè, F. (2009). The complex relationship between folate/homocysteine metabolism and risk of Down syndrome. *Mutat Res*, Vol. 682, No. 1, pp. 54-70. Epub 2009 Jun 11.

Czeizel, A.E., & Dudas, I. (1992). Prevention of the first occurrence of neural-tube defects by periconceptional vitamin supplementation. *N Engl J Med*, Vol. 327, No. 26, pp. 1832–1835.

Daly, L.E., Kirke, P.N., Molloy, A., Weir, D.G., & Scott, J.M. (1995). Folate levels and neural tube defects. Implications for prevention. *JAMA* Vol. 274, No. 21, pp. 1698–1702.

Daly, S., Mills, J.L., Molloy, AM., Conley, M., Lee, Y.J., Kirke, P.N., Weir, D.G., & Scott, J.M. (1997). Minimum effective dose of folic acid for food fortification to prevent neural-tube defects. *Lancet*, Vol. 350, No.9092, pp. 1666–1669.

Dávalos, I.P., Olivares, N., Castillo, M.T., Cantú, J.M., Ibarra, B., Sandoval, L., Morán, M.C., Gallegos, M.P., Chakraborty, R., & Rivas, F. (2000). The C677T polymorphism of the methylenetetrahydrofolate reductase gene in Mexican mestizo neural-tube defect parents, control mestizo, and native populations. *Ann Genet*, Vol. 43, No. 2, pp. 89-92.

de Bree, A., van Dusseldorp, M., Brouwer, I.A., van het Hof, K.H., & Steegers-Theunissen, R.P. (1997). Folate intake in Europe: recommended, actual and desired intake. *Eur J Clin Nutr*, Vol.51, No. 10, pp. 643-660.

De Marco, P., Calevo, M.G., Moroni, A., Arata, L., Merello, E., Finnell, R.H., Zhu, H., Andreussi, L., Cama, A., & Capra, V. (2002). Study of MTHFR and MS polymorphisms as risk factors for NTD in the Italian population. *J Hum Genet*, Vol. 47, No. 6, pp. 319-24.

Doolin, M.T., Barbaux, S., McDonnell, M., Hoess, K., Whitehead, A.S., & Mitchell, L.E. (2002). Maternal genetic effects, exerted by genes involved in homocysteine remethylation, influence the risk of spina bifida. *Am J Hum Genet*, Vol. 71, No. 5, pp. 1222-1226.

Doudney, K., Grinham, J., Whittaker, J., Lynch, S.A., Thompson, D., Moore, G.E., Copp, A.J., Greene, N.D., & Stanier, P. (2009). Evaluation of folate metabolism gene polymorphisms as risk factors for open and closed neural tube defects. *Am J Med Genet A*, Vol. 149A, No. 7, pp. 1585-1589.

Edwards, J.H. (1958). Congenital malformations of the central nervous system in Scotland. *Br J Prev Soc Med*, Vol.12, No.3, pp. 115-130.

Eichholzer, M., Tönz, O., & Zimmermann, R. (2006). Folic acid: a public-health challenge. Lancet, Vol. 367, No. 9519, pp. 1352-1361.

Eikelboom, J.W., Lonn, E., Genest, J Jr., Hankey, G., & Yusuf, S. (1999). Homocysteine and cardiovascular disease: a critical review of the epidemiologic evidence. *Ann Intern Med,* Vol. 131, No. 5, pp. 363-375.

Erdogan, M.O., Yildiz, S.H., Solak, M., Eser, O., Cosar, E., Eser, B., Koken, R., & Buyukbas, S. (2010). C677T polymorphism of the methylenetetrahydrofolate reductase gene does not affect folic acid, vitamin B12, and homocysteine serum levels in Turkish children with neural tube defects. *Genet Mol Res,* Vol. 9, No. 2, pp. 1197-1203.

Eser, B., Cosar, M., Eser, O., Erdogan, M.O., Aslan, A., Yildiz, H., Boyaci, G., Buyukbas, S., & Solak, M. (2010). 677C>T and 1298A>C polymorphisms of methylenetetrahydropholate reductase gene and biochemical parameters in Turkish population with spina bifida occulta. *Turk Neurosurg,* Vol. 20, No. 1, pp. 9-15.

Food and Drug Administration. (1996). Food Standards: Amendment of Standards of Identity for Enriched Grain Products to Require Addition of Folic Acid. *Federal Register,* Vol.61, No.44, pp. 8781-8797.

Friso, S., Choi, S.W., Girelli, D., Mason, J.B., Dolnikowski, G.G., Bagley, J., Olivieri, O., Jacques, P.F., Rosenberg, I.H., Corrocher, R., & Selhub, J. (2002). A common mutation in the 5,10-methylenetetrahydrofolate reductase gene affects genomic DNA methylation through an interaction with folate status. *Proc Nat Acad Sci USA,* Vol. 99, No.8, pp. 5606-5611.

Frosst, P., Blom, H.J., Milos, R., Goyette, P., Sheppard, C.A., Matthews, R.G., Boers, G.J., den Heijer, M., Kluijtmans, L.A., & van den Heuvel, L.P. (1995). A candidate genetic risk factor for vascular disease: a common mutation in methylenetetrahydrofolate reductase. *Nat Genet.* Vol. 10, No. 1, pp. 111-113.

García-Fragoso, L., García-García, I., de la Vega, A., Renta, J., & Cadilla, C.L. (2002). Presence of the 5,10-methylenetetrahydrofolate reductase C677T mutation in Puerto Rican patients with neural tube defects. *J Child Neurol,* Vol. 17, No. 1, pp. 30-32.

García-Fragoso, L., García-García, I., & Rivera, C.E. (2008). The use of folic acid for the prevention of birth defects in Puerto Rico. *Ethn Dis,* Vol.18, (2 Suppl 2), pp. 168-171.

García-Fragoso, L., García-García, I., Leavitt, G., Renta, J., Ayala, MA., & Cadilla, .CL. (2010). MTHFR polymorphisms in Puerto Rican children with isolated congenital heart disease and their mothers. *Int J Genet Mol Biol,* Vol. 2, No. 3. pp. 43-47.

Gaughan, D.J., Kluijtmans, LA., Barbaux, S., McMaster, D., Young, IS., Yarnell, JW., Evans, A., & Whitehead, AS. (2001). The methionine synthase reductase (MTRR) A66G polymorphism is a novel genetic determinant of plasma homocysteine concentrations. *Atherosclerosis,* Vol. 157, No. 2, pp. 451-456.

Gentili, A., Vohra, M., Vij, S., Kuan-Hua, D., & Siddiqi, W. Aug 24, 2009. Folic Acid Deficiency, In: *Medscape Reference,* Accessed Aug 3, 2011, Available from: http://emedicine.medscape.com/ article/200184-overview.

Gilbert, S.F. (2000). Formation of the neural tube, In: *Developmental Biology,* Sunderland (MA): Sinauer Associates. Retrieved from http://www.ncbi.nlm.nih.gov/books/NBK10080. ISBN-10:0-87893-243-7.

Godwin, K.A., Sibbald, B., Kuzeljevic, B., Lowry, R.B., & Arbour, L. (2008). Changes in frequencies of select congenital anomalies since the onset of folic acid fortification in a Canadian Birth defect registry. *Can J Public Health, Vol.*99, No. 4, pp. 271-275.

Goh, Y.I., Bollano, E., Einarson, T.R., & Koren, G. (2006). Prenatal multivitamin supplementation and rates of congenital anomalies: a meta-analysis. *J Obstet Gynaecol Can,* Vol.28, No. 8, pp. 680–689.

Green, T.J., Skeaff, C.M., Rockell, J.E., & Venn, B.J. (2005). Folic acid fortified milk increases blood folate and lowers homocysteine concentration in women of childbearing age. *Asia Pac J Clin Nutr,* Vol.14, No.2, pp. 173-178.

Greene, N.D.E., Stanier, P. & Copp, A.J. (2009) Genetics of neural tube defects. *Human Mol Gen,* Vol. 28, Review issue No. 2, pp. R113-R129.

Gupta, H. & Gupta, P. (2004). Neural tube defects and folic acid. *Indian Pediatr,* Vol. 41, No. 6, pp. 577-586.

Halsted, C.H. (1989). The intestinal absorption of dietary folates in health and disease. *J Am Coll Nutr,* Vol.8, No.6, pp. 650-658.

Hamner, H.C., Mulinare, J., Cogswell, M.E., Flores, A.L., Boyle, C.A., Prue, C.E., Wang, C.Y., Carriquiry, A.L., & Devine, O. (2009). Predicted contribution of folic acid fortification of corn masa flour to the usual folic acid intake for the US population: National Health and Nutrition Examination Survey 2001--2004. *Am J Clin Nutr,* Vol.89, No.1, pp. 305--315.

Harisha, P.N., Devi, B.I., Christopher, R., & Kruthika-Vinod, T.P. (2010). Impact of 5,10-methylenetetrahydrofolate reductase gene polymorphism on neural tube defects. *J Neurosurgery Pediatrics,* Vol. 6, No.4, pp. 364-367.

Herbert, V. (1999). Folic Acid. In: *Nutrition in Health and Disease.* Shils M, Olson J, Shike M, Ross AC, (Eds.), Williams & Wilkins, Baltimore, MD.

Hernández-Diaz, S., Werler, M.M., Walker, A.M., & Mitchell, A.A. (2000). Folic acid antagonists during pregnancy and the risk of birth defects. *N Engl J Med,* Vol. 343, No. 22, pp. 1608-1614.

Hertrampt, E., Cortés, F., Erickson, D., Cayazzo, M., Freire, W., Bailey, L.B., Howson, C., Kauwell, G.P., & Pfeiffer, C. (2003). Consumption of folic acid-fortified bread improves folate status in women of reproductive age in Chile. *J Nutr,* Vol.133, No. 10. pp. 3166-3169.

Hertrampt, E., & Cortés, F. (2008). National food-fortification program with folic acid in Chile. *Food Nutr Bull,* Vol.29, (2Suppl), pp. S231-237.

Hibbard, E.D., & Smithells, R.W. (1965). Folic acid metabolism and human embryopathy. *Lancet* Vol. 1, pp. 1254.

Higdon, J. (2003). *An evidence-based approach to vitamins and minerals: Health benefits and intake recommendations,* Thieme Medical Publishers Inc, New York.

Holmes, L.B., Driscoll, SG., & Atkins, L. (1976). Etiologic Heterogeneity of Neural-Tube Defects. *N Engl J Med,* Vol. 294, No.7, pp. 365-369.

Hoyme, H.E. (1990). Teratogenically Fetal Anomalies. *Clin Perinatol,* Vol. 17, No.3, pp. 547-567.

Institute of Medicine (IOM), Food and Nutrition Board. (1998). Dietary reference intakes for thiamin, riboflavin, niacin, vitamin $B_6$, folate, vitamin $B_{12}$, pantothenic acid, biotin, and choline / a report of the Standing Committee on the Scientific Evaluation of Dietary Reference Intakes and its Panel on Folate, Other B Vitamins, and Choline and Subcommittee on Upper Reference Levels of Nutrients, National Academy Press, Washington, DC. ISBN 0309065542.

Isotalo, P.A., Wells, G.A., & Donnelly, J.G. (2000). Neonatal and fetal methylenetetrahydrofolate reductase genetic polymorphisms: an examination of C677T and A1298C mutations .*Am J Hum Genet.* Vol. 67, No. 4, pp. 986-990.

Jacques, P.F., Bostom, A.G., Williams, R.R., Ellison, R.C., Eckfeldt, J.H., Rosenberg, I.H., Selhub, J., & Rozen, R. (1996). Relation between folate status, a common mutation in methylenetetra-hydrofolate reductase, and plasma homocysteine concentrations. *Circulation*, Vol. 93, pp. 7-9.

James, S.J., Pogribna, M., Pogribny, I.P., Melnyk, S., Hine, R.J., Gibson, J.B., Yi, P., Tafoya, D.L., Swenson, D.H., Wilson, V.L., & Gaylor, D.W. Abnormal folate metabolism and mutation in the methylenetetrahydrofolate reductase gene may be maternal risk factors for Down syndrome. *Am J Clin Nutr*, Vol.70, No.4, pp. 495-501.

Johnson, L.E. (2007). Folate, In: *Merck Manual.* Accessed July 25, 2011, Merck Sharp & Dohme Corp. Retrieved from
http://www.merckmanuals.com/professional/sec01/ch004/
ch004c.html#v884631.

Johnson, W.G., Stenroos, ES., Heath, SC., Chen, Y., Carroll, R., McKoy, VV., Chatkupt, S., & Lehner, T. (1999). Distribution of alleles of the methylenetetrahydrofolate reductase (MTHFR) C677T gene polymorphism in familial spina bifida. *Am J Med Genet,* Vol. 87, No. 5, pp. 407-12.

Junker, R., Kotthoff, S., Vielhaber, H., Halimeh, S., Kosch, A., Koch, H.G., Kassenböhmer, R., Heineking, B., & Nowak-Göttl, U. (2001). Infant methylenetetrahydrofolate reductase 677TT genotype is a risk factor for congenital heart disease. *Cardiovasc Res,* Vol. 51, No. 2, pp. 251-254.

Larroche, J.C., & Encha-Razavi, F. (1991). Central Nervous System Malformations, In: *Textbook of Fetal and Perinatal Pathology,* Wigglesworth, JS., & Singer, DB., eds, pp. 784-807, Blackwell Scientific Publications, Boston.

Leclerc, D., Campeau, E., Goyette, P., Adjalla, C.E., Christensen, B., Ross, M., Eydoux, P., Rosenblatt, D.S., Rozen, R., & Gravel, R.A. (1996). Human methionine synthase: cDNA cloning and identification of mutations in patients of the cblG complementation group of folate/cobalamin disorders. *Hum. Molec. Genet,* Vol. 5, pp. 1867-1874.

Leclerc, D., Wilson, A., Dumas, R., Gafuik, C., Song, D., Watkins, D., Heng, H.H.Q., Rommens, JM., Scherer, S.W., Rosenblatt, D.S., & Gravel, R.A. (1998). Cloning and mapping of a cDNA for methionine synthase reductase, a flavoprotein defective in patients with homocystinuria. *Proc Nat Acad Sci,* Vol. 95, Vol. 6, pp. 3059-3064.

Lin, J., Lee, I.M., Song, Y., Cook, N.R., Selhub, J., Manson, J.E., Buring, J.E., & Zhang, S.M. (2010). Plasma homocysteine and cysteine and risk of breast cancer in women. *Cancer Res,* Vol. 70, No. 6, pp. 2397-405.

Liu, S., West, R., Randell, E., Longerich, L., O'connor, K.S, Scott, H., Crowley, M., Lam, A, Prabhakaran, V., & McCourt, C. (2004). A comprehensive evaluation of food fortification with folic acid for the primary prevention of neural tube defects. *BMC Pregnancy Childbirth,* Vol. 27, No. 4, pp. 20.

Lonescu-Ittu, R., Marelli, A.J., Mackie, A.S., & Pilote, L. (2009). Prevalence of severe congenital heart disease after folic acid fortification of grain products: time trend analysis in Quebec. *BMJ,* Vol. 338, pp. b1673.

Martinelli, M., Scapoli, L., Pezzetti, F., Carinci, F., Carinci, P., Stabellini, G., Bisceglia, L., Gombos, F., & Tognon, M. (2001). C677T variant form at the MTHFR gene and CL/P: a risk factor for mothers? *Am J Med Genet*, Vol. 98, No. 4, pp. 357-360.

Martínez de Villarreal, L.E., Delgado-Enciso, I., Valdéz-Leal, R., Ortíz-López, R., Rojas-Martínez, A., Limón-Benavides, C., Sánchez-Peña, M.A., Ancer-Rodríguez, J., Barrera-Saldaña, H.A., Villarreal-Pérez, J.Z. (2001). Folate levels and N(5),N(10)-methylenetetrahydrofolate reductase genotype (MTHFR) in mothers of offspring with neural tube defects: a case-control study. *Arch Med Res*. Vol. 32, No. 4, pp. 277-282.

Matherly, L.H. & Goldman, D.I. (2003). Membrane transport of folates. *Vitam Horm*, Vol. 66, pp. 403–456.

McAndrew, P.E., Brandt, J.T., Pearl, D.K., Prior, T.W. (1996). The incidence of the gene for thermolabile methylene tetrahydrofolate reductase in African Americans. *Thromb Res*, Vol. 83, pp. 195-198.

Miller, J.R. (1962). A strain difference in response to the teratogenic effect of maternal fasting in the house mouse. *Can J Genet Cytol*, Vol.4, pp. 69–78.

Mills, J.L., McPartlin, J.M., Kirke, P.N., Lee, Y.J., Conley, M.R., Weir, D.G., & Scott, J.M. (1995). Homocysteine metabolism in pregnancies complicated by neural-tube defects. *Lancet*, Vol. 345, No. 8943, pp. 149-151.

Mosley, B.S., Cleves, M.A., Siega-Riz, A.M., Shaw, G.M., Canfield, M.A., Wallerm D.K., Werler, M.M., & Hobbs, C.A. (2009). National Birth Defects Prevention Study. Neural tube defects and maternal folate intake among pregnancies conceived after folic acid fortification in the United States. *Am J Epidemiol*, Vol. 169, No. 1, pp. 9-17.

MRC Vitamin Study Research Group. (1991). Prevention of neural tube defects: results of the Medical Research Council Vitamin Study. MRC Vitamin Study Research Group. *Lancet*, Vol. 338, No. 8760, pp. 131–137.

Mutchinick, O.M., López, M.A., Luna, L., Waxman, J., & Babinsky, V.E. (1999). High prevalence of the thermolabile methylenetetrahydrofolate reductase variant in Mexico: a country with a very high prevalence of neural tube defects. *Mol Genet Metab*, Vol. 68, No. 4, pp. 461-467.

Naushad, S.M., & Devi, A.R. (2010). Role of parental folate pathway single nucleotide polymorphisms in altering the susceptibility to neural tube defects in South India. *J Perinat Med*, Vol. 38, No. 1, pp. 63-69.

National Institutes of health (NIH). Office of Dietary Supplements. n.d. Dietary Supplement Fact Sheet: Folate, In: *Dietary Supplements Fact Sheets*, Accessed August 1, 2011, Available from http://ods.od.nih.gov/factsheets/folate.

Ogino, S., & Wilson, R.B. (2003). Genotype and haplotype distributions of MTHFR 677C-T and 1298A-C single nucleotide polymorphisms: a meta-analysis. *J Hum Genet*, Vol. 48, No. 1, pp. 1-7.

Olinger, E.J., Bertino, J.R., & Binder, H.J. (1973). Intestinal folate absorption. II. Conversion and retention of pteroylmonoglutamate by jejunum. *J Clin Invest*, Vol. 52, No. 9, pp. 2138-2145.

Ou, C.Y., Stevenson, R.E., Brown, V.K., Schwartz, C.E., Allen, W.P., Khoury, M.J., Rozen, R., Oakley, G.P., Jr., & Adams, M.J., Jr. (1996). 5,10 Methylenetetrahydrofolate reductase genetic polymorphism as a risk factor for neural tube defects. *Am J Med Genet,* Vol. 63, No. 4, pp. 610-614.

Parle-McDermott, A., Mills, J.L., Kirke, P.N., O'Leary, V.B., Swanson, D.A., Pangilinan, F., Conley, M., Molloy, A.M., Cox, C., Scott, J.M., & Brody, L.C. (2003). Analysis of the MTHFR 1298A-->C and 677C-->T polymorphisms as risk factors for neural tube defects. *J Hum Genet,* Vol. 48, No. 4, pp. 190-193.

Patterson, D. (2008). Folate metabolism and the risk of Down syndrome. *Downs Syndr Res Pract,* Vol. 12, No. 2, pp. 939-937.

Pfeiffer, C.M., Johnson, C.L., Jain, R.B., Yetley, E.A., Picciano, M.F., Rader, J.I., Fisher, K.D., Mulinare, J., & Osterloh, J.D. (2007). Trends in blood folate and vitamin B-12 concentrations in the United States, 1988--2004. *Am J Clin Nutr,* Vol. 86, No. 3, pp. 718--727.

Posey, D.L., Khoury, M.J., Mulinare, J., Adams, M.J, Jr, & Ou, C.Y. (1996). Is mutated MTHFR a risk factor for neural tube defects? *Lancet,* Vol. 347, No. 9002, pp. 686-687.

Prue, C.E., Hamner, H.C., & Flores, A.L. (2010). Effects of folic acid awareness on knowledge and consumption for the prevention of birth defects among Hispanic women in several US communities. *J Women's Health* Vol. 19, No. 4, pp. 689--698.

Puerto Rico Health Department. (2010). *Puerto Rico Birth Defects Surveillance System, 2010 annual report.* San Juan, Puerto Rico.

Rader, J.I., & Schneeman, B. (2006). Prevalence of neural tube defects, folate status, and folate fortification of enriched cereal-grain products in the United States. *Pediatrics,* Vol. 117, No. 4, pp. 1394-1399.

Rampersaud, E., Melvin, E.C., Siegel, D., Mehltretter, L., Dickerson, M.E., George, T.M., Enterline, D., Nye, J.S., Speer, M.C. & NTD Collaborative Group. (2003). Updated investigations of the role of methylenetetrahydrofolate reductase in human neural tube defects. *Clin Genet,* Vol. 63, No. 3, pp. 210-214.

Ray, J.G. (1998). Meta-analysis of hyperhomocystinemia as a risk factor for venous thromboembolic disease. *Arch Intern Med,* Vol. 158, No. 19, pp. 2101-2106.

Ray, J.G., Singh, G., & Burrows, R.F. (2004). Evidence for suboptimal use of periconceptional folic acid supplements globally. BJOG, Vol. 111, No. 5, pp. 399-408.

Relton, C.L., Wilding, C.S., Jonas, P.A., Lynch, S.A., Tawn, E.J., Burn, J. (2003). Genetic susceptibility to neural tube defect pregnancy varies with offspring phenotype. *Clin Genet,* Vol. 64, No. 5, pp. 424-428.

Relton, C.L., Wilding, C.S., Pearce, M.S., Laffling, A.J., Jonas, P.A., Lynch, S.A., Tawn, E.J., Burn, J. (2004). Gene-gene interaction in folate-related genes and risk of neural tube defects in a UK population. *J Med Genet,* Vol. 41, No.4, pp. 256-260.

Richter, B., Stegmann, K., Röper, B., Böddeker, I., Ngo, E.T., Koch, M.C. (2001). Interaction of folate and homocysteine pathway genotypes evaluated in susceptibility to neural tube defects (NTD) in a German population. *J Hum Genet,* Vol. 46, No. 3, pp 105-109.

Rofail ,D., Colligs, A., Abetz, L., Lindemann, M., & Maguire, L. (2011). Factors contributing to the success of folic acid public health campaigns. *J Public Health (Oxf),* 2011 Jul 3. [Epub ahead of print].

Rosenberg, N., Murata, M., Ikeda, Y., Opare-Sem, O., Zivelin, A., Geffen, E., & Seligsohn, U. (2002) The frequent 5,10-methylenetetrahydrofolate reductase C677T polymorphism is associated with a common haplotype in whites, Japanese, and Africans. *Am J Hum Genet,* Vol. 70, No. 3, pp.758-762.

Saitoh, A., Hull, A.D., Franklin, P., & Spector, S.A. (2005). Myelomeningocele in an infant with intrauterine exposure to efavirenz. J Perinatol, Vol. 25, No.8, pp. 555-556.

Sandford, M.K., Kissling, G.E., & Joubert, P.E. (1992). Neural Tube Defect Etiology: new evidence concerning maternal hyperthermia, health and diet. *Dev Med Child Neurol,* Vol. 34, No.8, pp. 661-675.

Schneider, J.A., Rees, D.C., Liu, Y.T., & Clegg, J.B. (1998). Worldwide distribution of a common methylenetetrahydrofolate reductase mutation. (Letter). *Am J Hum Genet,* Vol. 62, pp.1258-1260.

Sedhadri, S., Beiser, A., Selhub, J., Jacques, P.J., Rosenberg, I.H. , D 'Agostino, R.B., Wilson, P.W.F., & Wolf, P.A. (2002). Plasma homocysteine as a risk factor for dementia and Alzheimer's disease. *N Engl J Med,* Vol. 346, No. 7, pp. 476-83.

Seller, M.J. (1983). Maternal nutrition factors and neural tube defects in experimental animals. In: *Prevention of spina bifida and other neural tube defects,* Dobbing J, ed, pp.1-23, Academic Press, New York, NY.

Shaw, G.M., Lu, W., Zhu, H., Yang, W., Briggs, F.B.S., Carmichael, S.L., Barcellos, L.F., Lammer, E.J., & Finnell, R.H. (2009). 118 SNPs of folate-related genes and risks of spina bifida and conotruncal heart defects. *BMC Medical Genetics,* Vol. 10, No. 49, pp. 1-11.

Shils, M.E., Shike, M., Ross, A.C., Caballero, B., & Cousins, R.J. (2006). *Modern Nutrition in Health and Disease,* Lippincott Williams & Wilkins, Maryland.

Siebert, J.R., Lemire, R.J., & Cohen, M.M. (1990). Aberrant morphogenesis of central nervous system. *Clin Perinatol,* 17, No. 3, pp. 569-595.

Smithells, R.W., Sheppard, S., & Sehorah, C.J. (1959). Vitamin levels and neural tube defects. *Arch Dis Child,* Vol. 51, pp. 944-950.

Smithells, R.W., Nevin, N.C., Seller, M.J., Sheppard, S., Harris, R., Read ,A.P., Fielding, D.W., Walker, S., Schorah, C.J., & Wild, J. (1983). Further experience of Vitamin Supplementation for Prevention of Neural Tube Defect Recurrences. *Lancet,* Vol. 1, No. 8332, pp. 1027-1031.

Steegers-Theunissen, R.P., Boers, G.H., Trijbels, F.J., Finkelstein, J.D., Blom, H.J., Thomas, C.M., Borm, G.F., Wouters, M.G., & Eskes, T.K. (1994). Maternal hyperhomocysteinemia: a risk factor for neural-tube defects? *Metabolism,* Vol. 43, No. 12, pp. 1475-1480.

Stegmann, K., Ziegler, A., Ngo, E.T.K.M., Kohlschmidt, N., Schröter, B., Ermert, A., and Koch, M.C. (1999). Linkage disequilibrium of MTHFR genotypes 677C/T-1298A/C in the german population and association studies in probands with neural tube defects (NTD). *Am J Med Genet,* Vol. 87, pp. 23-29.

Stein, Z., & Susser, M. (1976). Maternal starvation and birth defects. In: *Birth defects: Risk and Consequences.* Kelly, S., Hook, E., Janerich, D., et al, eds, pp. 205-220, Academic Press Inc, New York, NY.

Stevenson, R.E., Schwartz, C.E., Du, Y.Z., & Adams, M, Jr. (1997). Differences in methylenetetra-hydrofolate reductase genotype frequencies, between whites and blacks. (Letter). *Am J Hum Genet,* Vol. 60, No. 1, pp. 229-230.

Stevenson, R.E., Allen, W.P., Pai, G.S., Best, R., Seaver, L.H., Dean, J., & Thompson, S. (2000). Decline in prevalence of neural tube defects in a high-risk region of the United States. *Pediatrics,* Vol. 106, No.4, pp. 677-683.

Suitor, C.W., & Bailey, L.B. (2000). Dietary folate equivalents: interpretation and application. J Am Diet Assoc, Vol. 100, No. 1, pp. 88-94.

Talaulikar, V.S., & Arulkumaran, S. (2011). Folic Acid in obstetric practice: a review. *Obstet Gynecol Surv,* Vol. 66, No. 4, pp. 240-247.

Thiersch, J.B. (1952). Therapeutic abortions with a folic acid antagonist, 4-aminopteroyl glutamic acid (4-amino PGA) administered by the oral route. *Am J Obstet Gynecol,* Vol. 63, No. 6, pp. 1296-1304.

U.S. Preventive Services Task Force (USPSTF). (2009). Folic acid for the prevention of neural tube defects: U.S. Preventive Services Task Force recommendation statement. , Vol. 150, No. 9, pp.6266-31.

van Beynum, I.M., Kapusta, L., den Heijer, M., Vermeulen, S.H., Kouwenberg, M., Daniëls, O., & Blom, H.J. (2006). Maternal MTHFR 677C>T is a risk factor for congenital Herat defects: effect modification by periconceptional folate supplementation. *Eur Heart J,* Vol. 27, No. 8, pp. 981-987.

van der Linden, I.J., Afman, LA., Heil, SG., & Blom HJ. (2006a). Genetic variation in genes of folate metabolism and neural-tube defect risk. *Proc Nutrition Soc,* Vol. 65, No. 2, pp. 204-215.

van der Linden, I.J., den Heijer, M., Afman, LA., Gellekink, H., Vermeulen, S.H., Kluijtmans, L.A., & Blom, H.J. (2006b).The methionine synthase reductase 66A>G polymorphism is a maternal risk factor for spina bifida. *J Mol Med (Berl),* Vol. 84, No. 12, pp. 1047-1054.

van der Put, N.M., Steegers-Theunissen R.P., Frosst, P., Trijbels, F.J., Eskes T.K., van den Heuvel, L.P., Mariman, E.C., den Heyer, M., Rozen, R., & Blom, H.J. (1995). Mutated methylenetetrahydro-folate reductase as a risk factor for spina bifida. *Lancet,* Vol. 346, No. 8982, pp. 1070-1071.

van der Put, N.M., Eskes, T.K., Blom, H.J. (1997). Is the common 677C-->T mutation in the methylenetetrahydrofolate reductase gene a risk factor for neural tube defects? A meta-analysis. *Quarterly J Med,* Vol. 90, No. 2, pp. 111-115.

Vaughn, J.D., Bailey, L.B., Shelnutt, K.P., Dunwoody, K.M., Maneval, D.R., Davis, S.R., Quinlivan, E.P., Gregory, J.F. 3rd, Theriaque, D.W., Kauwell, G.P. (2004). Methionine synthase reductase 66A->G polymorphism is associated with increased plasma homocysteine concentration when combined with the homozygous methylenetetrahydrofolate reductase 677C->T variant. *J Nutr,* Vol. 134, No. 11, pp. 2985-2990.

Volpe, J.J. (1994). *Neurology of the Newborn,* pp. 3-42, W.B. Saunders Company, Philadelphia.

Watkins M.L. Efficacy of folic acid prophylaxis for the prevention of neural tube defects. (1998). *MRDD Research Reviews,* Vol. 4, pp. 282-290.

Weisberg, I., Tran, P., Christensen, B., Sibani, S., Rozen, R. (1998). A second genetic polymorphism in methylenetetrahydrofolate reductase (MTHFR) associated with decreased enzyme activity. *Mol Genet Metab,* Vol. 64, No. 3, pp. 169-172.

Whitehead, A.S., Gallagher, P., Mills J.L., Kirke, P.N., Burke H., Molloy, A.M., Weir, D.G., Shields, D.C., & Scott, J.M. (1995). A genetic defect in 5,10 methylenetetrahydrofolate reductase in neural tube defects. *Q J M,* Vol. 88, No. 11, pp. 763-766.

Wilcox, A.J., Lie, R.T., Solvoll, K., Taylor, J., McConnaughey, D.R., Abyholm, F., Vindenes, H., Vollset, S.E., & Drevon, C.A. (2007). Folic acid supplements and risk of facial clefts: national population based case-control study. BMJ, Vol. 334, No. 7591, pp. 464.

Wilson, A., Leclerc, D., Rosenblatt, D.S., & Gravel, R.A. (1999a). Molecular basis for methionine synthase reductase deficiency in patients belonging to the cblE complementation group of disorders in folate/cobalamin metabolism. *Hum Molec Genet,* Vol. 8, pp. 2009-2016.

Wilson, A., Platt, R., Wu, Q., Leclerc, D., Christensen, B., Yang, H., Gravel, R.A., & Rozen, R. (1999b). A common variant in methionine synthase reductase combined with low cobalamin (vitamin B12) increases risk for spina bifida. *Molec Genet Metab,* Vol. 67, No. 4, pp. 317-323.

Wong, L.Y. & Paulozzi, L.J. (2001). Survival of infants with spina bifida: a population study, 1979-94. *Paediatr Perinat Epidemiol,* Vol. 15, No. 4, pp. 374-378.

# 2

# Strategies for Prevention of Neural Tube Defects

Hiroko Watanabe[1] and Tomoyuki Takano[2]
[1]*Department of Clinical Nursing,*
[2]*Department of Pediatrics, Shiga University of Medical Science*
*Japan*

## 1. Introduction

Neural tube defects (NTDs) are congenital malformations of the brain and spinal cord caused by the failure of neural tubes to close between 21 and 28 days after conception (Sadler, 2005). Any disruption of neurulation during or prior to this time may result in a defect or failure of neural tube closure. Non-invasive prenatal diagnostic testing by ultrasound and maternal serum screening, which should be offered at 16 to 20 weeks gestation and 15 to 20 weeks gestation, respectively, will identify 95% of spina bifida and 100% of anencephaly cases. After 15 weeks of pregnancy, invasive prenatal diagnostic testing with ultrasound-guided amniocentesis can evaluate the fetal karyotype and measure amniotic fluid alpha-fetoprotein and acetylcholinesterase, to assist in differentiating between open or closed lesions (Chodirker et.al., 2001). The majority of cases can be categorized as either anencephaly (lack of closure in the region of the head) or spina bifida (lack of closure below the head).

Folate deficiency before conception and during early pregnancy is one potential cause of NTDs. Folate is the general term for water soluble B vitamin predominantly found in green leafy vegetables. Adequate folate intake is required for normal metabolism, cell division, neural function and growth. Humans are unable to synthesize folate and depend on an adequate and constant intake. Both observational and interventional studies, including randomized, controlled trials, have demonstrated that adequate consumption of folic acid periconceptionally can prevent 50-70% of NTDs (Czeizel & Dudas, 1992).

Currently, 57 countries have regulations for mandatory fortification of wheat flour with folic acid, (Flour Fortification Initiative, 2009) and health agencies in many countries have officially recommended the periconceptional consumption of folic acid in the range of 400 to 500 μg in young women of reproductive age who are capable of conceiving or planning to conceive (Centers for Disease Control and Prevention [CDC], 1992; Bower et al., 1995). The prevalence of spina bifida and anencephaly in the United States has declined significantly since the onset of fortification of enriched grain products with folic acid. The latest prevalence of spina bifida and anencephaly rates in the United States, reported in 2006, was 3.05 and 1.56 per 10,000 live births, respectively (Neural tube defect ascertainment project, 2010). On the other hand, the incidence of spina bifida in countries in which the fortification of enriched grain product with folate is not compulsory or endorsed officially, was 5.32 per 10,000 live births (Annual report 2007 with data 2005, 2009). The primary objective of this review article is to discuss the strategies for prevention of NTDs.

## 2. Definition and classification

NTDs are common and severe congenital malformations of the central nervous system occurring secondary to a lack of closure of the neural tube. The following three groups are categorized based on the severity of the defects (Copp & Harding, 2004).

### 2.1 Severe form

The severe form of the NTD spectrum includes open defects resulting from the failure of neural tube closure, in which the interior of the brain or spinal cord communicates directly with outside, and includes the following:

- *Craniorachischisis:* There is an almost complete absence of neural tube closure, affecting both the brain and spine. This malformation results from a failure of the initiating event of neurulation in the early embryo.
- *Excencephaly:* This is a brain defect resulting from a failure of cranial neural tube closure. Although this appearance is seen only in embryos and early fetuses, the persistently open cranial neural folds have an everted appearance.
- *Anencephaly:* Exposed cranial neural folds may degenerate with advancing gestation. This is a catastrophic malformation in which the brain is severely degeneratd and the skull vault is absent.
- *Myelomeningocele:* This results from a failure of the closure of the spinal neural tube, most often in the lumbosacral region. In *spina bifida cystica*, a meningeal sac containing the open spinal cord herniates through a vertebral defect. In *myeloceles*, the open spinal cord is directly exposed as a flat open lesion.

### 2.2 Moderate form

The moderate form of NTD includes *encephaloceles* and *meningoceles*. These defects result from herniation of the brain or meninges through an opening in the skull or vertebral column, respectively. These defects appear to be primary abnormalities of skeletal development, not neural tube closure, as the brain and spinal cord appear to have closed normally prior to herniation.

### 2.3 Mild form

The mild end of the NTD spectrum is represented by a third group of dysraphic defects in which there are closed abnormalities of the spinal cord, usually in the low lumbar and sacral regions. The following types are included:

- *Diplomyelia:* This is a side-by-side or anteroposterior duplication of the spinal cord.
- *Diastematomyelia:* A midline septum divides the spinal cord longitudinally into two usually unequal portions extending up to 10 thoracolumbar segments.
- *Hydromyelia:* The central canal is overdistended (Fig. 1).

- *Lipomeningocele:* The dysraphic spinal cord is accompanied by fatty tissue deposits.
- *Spina bifida occulta:* This is defined as a defect in the posterior bony components of the vertebral column without involvement of the cord or meninges.

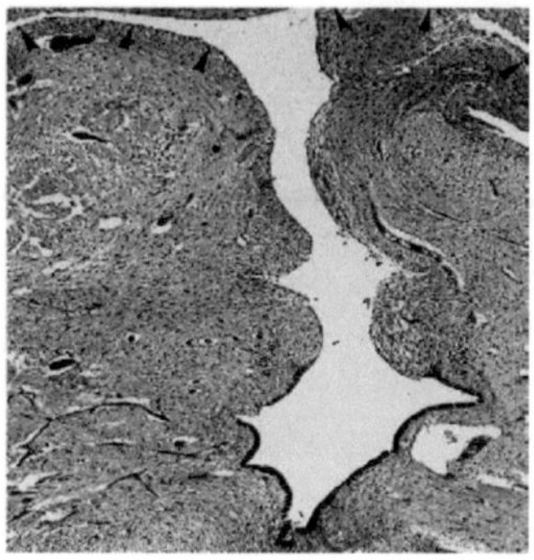

Source; Modified from Takano, T. & Becker, L.E. (1997).

Fig. 1. A coronal section of the spinal cord in a patient with a meningomyelocele. Note the overdistended and deformed central canal showing hydromyelia. Hematoxylin and eosin staining.

## 3. Clinical features and management

### 3.1 Craniorachischisis, excencephaly and anencephaly

These malformations are incompatible with survival beyond birth and today are observed almost exclusively on ultrasound examination during pregnancy.

### 3.2 Myelomeningocele

Myelomeningoceles involve all of the underlying layers, including the spinal cord, nerve roots, meninges, vertebral bodies and skin. The spinal cord may be exposed because of a complete failure of neural closure, or may be covered by a membrane. Although myelomeningocele may be situated at any longitudinal level of the neuroaxis, lumbosacral involvement is the most common (Fig. 2). Varying degrees of paresis of the legs, usually profound, and sphincter dysfunction are the major clinical manifestations. Fifty to seventy percent of neural tube defects can be prevented if a woman consumes sufficient folic acid daily before conception and throughout the first trimester of her pregnancy (Gleeson et al., 2006). Maternal serum alpha-fetoprotein determination and ultrasound examination are now routinely used to identify fetuses that have or are likely to have spina bifida or anencephaly (Drugan et al., 2001). Alpha-fetoprotein is a component of the fetal cerebrospinal fluid, and it may leak into the amniotic fluid from the open neural tube. Closed lesions often do not lead to increased alpha-fetoprotein concentrations. The management of a child with a myelomeningocele requires the concerted efforts of a multidisciplinary team involving many specialists. Treatment includes surgical reduction of the myelomeningocele and other associated defects, prevention of infection, covering of the myelomeningocele, control of hydrocephalus, management of urinary dysfunction, and treatment of the paralysis and abnormalities of the hips and feet (Gleeson et al., 2006).

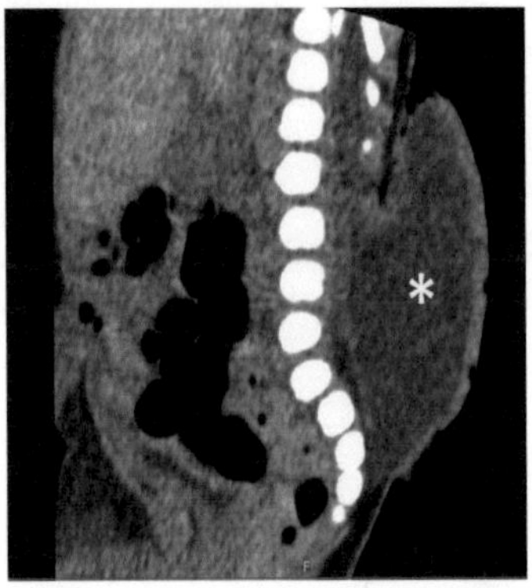

Fig. 2. A lumbar myelomeningocele in a newborn, showing a large meningeal sac (asterisk). The midline sagittal view from a computed tomography study.

### 3.3 Meningocele

A meningocele is a protrusion of the meninges without accompanying nervous tissue, and it is not associated with neurological deficits. The mass usually is evident as a fluid-filled protrusion covered by skin or a membrane in the midline. When careful examination of patients with a suspected meningocele reveals significant neurological abnormalities such as the equinovarus deformity, gait disturbance or abnormal bladder function, the diagnosis of a meningomyelocele is appropriate. A meningocele can be found in the cranial (Fig. 3) or high cervical area.

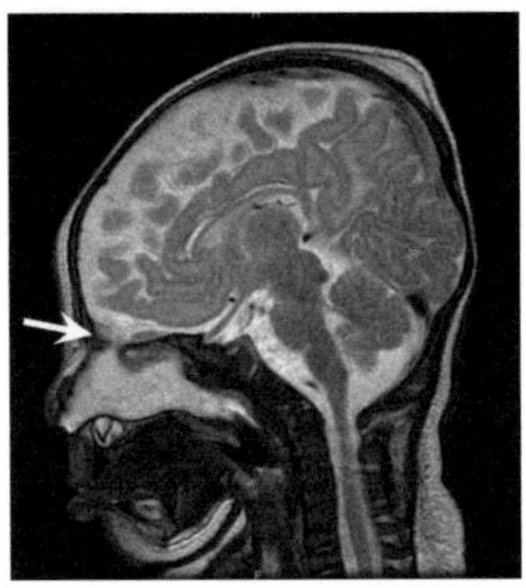

Fig. 3. A cranial meningocele in a newborn. Note the meningeal herniation through a small opening of the frontal skull (arrow) into the nasal cavity. The midline sagittal view from a magnetic resonance imaging study.

### 3.4 Encephalocele

An encephalocele is a herniation of the intracranial contents through a midline skull defect. The cranial meningoceles contain only leptomeninges and cerebrospinal fluid, whereas encephaloceles also contain brain parenchyma. The amount of compromised and deformed neural tissue and the degree of resultant microcephaly determine the extent of cerebral dysfunction (Gleeson et al., 2006). Severe intellectual and motor delays typically occur in association with microcephaly. A prenatal diagnosis of encephaloceles may be established by the determination of an increased amniotic alpha-fetoprotein content and ultrasound studies (Graham et al., 1982). Surgical corrections of all but the smallest encephaloceles are necessary.

### 3.5 Diplomyelia

This malformation is compatible with normal spinal function, and neurological deterioration suggests the presence of diastematomyelia or tethering.

### 3.6 Diastematomyelia

Patients with diastematomyelia present with congenital scoliosis, hydrocephalus, or cutaneous lesions such as hairy patch, dimple, hemangioma, subcutaneous mass, or teratoma (Kothari & Bauer, 1997). A progressive myelopathy, with deformities of the feet, scoliosis, kyphosis, or discrepancy in leg length, also may develop. Resection of the spur in diastematomyelia frequently does not result in any clinical improvement.

### 3.7 Spina bifida occulta

This occurs in at least 5% of the population, but most often is asymptomatic. This defect is often found incidentally on radiographic studies or is diagnosed because of a subtle clinical finding, such as a tuft of hair or a cutaneous angioma or lipoma in the midline of the back marking the location of the defect (Guggisberg et al., 2004).

## 4. The mechanism of folate deficiency and NTDs

In 1976, Smithells et al. (1976) suggested that folate deficiency was a cause of NTDs because women with NTDs infants had low blood folate levels. Later, they reported that periconceptional vitamin supplementation, including folic acid, reduced the recurrence of NTDs (Smithells et al., 1983). Further studies provided a growing body of evidence. Folic acid exists as polyglutamates in green leafy vegetables and other natural sources. It consists of a pteridine ring, p-aminobenzoic acid, and glutamine acid. Although folate deficiency is an established risk factor for NTDs, the exact mechanism is not clear.

Beaudin and Storver (2007) showed the pathway linking alterations in folate status with NTDs (Fig. 4). They summarized that disruption of folate metabolism could result in homocysteine accumulation, impaired nucleotide biosynthesis, and impaired cellular methylation. These metabolic impairments evoke genomic responses such as alterations in gene expression, genomic instability, reduced mitotic rates, and impaired DNA repair. Impairments in metabolism and/or genomic responses may influence cellular responses critical to proper neural tube closure, including cell proliferation, survival, differentiation, and migration. SNPs in folate-related genes can influence both maternal and infant folate status, or alternatively, Aminopterin (4-aminopteroic acid; APN) can also directly disrupt metabolism. APN is an antineoplastic drug with immunosuppressive properties used in chemotherapy and a synthetic derivative of pterin, and works as an enzyme inhibitor by competing for the folate binding site of the enzyme dihydrofolate reductase. Its binding affinity for dihydrofolate reductase effectively blocks tetrahydrofolate synthesis. This results in the depletion of nucleotide precursors and inhibition of DNA, RNA, and protein synthesis.

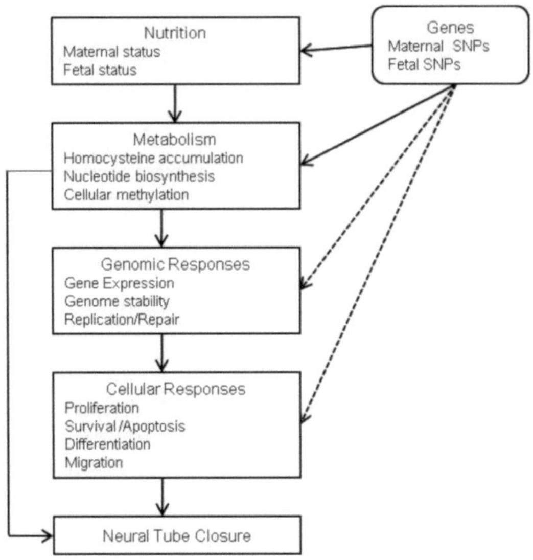


Source: Beaudin, A.E. & Stover, P.J. (2007)

Fig. 4. Pathway linking alterations in folate status with NTDs

## 5. Strategies for prevention of NTDs

The prevalence of NTDs has declined considerably during the past three decades, due to advances in the refined resolution of ultrasonography for fetal examination, the clinical availability of serum alpha-fetoprotein measurements, termination of affected pregnancies, and the consumption of folic acid supplements among reproductive-aged women. Included in these factors, successful mandatory fortification programs have been documented in several countries, including the United States, Canada, and Australia (Abeywardana et al., 2010; De Wals et al., 2008; Pfeiffer et al., 2008).

### 5.1 Countries of fortification of enriched grain product with folate

#### 5.1.1 Mandated folic acid fortification programs

In 1992, the U.S. Public Health Service recommended that all women of reproductive age in the United States who were capable of becoming pregnant should consume 400 µg of synthetic folic acid daily from fortified foods and/or supplements and that they should consume a balanced, healthy diet of folate-rich food in order to reduce the risk of NTDs (CDC, 1992). The Food and Drug Administration mandated the addition of folic acid to all enriched cereal grain products by January 1998 (Food and Drug Administration, 1996). In 2009, the U.S. Preventive Services Task Force (2009) published updated guidelines reinforcing these recommendations.

Canada introduced a fortification program in 1998, mandating the folic acid fortification of enriched white flour, as well as some corn and rice products, with ranges from 95 to 309 µg/100 g for different products (Ray et al., 2002). In Australia, the Australian National Health and Medical Research Council recommended a periconceptional daily supplement intake of 500 µg folic acid for women of childbearing age in 1993, and voluntary folic acid fortification of certain foods was permitted (National Health and Medical Research Council,

1994). In June 2007, the Australian Food Regulatory Ministerial Council agreed to mandatory fortification of bread-making flour with folic acid. The standard, September 2009, requires the mandatory addition of 200-300 µg folic acid per 100 grams of bread-making flour (Food Liaison, 2007).

The percentage of the world's wheat flour produced in large roller mills that is fortified has increased from 18% to 30%. By 2015, the target date of the World Health Organization millennium Development Goals, the Flour Fortification Initiative goal is for 80% of the world's roller-mill wheat flour to be fortified (CDC, 2010).

### 5.1.2 The effect of fortification

According to the Morbidity and Mortality Weekly Report, if 50%-70% of NTDs can be prevented through daily consumption of 400 µg of folic acid, assuming an annual prevalence of 300,000 NTDs, worldwide folic acid fortification could lead to the prevention of 150,000 - 210,000 NTDs per year (CDC, 2010).

Numerous studies have evaluated the effect of folic acid fortification on primary prevention of NTDs. A significant, worldwide decline in the prevalence of NTDs was noted in the period following folic acid fortification. In the United States, during 1995-1996, an NTD affected approximately 4,000 pregnancies. The number declined to 3,000 pregnancies in 1999-2000, following the mandated fortification of enriched cereal grain products with folic acid (CDC, 2004). From the prefortification period of 1996-1996 to the early postfortification of 1999-2000, the prevalence of spina bifida and anencephaly decreased dramatically (CDC, 2008). The latest prevalence of spina bifida and anencephaly rates in the United States, reported in 2006, was 3.05 and 1.56 per 10,000 live births, respectively, based on birth defects surveillance data (Neural tube defect ascertainment project, 2010) (Fig. 5).

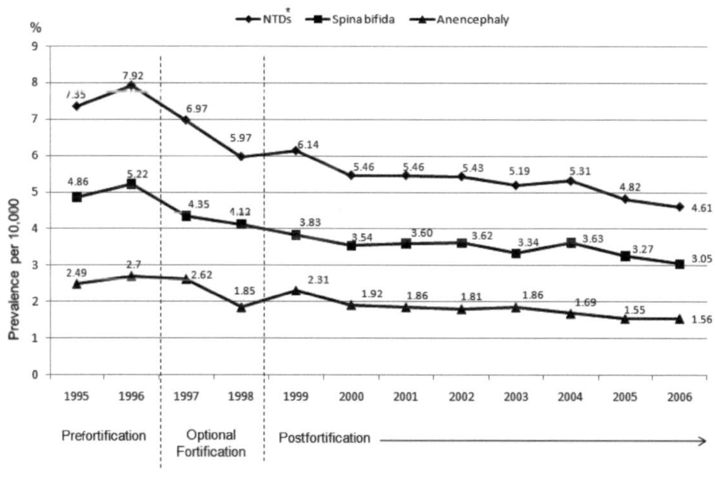


Source by neural tube defect ascertainment project of the National Birth Defects Prevention Network at Centers for Disease Control and Prevention.
*NTDs: Spina bifida + Anencephaly

Fig. 5. Prevalence of spina bifida and anencephaly in the United States, 1995-2006

Australia presented similar findings. The prevalence of NTDs dramatically declined from 20 per 10,000 births in the prefortification period to 5 per 10,000 births in the postfortification period. A declining trend of 26% was seen during this period (Abeywardana et al., 2010). Chan et al. (2008) reported a decline in the total prevalence of NTDs from 2.06 per 1,000 births in the prefortification period to 1.23 per 1,000 births in the mandatory fortification period (RR: 0.60, 95% confidence interval (CI): 0.48-0.74; $p<0.001$). Sayed et al. (2008) showed that the prevalence of spina bifida decreased from 1.41 per 1,000 births in the prefortification period to 0.98 per 1,000 births in the mandatory fortification period (RR: 0.69, 95% CI: 0.49-0.98). Ten studies suggested that food fortification could reduce the incidence of NTDs by 20 to 50%.

The effect of folic acid fortification on the incidence of NTDs has also reported in Jordan. Seventy-eight NTDs were recorded among 61,447 births between 2000 and 2006 at a Jordan hospital. Of the cases, spina bifida was the most common type of anomaly (87.2%), followed by encephalocele (11.5%), and anencephaly (1.3%). The incidence of NTDs decreased from 1.85 (95% CI; 1.2-2.4)per 1000 births before fortification (2000-2001) to 1.07 (95% CI; 0.7-1.5) during the fortification period (2002-2004), and to 0.95 (95% CI; 0.5-1.5) after full fortification (2005-2006), a 49% reduction (Amarin & Obeidat, 2011). Thus, the folic acid fortification strategy was clearly successful in some countries.

### 5.1.3 Blood folate levels after fortification

The mandatory fortification of standardized enriched cereal grain products in the United States has resulted in a substantial increase in blood folate concentrations. The percentage of the population with low serum folate (<3 ng/mL) declined from 21% in the period before fortification (1988-1994) to <1% of the total population in the period immediately following fortification (1999-2000) (Pfeiffer et al., 2008). In a study based on data from the National Health and Nutrition Examination Survey (NHANES), the mean serum folate concentration for women aged 15-44 years who did not use supplements increased from 10.7 nmol/L to 28.6 nmol/L shortly after the initiation of fortification in the United States, representing an almost threefold increase (CDC, 2000). In the most recent analysis of NHANES data, the CDC reported a 16% decline in serum folate concentrations among women aged 15-44 years from 1999-2000 to 2003-2004; red blood cell folate concentrations decreased 8% over the same time periods (CDC, 2007). The reason of these different decreased rate may that red blood cell folate concentrations reflect body stores at the time of red cell synthesis and are considered a better measure of long-term folate status (>3 months) than serum folate concentrations, which reflect recent dietary intake (Scientific Advisory Committee on Nutrition, 2006).

In Australia, researchers examined the impact of mandatory fortification of flour with folic acid on the blood folate levels in 20,592 Australians, including in women of childbearing age between 2009 and 2010. In 2010, there was a 31% increase in mean serum folate levels (from 17.7 nmol/L to 23.1 nmol/L), and a 22% increase in mean red blood cell (RBC) folate levels (from 881 nmol/L to 1071 nmol/L) after mandatory fortification with folic acid of wheat flour used in bread making among women of childbearing age (Brown et al., 2011). The introduction of mandatory fortification with folic acid has significantly reduced the prevalence of folate deficiency.

## 5.2 Countries with voluntary fortification of enriched grain products with folate

Countries where the fortification of enriched grain products with folate is not compulsory or officially endorsed report low folate status among reproductive-aged women and high incidences of NTDs. Japan is one such country, although 440 μg of dietary folate with balanced meals was recommended to all Japanese women of reproductive age by the Ministry of Health (2000) to prevent birth defects. In 2008, the National Nutrition Survey in Japan reported that the mean dietary intake of folate, vitamin $B_6$, and vitamin $B_{12}$ of non-pregnant women aged 18-29 years was less than the recommended dietary allowance (RDA) (Ministry of Health, Labour and Welfare, 2008). Another study showed (Mito et al., 2007) that more than 80% of Japanese women aged between 17 and 41 had inadequate (i.e., less than the RDA of 240 μg/d) folate intake in 2002. This failure of women to meet the RDA for folate intake may have lead to the increase in the prevalence of spina bifida from1.96 per 10,000 live births (1974-1980) to 5.32 (2001-2005) (Annual report 2007 with data 2005, 2009).

In China, women who are planning marriage or pregnancy are advised to take 400 μg of supplemental folic acid every day, starting before conception, through to the end of the first trimester of pregnancy, but this is not mandatory (Ren et al., 2006). Northern China has one of the highest reported NTD birth prevalence rates in the world. The prevalence of NTDs was 4.5 per 1,000 in 2002 (Zhang & Wang, 2004), and only 35.8% of the affected population was aware of folic acid; fewer than 15% of women reported taking folic acid periconceptionally, with the percentage being significantly lower than the average among rural farming women with less education (Ren et al., 2006). The low level of awareness as well as the low reported rate of periconceptional supplementation may explain the high prevalence of NTDs.

## 6. Feature approaches

There have been three main approaches to reduce the incidence of NTDs: health promotion to improve the knowledge and awareness of folic acid, ensuring the use of fortified folic acid and folic acid supplements, and reducing the number of obese women, which is also a known environmental factor (Waller et al., 1994; Werler et al., 1996).

### 6.1 Health promotion to improve knowledge and awareness regarding folic acid

The USA, Canada, and Australia have implemented food fortification programs successfully with resultant improvement in serum folate levels and reduction in incidences of NTDs. Education campaigns can be effective and public health campaigns aimed at informing and influencing behavioral change in all individuals. Rofail et al. (2011) examined pre- and post-campaign awareness, knowledge, and consumption data for women of reproductive-age in Australia. Awareness of folic acid improved post-campaign, with the percentage improvement between pre- and post-campaigns ranging from 6 to 41%. Women's knowledge of the association between folate and spina bifida increased from 8% before the program began to 67% two-and-a-half years later. The proportion of women taking periconceptional folic acid supplements increased from 13% to 30% over the same period (Bower et al., 1997). Since the introduction of this promotion, the prevalence of NTDs in Western Australia, which was about two per 1,000 births from 1980 until 1995, fell by 30% in 1996 (Bower et al., 2002). The estimated increase in mean serum folate concentration was 19% after educational campaigns to increase periconceptional folic acid use (Metz et al., 2002). The ultimate goal of any folic acid awareness campaign is to promote use of folic acid supplements, to increase the blood folate levels of women, and to prevent the occurrence of NTDs.

An U. S. national survey showed differences in folic acid awareness and knowledge among age groups (CDC, 2008). In 2007, approximately 61% of women aged 18-24 years reported being aware of folic acid, compared to 87% of women aged 25-34 years and 89% of women aged 35-45 years. Women aged 18-24 years were also less knowledgeable about the need for folic acid consumption before pregnancy (6%), compared to women aged 35-45 years (16%). In addition, approximately 33% of women who were aware of folic acid had received the information about folic acid from their health-care providers, followed by finding information in a magazine or newspaper (31%) and receiving it through radio or television (23%). Official health education initiatives have promoted folic acid supplementation and a diet rich in folates through mass media, including TV, newspapers, and magazine articles worldwide (CDC, 2010). Special attention and targeted approaches must concentrate on this age group. Public health campaigns aimed at increasing awareness, knowledge, and periconceptional use of folic acid should concentrate on using appropriate intervention methods worldwide.

### 6.2 Encouragement to increase women's dietary intake of folic acid and use of folic acid supplements

Many women of childbearing age in the United States do not maintain a healthy diet prior to, during, or after pregnancy. Numerous studies have reported that women in the United States do not consume the recommended 400 µg of folic acid (Hilton, 2007; Rinsky-Eng & Miller, 2002). In Japan, more than 80% of Japanese women between 17 and 41 years of age had inadequate folate intake - less than the recommended daily allowance of 240 µg/d (Mito et al., 2007; Watanabe et al., 2008). Other studies have also shown that most women of reproductive age in the U.S. are not getting enough vitamin C or B6, in addition to folic acid (Cena et al., 2008 ; Yang et al., 2007).

As previously indicated, consuming folate-rich foods or ingesting folic acid, a synthetic compound available through dietary supplements and through fortified foods, can increase folate levels. Folic acid is approximately 1.7 times more bio-available than folate, and therefore, has a greater efficiency in making an impact on folate levels (Neuhouser & Beresford, 2001).

In the U.S, the percentage of women of childbearing age who took daily supplements containing folic acid increased from 28% in 1995 (prefortification) to 32% in 2003 (postfortification) (Green-Raleigh et al., 2006), and to 40% in 2007 (US Department of Health and Human Services [USDHHS], 2010). One of the Healthy People 2010 objectives was to increase to 80% the proportion of all women of childbearing age who consume 400 µg of folic acid daily to reduce the risk for serious birth defects (USDHHS, 2010). Although a worldwide campaign contributed to progress toward this goal, approximately 60% of childbearing-aged women are still not consuming a daily supplement containing folic acid.

One should note that supplementation alone is not an effective approach because one-third to one-half of all pregnancies in the Unites States is unplanned (Custer et al., 2008). Women often do not know that they are pregnant during the crucial first 4 to 8 weeks of pregnancy. Neural tube development occurs during this time, hence the importance of ensuring adequate folic acid intake. Women aged 18-24 years have the highest rate of unintended pregnancies in the United States (Finer & Henshaw, 2006) but remain the least aware of and knowledgeable about folic acid; they are also the least likely to report consuming a supplement containing folic acid. Recent studies have indicated that only 39% of southern Australian subjects (Chan et al., 2008), and 13.5% of Canadian subjects (French et al., 2003), knew they should take folic acid before pregnancy. Fortifying foods with folic acid has been a highly effective and uniform intervention, because fortification makes folic acid accessible to all women of childbearing age, without requiring substantial behavioral changes.

### 6.3 Reduce the number or obese or overweight women

Overweight status and obesity have become serious global public health issues. Nearly two thirds of reproductive-aged women in the United States are currently overweight or obese (≥25 $kg/m^2$). In the NHANES, the prevalence of obesity (BMI ≥30 $kg/m^2$) in women aged 20-49 years continues to be high, exceeding 30% after 1999 (Flegal et al., 2010). In the latest NHANES data from 2007-2008 of 877 women aged 20-39 years, the prevalence of overweight status (BMI ≥25 $kg/m^2$) and obesity were 59.5% and 34.0%, respectively.

The worldwide trend of increasing obesity may lead to increasing the incidences of NTDs. A population-based case-control study by Shaw et al. (1996) indicated an increased risk for NTD-affected pregnancies among obese women with BMIs >29 $kg/m^2$, compared to women of normal pre-pregnancy BMIs (OR: 1.9, 95% CI: 1.3-2.9), when adjusted for maternal age, education, gravidity, use of vitamins, and use of alcohol. Rasmussen et al. (2008) conducted a metaanalysis of 12 published reports, including 4 cohort and 8 case-control studies conducted from 2000 through 2007, on the relationship between maternal obesity and the risk of NTDs. Unadjusted odds ratios for an NTD-affected pregnancy were 1.22 (95% CI: 0.99-1.49), 1.70 (95% CI: 1.34-2.15), and 3.11 (95% CI: 1.75-5.46) among overweight, obese, and severely obese women, respectively, compared with normal-weight women. Based on the results of this metaanalyisis, maternal obesity was associated with a 1.7-fold increased risk of NTDs, and severe obesity was associated with a >3-fold increased risk. A possible mechanism may involve problems with glucose metabolism, because obese women are more likely to have pre-pregnancy diabetes mellitus, which is a well-known risk factor for NTDs (Becerra et al., 1990; Werler et al., 1996). However, the reasons for this association are not yet known.

The risks associated with high BMI are best addressed before conception because weight loss during pregnancy is not recommended. Counseling to support improvements in diet and physical activity is a first-step intervention. All women with a BMI of 25 $kg/m^2$ or greater should be offered specific strategies to improve the balance and quality of their diets, to decrease caloric intake, and to increase physical activity.

## 7. Conclusion

NTDs are life threatening and cause life-long disabilities. They are a worldwide problem, affecting an estimated 300,000 or more fetuses or infants each year. Experimental and epidemiological evidence has shown that periconceptional dietary supplementation with folic acid can result in an estimated 50-70% decrease in the prevalence of NTDs. To reduce more incidences of NTDs, each reproductive-aged woman must try to consume food fortified with folic acid and folic acid supplements and maintain adequate BMIs before conception. Special attention or renewed educational approaches must target reproductive-aged women. Public health campaigns aimed at increasing awareness, knowledge, and periconceptional use of folic acid using appropriate intervention methods worldwide continues to be the most effective strategy.

## 8. References


Abeywardana, S.; Bower, C.; Halliday, J.; Chan, A. & Sullivan, E.A. (2010). Prevalence of neural tube defects in Australia prior to mandatory fortification of bread-making flour with folic acid. *Aust NZ J Public Health*, Vol. 34(4): 351-5.

Amarin, Z.O. & Obeidat, A.Z. (2011). Effect of folic acid fortification on the incidence of neural tube defects, *Paediatrd Perinat Epidemiol*, Vol. 24(4): 349-51.

Annual report 2007 with data 2005. (2009). The International Centre on Birth Defects-ICBDSR Center, Roma, pp. 191-2.

Beaudin, A.E. & Stover, P.J. (2007). Folate-mediated one-carbon metabolism and neural tube defects: balancing genome synthesis and gene expression. *Birth Defects Res C Embryo Today*, Vol. 81(3): 183-203.

Becerra, J.E.; Khoury, M.J.; Cordero, J.F. & Erickson, J.D. (1990). Diabetes mellitus during pregnancy and the risks for specific birth defects: a polulation-based case-control study. *Pediatrics*, Vol. 85(1): 1-9.

Bower, C.; Blum, L.; Ng, M.L.; Irvin, C. & Kurinczuk, J. (1995). Folate and the prevention of neural tube defects: evaluation of a health promotion project in Western Australia. Health promotion International, Vol. 11(3): 177-87.

Bower, C.; Blum, L.; O'Daly, K.; Higgins, C.; Loutsky, F. & Kosky, C. (1997). Promotion of folate for the prevention of neural tube defects: knowledge and use of periconceptional folic acid supplements in Western Australia, 1992-1995. *Aust NZ J Public Health*, Vol. 21(7): 716-21.

Bower, C.; Ryan, A.; Rudy, E. & Miller, M. (2002). Trends in neural tube defects in Western Australia. *Aust NZ J Public Health*, Vol. 26(2): 150-1.

Brown, R.D.; Langshaw, M.R.; Uhr, E.J.; Gibson, J.N. & Joshua, D.E. (2011). The impact of mandatory fortification of flour with folic acid on the blood folate levels of an Australian population. *Med J Aust*, Vol. 194(2): 65-7.

Cena, E.R.; Joy, A.B.; Heneman, K.; Espinosa-Hall, G.; Garcia, L.; Schneider, C.; Wooten Swanson, P.C.; Hudes, M. & Zidenberg-Cherr, S. (2008). Folate intake and food-related behaviors in nonpregnant, low-income women of childbearing age. *J Am Diet Assoc*, Vol. 108(8): 1364-8.

Centers for Disease Control and Prevention (CDC). (1992). Recommendations for the use of folic acid to reduce the number of cases spina bifida and other neural tube defects. *MMWR Recomm Rep*, Vol. 41 (RR-14): 1-7.

CDC. (2000). Folate status in women of childbearing age-United States, 1999. *MMWR Morb Mortal Wkly Rep*, Vol. 49(42): 962-5.

CDC. (2004). Spina bifida and anencephaly before and after folic acid mandate-United States, 1995-1996 and 1999-2000. *MMWR Morb Mortal Wkly Rep*, Vol. 53(17): 362-5.

CDC. (2007). Folate status in women of childbearing age, by race/ethnicity-United States, 1999-2000, 2001-2002, and 2003-2004. *MMWR Morb Mortal Wkly Rep*, Vol. 55(51-52): 1377-80.

CDC. (2008). Use of supplements containing folic acid among women of childbearing age-United States, 2007. *MMWR Morb Mortal Wkly Rep*, Vol. 57(1): 5-8.

CDC. (2010). CDC grand rounds: additional opportunities to prevent neural tube defects with folic acid fortification. *MMWR Morb Mortal Wkly Rep*, Vol. 59(13): 980-4.

Chan, A.C.; van Essen, P.; Scott, H.; Haan, E.A.; Sage, L.; Scott, J.; Gill, T.K. & Nguyen, A.M. (2008). Folate awareness and the prevalence of neural tube defects in South Australia, 1996-2007. *Med J Aust*, Vol. 189(10): 566-9.

Chodirker, B.N.; Cadrin, C.; Davies, G..A.; Summers, A.M.; Wilson, R.D.; Winsor, E.J. & Young, D. (2001). Canadian guidelines for prenatal diagnosis, genetic indications for prenatal diagnosis. *J SOGC*, Vol. 23(5): 523-31.

Copp, A.J. & Harding, B.N. Neural tube defects In: Pathology and Genetics: Developmental neuropathology, Golden, J. A. & Harding, B.N. (eds). (2004). pp 2-13, ISN Neuropath Press, Basel.

Custer, M.; Waller, K.; Vernon, S. & O'Rourke, K. (2008). Unintended pregnancy rates among a US military population. *Paediatr Perinat Epidemiol*, Vol. 22(2): 195-200.

Czeizel, A.E. & Dudas, I. (1992). Prevalence of the firs occurrence of neural tube defects by periconceptional vitamin supplementation. N Engl J Med, Vol. 327(26): 1832-5.

De Wals, P.; Tairou, F.; Van Allen, M.I.; Lowry, R.B.; Evans, J.A.; Van den Hof, M.C.; Crowley, M.; Uh, S.H.; Zimmer, P.; Sibbald, B.; Fernandez, B.; Lee, N.S. & Niyonsenga, T. (2008). Spina bifida before and after *folic acid fortification in Canada. Birth Defects Res A Clin Mol Teratol, Vol. 82(9):622-6.*

Drugan, A.; Weissman, A. & Evans, M.I. (2001). Screening for neural tube defects. *Clin Perinatol*, Vol. 28(2): 279-87.

Finer, L.B. & Henshaw, S.K. (2006). Disparities in rates of unintended pregnancy in the United States, 1994 and 2001. *Perspect Sex Reprod Health* , Vol. 38(2): 90-6.

Flegal, K.M.; Carroll, M.D.; Ogden, C.L. & Curtin, L.R. (2010). Prevalence and trends in obesity among US adults, 1999-2008. *JAMA*, Vol. 303(3): 235-41.

Flour Fortification Initiative. (2009). (Access on August 10, 2011), Available from http://www.sph.emory.edu/wheatflour/countrydata.php

Food and Drug Administration. (1996). Food standards: amendment of standards of identify for enriched grain products to require addition of folic acid. *Federal Register*, Vol. 61: 8781-97.

Food Liaison [FOODfine page on the Internet]. *Canberra ( AUST ): Food Liaison Pty Ltd; 2007.* Australia New Zealand Food Law on Disc® Australia and New Zealand. Version 51. (Access on August 8, 2011), Available from http://www.foodliaison.com.au/amendments/notes51.pdf

French, M.R.; Barr, S.I. & Levy-Milne, R. (2003). Folate intake and awareness of folate to prevent neural tube defects: a survey of women living in Vancouver, Canada. J *Am Diet Assoc*, Vol. 103(2): 181-5.

Gleeson, J.G.; Dobyns, W.B.; Plawner, L. & Ashwal, S. (2006). Congenital structural defects In: *Pediatric Neurology: principles and practice*, Swaiman, K.F., Ashwal, S. & Ferriero, D.M.(eds.). (2006). pp. 363-490, Mosby Elsevier, Philadelphia.

Graham, D.; Johnson, T.R Jr.; Winn, K. & Sanders, R.C. (1982). The role of sonography in the prenatal diagnosis and management of encephalocele. *J Ultrasound Med*, Vol. 1(3): 111-5.

Green-Raleigh, K.; Carter, H.; Mulinare, J.; Prue, C. & Petrini, J. (2006). Trends in folic acid awareness and behavior in the United States: the Gallup Organization for the March of Dimes Foundation surveys, 1995-2005. *Matern Child Health J*, Vol. 10(5 suppl): S177-82.

Guggisberg, D.; Hadj-Rabia, S.; Viney, C.; Bodemer, C.; Brunelle, F.; Zerah, M.; Pierre-Kahn, A.; de Pros, Y. & Hamel-Teillac, D. (2004). Skin markers of occult spinal dysraphism in children: a review of 54 cases. *Arch Dermatol*, Vol. 140(9): 1109-15.

Hilton, J.J. (2007). A comparison of folic acid awareness and intake among young women aged 18-24 years. *J Am Acad Nurse Pract*, Vol. 19(10): 516-22.

Kothari, M.J. & Bauer, S.B. (1997). Urodynamic and neurophysiologic evaluation of patients with diastematomyelia. *J Child Neurol*, Vol. 12(2): 97-100.

Metz, J.; Sikaris, K.A.; Maxwell, E.L. & Levin, M.D. (2002). Changes in serum folate concentration following voluntary food fortification in Australia. *Med J Aus*, Vol. 176(2); 90-1.

Ministry of Health: Department of Maternal and Child Health, Bureau of Children and Families. (2000). Information on promoting intake of folic acid in order to reduce children afflicted with neural tube defects among young women who are capable of becoming pregnant (in Japanese).

Ministry of Health, Labour and Welfare: Department of Nutrition. (2008). National nutrition survey results. Available from: www.mhlw.go.jp/houdou/2009/11/dl/h1109-1b.pdf (Access on August 5, 2011).

Mito, N.; Takimoto, H.; Umegaki, K.; Ishiwaki, A.; Kusama, K.; Fukuoka, H.; Ohta, S.; Abe, S.; Yamawaki, M.; Ishida, H. & Yoshiike, N. (2007). Folate intakes and folate biomarker profiles of pregnant Japanese women in the first trimester. *Eur J Clin Nutr*, Vol. 61(1):83–90.

National Health and Medical Research Council. (1994). Revised statement on the relationship between dietary folic acid and neural tube defects such as spina bifida. *J Paediatr Child Health*, Vol. 30(6): 476-7.

Neuhouser, M.L. & Beresford, S.A. (2001). Folic acid: are current fortification levels adequate? *Nutrition*, Vol. 17(10): 868-72.

Neural tube defect ascertainment project. (2010). (Access on August 1, 2011), Available from http://www.nbdpn.org/current/2010pdf/NTD%20fact%20sheet%2001-10%20for%20 website.pdf

Pfeiffer, C.M.; Johnson, C.L,; Jain, R.B.; Yetley, E.A.; Picciano, M.F,; Rader, J.I.; Fisher, K.D.; Mulinare, J. & Osterloh, J.D. (2008).Trends in blood folate and vitamin B-12 concentrations in the United States, 1988-2004. *Am J Clin Nutr*, Vol. 86(3): 718-27.

Rasmussen, S.A.; Chu, S.Y.; Kim, S.Y., Schmid, C.H. & Lau, J. (2008). Maternal obesity and risk of neural tube defects: a metaanalysis. *Am J Obstet Gynecol*, Vol.198(6): 611-9.

Ray, J.G.; Vermeulen, M.J.; Boss,S.C. & Cole, D.E. (2002). Declining rate of folate 43
insufficiency among adults following increased folic acid food fortification in 44
Canada. *Can J Public Health*, Vol. 93(4): 249-53.

Ren, A.; Zhang, L.; Li, Z.; Hao, L.; Tian, Y. & Li, Z. (2006). Awareness and use of folic acid, and blood folate concentrations among pregnant women in northern China-An area with a high prevalence of neural tube defect. *Reprod Toxicol*, Vol. 22(3): 431-6.

Rinsky-Eng, J. & Miller, L. (2002). Knowledge, use, and education regarding folic acid supplementation: continuation study of women in Colorado who had a pregnancy affected by a neural tube defect. *Teratology*, Vol. 66 (Suppl 1): S29-31.

Rofail, D.; Colligs, A.; Abetz, L.; Lindemann, M. & Maguire, L. (2011). Factors contributing to the success of folic acid public health campaigns. *J Public Health (Oxf)*, [E pub ahead of print].

Sadler, T.W. (2005). Embrology of neural tube development: embryology of neural tube development. *Am J Med Genet C Semin Med Genet*, Vol. 135C(1): 2-8.

Sayed, A.R.; Bourne, D.; Pattinson, R.; Nixon, J. & Henderson, B. (2008). Decline in the prevalence of neural tube defects following folic acid fortification and its cost-benefit in South Africa. *Birth Defects Res A Clin Mol Teratol*, Vol. 82(4): 211-6.

Scientific Advisory Committee on Nutrition. (2006). Folate and disease prevention. Norwich: The Stationery Office.

Shaw, G.M.; Velie, E.M. & Schaffer, D. (1996). Risk of neural tube defect-affected pregnancies among obese women. *JAMA*, Vol. 275(14): 1093-6.

Smithells, R.W.; Sheppard, S. & Schorah, C.J. (1976). Vitamin deficiencies and nerural tube defects. Arch Dis Childh, Vol. 51(12): 944-50.

Smithells, R.W.; Nevin, N.C.; Seller, M.J.; Sheppard, S.; Harris, R.; Read, A.P.; Fielding, D.W.; Walker, S.; Schorah, C.J. & Wild, J. (1983). Further experience of vitamin supplementation for prevention of neural tube defect recurrences. *Lancet*, Vol. 1(8332): 1027-31.

Takano, T. & Becker, L.E. (1997). Overexpression of nestin and vimentin in the ependyma of spinal cords from hydrocephalic infants. *Neuropathol Appl Neurobiol*, Vol. 23(1): 3-15.

US Department of Health and Human Services. Healthy people 2010 (conference ed, in 2 vols). Washington, DC: US Department of Health and Human Services; 2000. (Access on August 5, 2011), Available from http://www.health.gov/healthypeople

U.S. Preventive Services Task Force. (2009). Folic acid for the prevention of neural tube defects: U.S. Preventive Services Task Force recommendation statement. *Ann Intern Med*, Vol. 150(9): 626-31.

Waller, D.K.; Mills, J.L.; Simpson, J.L.; Cunningham, G.C.; Conley, M.R.; Lassman, M.R. & Rhoads, G.G. (1994). Are obese women at higher risk for producing malformed offspring?, *Am J Obstet Gynecol*, Vol. 170(2): 541-8.

Watanabe, H.; Fukuoka, H.; Sugiyama, T.; Nagai, Y.; Ogasawara, K. & Yoshiike, N. (2008). Dietary folate intake during pregnancy and birth weight in Japan. *Eur J Nutr*, Vol. 47(6): 341-7.

Werler, M.M.; Louik, C.; Shapiro, S. & Mitchell, A.A. (1996). Prepregnant weight in relation to risk of neural tube defects. *JAMA*, Vol. 275(14): 1089-92.

Yang, Q.H,; Carter, K.; Mulinare, J.; Berry, R.J.; Friedman, J.M. & Erickson, J.D. (2007). Race-ethnicity differences in folic acid intake in women of childbearing age in the United States after folic acid fortification: findings from the National Health and Nutrition Examination Survey, 2001-2002. *Am J Clin Nutr*, Vol. 85(5): 1409-16.

Zhang, X. & Wang, L. (2004). Analysis of birth defects surveillance, 1966-2002. *Matern Child Health Care China*, Vol. 19: 93-4 (in Chinese).

# 3

# Primary Prevention of Neural Tube Defects

Claudine Nasr Hage and Grace Abi Rizk
*Saint Joseph school of medicine*
*Lebanon*

## 1. Introduction

Neural tube defects (NTD) are serious birth defects of the brain and spine, occurring when the neural tube doesn't form or close completely. They are among the most frequent congenital malformations, affecting 300,000 pregnancies worldwide. Two forms of NTDs, spina bifida and anencephaly, account for 90% of all cases (Centers for Disease Control, CDC, 1989).

Studies had proven that supplementation of women of childbearing age with folic acid can prevent up to 70% of all cases of NTDs (Laurence et al 1981, MRC Vitamin Study Research Group 1991). These researches led to international recommendations that all women of childbearing age consume 400 micrograms of folic acid daily for the prevention of neural tube defects at least 1 month before and throughout the first trimester of pregnancy (CDC 1992, Institutes of Medicine 1998, WHO 2002). Three potential approaches were advocated to increase level of folic acid consumption among the general population: fortification of food supply, improvement of dietary habits and use of dietary supplements (CDC, 1992). In some countries such as Canada and the USA, these recommendations led to the fortification of all enriched grain products with folic acid. This action decreased the occurrence of spina bifida by 31% and anencephaly by 16% (CDC 2004) and thus was considered as a partial success. As for the change in eating habits, meeting dietary recommendations for grain intake is an important step to achieving the recommended daily intake for folic acid. Studies have shown that non pregnant women of childbearing age reported an average daily consumption of 128 mcg of folic acid, representing only 32 percent of the daily recommended amount (Yang et al. 2007). These facts imply that most women still need to daily consume a dietary supplement containing folic acid at the recommended dose (400 µg) in order to prevent pregnancies with NTDs. Despite all this, several studies have shown a low consumption of folic acid supplements worldwide: numbers vary from prevalence as low as 7.5% in Lebanon (Nasr Hage et al 2011) to the highest percentage of 40 % in Canada and the USA (Morin et al. 2002; Petrini et al, 2008). These percentages remain far from the "Healthy people 2010" goal aiming that a minimum of 80% of women of childbearing age consume at least 400 mcg of folic acid daily in the periconception period. Levels of awareness and knowledge have been studied extensively in women of childbearing age in order to explain the low prevalence of folic acid intake with variable results in different countries. Although these levels of awareness and knowledge were thought to explain low levels of folic acid consumption, a systematic review of the literature showed that variable interventions on folic acid increased women's awareness from 60% to 72% and knowledge from 21% to 45%. At the same time, levels of folic acid consumption increased only from 14% to 23% showing a positive but suboptimal impact (Chivu et al. 2007). As Green and Kreuter say "changes in knowledge and awareness alone cannot be assumed to translate into changes in behavior" (Green and Kreuter, 1991). There is still a gap between awareness and behavior on one side and usage of folic acid on the other side. This gap could be explained by determinants of behavioral change such as unplanned pregnancies, perceived barriers for taking folic acid pills, lack of time, level of education, age group and culture.

This chapter will discuss the preventive role of folic acid in the development of neural tube defects and the recommendations concerning its consumption. Factors related to folic acid knowledge, attitude and behavior will be analyzed as well as suggestions made for effective strategies aiming to improve its usage among women of childbearing age.

## 2. Role of folic acid in the prevention of NTDs

### 2.1 Folic acid as a vitamin

Folate, also known as vitamin B9, is a water-soluble B vitamin that occurs naturally in food. It is an essential nutrient that humans can not synthesize. Folic acid is the synthetic form of folate that is found in supplements and added to fortified foods. Folate is found naturally in a wide variety of foods particularly leafy green vegetables such as spinach, asparagus and lettuce, grains such as beans, peas and lentils, fruits such as orange, cantaloupe and melon, kidney, liver, egg yolk and yeast. Most folates have many molecules of glutamic acid; they have to be converted to monoglutamate to be absorbed in the intestine. The synthetic form has one molecule of glutamic acid making it more bioavailable than the natural form. Folate is critically important for fetal development. It has a role in DNA synthesis, acts as a cofactor for many essential cellular reactions and is implicated in the metabolism of several amino acids especially in the conversion of homocysteine to methionine; thus, the need for folate increases during periods of rapid tissue growth such as in pregnancy. When folate is insufficient, DNA synthesis is impaired and cells are unable to successfully achieve mitosis. In addition, the methylation process of proteins, lipids and myelin is inhibited (Rosenblatt, 1995).

### 2.2 Mechanism of NTD prevention with folic acid

The mechanism by which folic acid prevents NTDs remains unknown. Many theories have been proposed. Genetic, nutritional, environmental factors or a combination of these play a role in the development of NTDs. The genetic theory of methylation was proposed by Blom et al (Blom et al, 2006). Problems during embryogenesis in the methylation of DNA, proteins and lipids are related to the development of NTDs. A mutation in the gene coding for the methylenetetrahydrofolate reductase enzyme, responsible of the generation of a methyl group essential for biosynthesis of methionine and nucleotides, is believed to contribute to fetal nervous system malformation such as spina bifida (Mills et al, 1995). This mutation accounts for one-fourth of NTDs suggesting that the protective effect of folate, reaching a 70% reduction in NTDs, involves other environmental factors or gene-environment interactions (Posey et al, 1996). Other genes involved in the methylation cycle through remethylation or transsulfuration of homocysteine were also involved in the development of NTDs (Boyles et al, 2005). Besides the methylation theory, two other theories were proposed as genetic explanations for the relationship between folic acid and NTDs: the role of the genes codifying to enzymes needed for nucleotide biosynthesis such as the polymorphism in methylenetetrahydrofolate dehydrogenase, and the role of the genes codifying proteins involved in the transport, capture and cell retention of folate (DeMarco et al, 2006; Beaudin and Stover, 2009). The role of nutrition in the development of NTDs has been studied. The relationship between folic acid deficiency and NTDs may be linked to lower gene expressions due to alteration in the methylation and synthesis of DNA (Zeisel, 2009). The daily consumption of folic acid reduced the level of homocysteine, a risk factor in the development of NTDs (Boyles et al, 2005).

### 2.3 Evidence for prevention of NTDs with folic acid

Early studies in the sixties and seventies suggested a role for diet in NTDS (Hibbard and Smithells 1965; Knox, 1972; Smithells et al 1976). In early eighties, two randomized controlled trials showed a reduction in the recurrence of NTDs with folic acid supplementation but these studies were criticized for their methodological limitations (Laurence et al 1981; Smithells et al, 1980). Further observational studies conducted in the eighties suggested that the consumption of folic acid by women of childbearing age is protective against NTDs in newborns (Bower and Stanley, 1989; Milunsky et al, 1989; Mulinar et al, 1988). This was confirmed by a randomized multicenter controlled trial showing that daily supplementation of women in childbearing age with folic acid reduced by 72% the risk of recurrence of NTDs (MRC Vitamin Study Research Group 1991). The conclusive proof of the preventive effect of folic acid for women with no NTD history came from a randomised controlled study conducted in Hungary that showed no NTD cases occured among 2104 women taking folic acid as compared with six cases among 2052 pregnancies in the group not taking folic acid (Czeizel and Dudas, 1992). A meta-analysis study published in 2010 reviewed all observational and randomized studies evaluating the first occurrence and recurrence of NTDs and related mortalities in pregnancy. It concluded that folic acid intake reduced the recurrence of NTDs by 70% and the first occurrence of NTD by 62% (Blencowe et al, 2010).

### 2.4 Recommendations for folic acid consumption in pregnancies

All the data confirming the protective effect of folic acid against NTDs led to international recommendations concerning folic acid consumption in women of childbearing age. The Institutes of Medicine and CDC recommend the maternal consumption of 400 micrograms of synthetic folic acid daily at least 1 month before conception and during the first few months of pregnancy (CDC, 1992; Institute of Medicine, 1998). The Canadian college of medical geneticists recommended that a minimum dose of 0.8 mg/day of folic acid along with a well-balanced diet should be prescribed for women planning a pregnancy, starting before conception and for at least 10-12 weeks of pregnancy (Van Allen et al, 1993). Similar guidelines were issued by the Canadian college of obstetricians and gynecologists.

The EUROCAT published a report about the "prevention of neural tube defects by periconceptional folic acid supplementation in Europe" (EUROCAT special report, updated version December 2009). In most European countries where a policy exists, periconceptional folic acid supplements are recommended at a daily dose of 0.4 to 0.5 mg and the dose of 4 to 5 mg is reserved for women who have had a previous pregnancy complicated with NTDs. Table 1 (adapted from the EUROCAT report) summarizes periconceptional folic acid supplementation policies around Europe.

Because half of all pregnancies in the United States are unplanned (Finer and Henshaw 2006), and because NTDs occur often before a woman knows she is pregnant, the Centers for Disease Control and Prevention (CDC) recommends that all women who can become pregnant consume the recommended amount of folic acid daily, regardless of their pregnancy intentions (CDC, 2004).

| Country | Folic acid policy | |
|---|---|---|
| | Status | Year current policy introduced |
| Austria | Unofficial | 1998 |
| Belgium | Unofficial | - |
| Croatia | Unofficial | - |
| Denmark | Official | 1997 |
| Finland | Official | 2004 |
| France | Official | 2000 |
| Germany | Unofficial | 1994 |
| Hungary | Official | 1996 |
| Ireland | Official | 1993 |
| Italy | Official | 2004 |
| Malta | Dietary | 1994 |
| Netherlands | Official | 1993 |
| Norway | Official | 1998 |
| Poland | Official | 1997 |
| Portugal | Official | 1998 |
| Slovenia | Official | 1998 |
| Spain | Official | 2001 |
| Sweden | Official | 1996 |
| Switzerland | Official | 1996 |
| UK | Official | 1992 |
| Ukraine | Official | 2002 |

Table 1. Folic acid supplementation policy in European countries (until December 2007)

## 3. Community interventions to increase folate intake

Three ways were advocated in order to increase folate intake in women of childbearing age: improvement of dietary habits, fortification of food supply with folic acid and the use of folic acid supplements (CDC, 1992)

### 3.1 Improvement of dietary habits

Studies have shown that the average consumption of folate by women is not more than 200μg/day (Gregory et al, 1990; Subar et al, 1989). Yang and colleagues calculated the average daily dietary intake of folate and folic acid by women of childbearing age in the

USA in 2001-2002. They found that the average daily consumption was 128 µg/day, representing 32% of the daily recommended amount (Yang et al, 2007). Knowing the importance of grain intake in achieving the recommended intake for folic acid, Briefel and Johnson reviewed national data in the USA on grain intake; they found that, in 1999-2000, only 24% of the population met the recommendation for daily servings of grains (Briefel and Johnson, 2004). The German Nutrition Report 2004 stated that the average daily intake of all women in Germany was 215µg/day, still below the reference value of 400µg/day (EUROCAT, 2009). Another study done by Heinz showed that 81% of women 18-40 years of age had a daily folic acid consumption of less than 150µg (Heinz et al, 2001 as in EUROCAT, 2009). In Hungary, a dietary survey conducted in 2003-2004 showed that the average daily folic acid intake is 132.3µg/day (EUROCAT, 2009).The average daily natural folate intake of most women in different European countries ranges from 230 to 280 µg /day (Flynn et al, 2009). A review done by Kumaniyka and his colleagues in 2000 on dietary behavioral changes in relation with nutrients such as fruits, vegetables and grains highlighted the difficulty of sustaining these behavioral modifications (Kumaniyka et al, 2000). These studies show that achieving the recommendations for folic acid consumption by food folates alone requires major dietary modifications unlikely to be achieved by women of childbearing age. Furthermore, one study tried to compare the effectiveness of the 3 suggested interventions for meeting the recommendations on folic acid. A 12-week trial evaluated the changes in red blood cell folate in response to one of the following interventions: folic acid supplementation (400µg/day), natural food folates (400µg/day), fortified food (400µg/day), qualitative dietary advice and control diet. The study showed that the only interventions increasing significantly blood folate were food fortification and folic acid supplements. The increase in natural food folates did not translate into higher levels of blood folate, most probably because of the low bioavailability and stability of natural folates compared to the synthetic form (Cuskelly et al, 1996).

### 3.2 Fortification of food with folic acid

Regulations for mandatory food fortification with folic acid are currently in place in 53 countries (CDC, 2010). In 1996, the United States Food and Drug Administration (FDA) issued a mandate to fortify all enriched grain products with folic acid, to be fully implemented in 1998. Food items covered by this mandate were mainly flour, corn meal, pasta and rice and they were fortified with 140µg/100g of cereal grains. At this level of fortification, women are expected to consume an average of 100µg daily of folic acid from fortified cereal grain products (FDA, 1996). Folic acid food fortification became mandatory in Canada and Costa Rica in 1998, with the fortification respectively of 150µg and 180µg /100g of enriched flour and uncooked cereal grains (Chen and Rivera, 2004; Ray, 2004). In 2000, the Chilean ministry of health mandated that folic acid should be added at a level of 2.2mg/kg to wheat flour (Hertrampf and Cortés, 2004). In June 2004, the Brazilian government introduced mandatory fortification of wheat and maize flour with 150µg/100 g (Almeida and Cardoso, 2010). A number of Middle Eastern countries, as well as Indonesia now fortify their flour. South Africa issued a mandate on food fortification in 2003 with 150 µg of folic acid added to 100g of cereal grains (Sayed et al, 2008).The Australian government had agreed to fortification of flour and bread with folic acid, starting September 2009. In Europe mandatory fortification of a staple food with folic acid has been seriously considered in 8 countries (Denmark, Germany, Ireland, Northern Netherlands, Norway, Poland,

Switzerland and the UK), but debates are still going on. Until now, no European country has agreed to mandatory food fortification with folic acid (EUROCAT, 2009). At the same time, food voluntarily fortified with folic acid (such as breakfast cereals) is available in many European countries. These countries do not implement mandatory folic acid supplementation because, according to them, expected additional health benefits are not scientifically proven in clinical trial, because of feared health consequences and because of the issue of freedom of choice (Eichholzer et al, 2006).

Studies have shown a positive impact of food fortification on blood folate concentrations and a reduction in the prevalence of NTDs in the USA (Boulet et al, 2008), in Canada (Godwin et al, 2008) and in Chile (Nazer et al, 2007).

Measuring blood folate concentrations constitutes one way to evaluate the effect of food fortification programs. Folate deficiency is defined as a serum folate concentration <7nmol/l (3ng/ml) or a red blood cell folate concentration <315nmol/l (140ng/ml) (Crider et al, 2011). In The USA, median serum folate increased from 12.6µg/l in 1994 to 18.7 µg/l in 1998 after food fortification (Lawrence et al, 1999). In Canada, a study conducted on 38,000 women in Ontario showed an increase in red blood cell folate from 527nmol/l to 741 nmole/l after food fortification ($p<0.001$) (Ray et al, 2002). In Chile, the mean serum concentrations and red blood cell folate increased respectively from 9.7 and 290nmol/l to 37.2 and 707nmol/l ($p<0.0001$) after mandatory fortification (Hertrampf et al, 2003).

The main purpose for folic acid fortification was to reduce the occurence of NTDs and the associated mortality and morbidities. Many studies around the world evaluated the impact of food fortification on the prevalence of NTDs. In the USA, a report published by the CDC in 2004 found a reduction of 27% in spina bifida and anencephaly between 1995-1996 and 1999-2000 (CDC, MMWR 2004). Different studies in the USA with different methodologies showed a decrease in the prevalence of NTDs between 19-32% after mandatory food fortification, reaching 23 to 54% for spina bifida and 11% to 16% for anencephaly (Boulet et al, 2008; Honein et al, 2001; Mathews, 2008; Williams et al, 2002). In Canada, studies have shown an even greater impact of food fortification than the impact shown in the USA. De Wals and collegues examined the NTD trends before and after food fortification in seven of ten Canadian provinces (De Wals et al, 2007, 2008). They showed a 46% reduction of NTDs and the magnitude of the decrease was higher for spina bifida (53%) than for anencephaly (38%) (De walls et al, 2007). Similar results were found in Chile, Argentina and Brazil with a reduction in the prevalence of NTDs by 19 to 55 % (Lopez-Camelo et al, 2010). In South Africa, Sayed and his collegues found a significant decline of 30.5% in the prevalence of NTDs (41.6% for spina bifida and 10.9% for anencephaly) following food fortification in 2003 (Sayed et al, 2008). The differences found in the magnitude of the decline in NTD prevalence after food fortification among different countries depend on many factors such as the initial prevalence of NTDs, the initial folate status of the population, the consumption of fortified food by the population and the presence of birth defects surveillance systems (Crider et al, 2011).

### 3.3 Folic acid supplements

The third way suggested for increasing women consumption of folic acid is the use of supplements. In order to be effective, these supplements should be taken at least 1 month before conception. This fact constitutes a limitation for the reliance on supplements as a primary public health program since in many countries, a high level of pregnancies are unplanned such as in the USA where up to 50% of pregnancies are unplanned. International studies have shown a low level of compliance with folic acid supplements intake. In the USA, the percentage of women of childbearing age who consume folic acid supplements is low, slightly increasing from 28% in 1995 to 33% in 2005, up to 40% in 2007 (CDC, 2008). Even in the Netherlands, where the percentage of planned pregnancies is estimated at 85%, only 36% of women take folic acid supplements during the periconceptional period (Meijer and De Walle, 2005). These low levels of intake were seen in different countries with the highest percentage of intake seen in Canada and the USA (40%) and the lowest percentages in Korea (10.3%), Thailand (9.7%) and Lebanon (7.5%) (Kim et al, 2009; Morin et al, 2002; Nasr Hage et al, 2011; Nawapun and Phupong, 2007; CDC, 2008).

## 4. Women's knowledge and awareness concerning folic acid

Of interest is the relationship between knowledge, awareness and adequate intake of folic acid. Awareness concerning folic acid is usually evaluated in response to the question "have you ever heard or read anything about folic acid?"; levels of awareness reported in the literature are very variable. In the USA, the March of Dimes Birth Defects Foundation reported national levels of awareness of 52% in 1995, increasing to 84% in 2005 (March of Dimes Birth Defects Foundation, 2005). The analysis done by the CDC showed that from 2003 to 2007, levels of awareness were stagnant around 80% (79% in 2003 and 81% in 2007) (CDC, 2008). In Canada, awareness reached a percentage of 95% (French et al, 2003). Even in countries were folic acid intake is very low, women have usually high levels of awareness such as in Lebanon where 60% of women knew about folic acid but only 7.5% of them were using supplements adequately (Nasr Hage et al, 2011). Still in some countries, the number of women who have heard of folic acid is low, reaching 18% in Turkey (Turgul et al, 2009). Even though levels of awareness are acceptable in general with some exceptions, the gap lies in knowledge concerning the benefits of folic acid in NTDs prevention, the nutritional source of natural and synthetic folates and the adequate period of folic acid intake. National percentages in the USA showed that in 1995 only 4% of American women knew that folic acid help reduce the risk of birth defects. These numbers reached 24% in 2004 before decreasing to 19% in 2005. The same report stated that only 2% of American women identified the adequate period for folic acid intake, percentages reaching 12% in 2004 and dropping to 7% in 2005 (March of Dimes Birth Defects Foundation, 2005). A CDC report showed that knowledge concerning the adequate period of intake raise slightly to 12% in 2007 (CDC, 2008). In Canada where the levels of awareness and intake are relatively high, only 25% of women studied in Vancouver knew that folic acid could prevent birth defects (French et al, 2003). As expected, low levels of knowledge were also found in countries with low levels of folic acid intake such as in Thailand where 25% of surveyed women knew that folic acid was something important and in Lebanon where 14% knew about the role of folic acid in NTD prevention and 25% knew about the adequate period for supplementation (Nasr Hage et al, 2011; Nawapun and Phupong, 2007). These numbers show that low intake of folic acid supplements is, at least partially related to lack of knowledge. This relationship was suggested by French and colleagues showing that 78% of the women in their study indicated that, with knowledge of the benefits of folate, they would use folic acid supplements to reduce the risk of birth defects (French et al, 2003). Another survey done in 2009 by the Gallup organization showed that when women were told the health benefits of taking a multivitamin with folic acid, 66% stated they were "willing" to buy and take a multivitamin and 22% stated they were "somewhat willing" (North Carolina Folic acid Council, 2009). A systematic review of the literature showed that variable interventions on folic acid increased women's awareness from 60% to 72% and knowledge from 21% to 45%. At the same time, levels of folic acid consumption increased only from 14% to 23% showing a positive but suboptimal impact (Chivu et al. 2007).

## 5. Folic acid intake

### 5.1 Determinants of folic acid intake

Studies measuring levels of folic acid intake looked for the factors related to behavior in order to explain low levels of usage. Daily folic acid intake is shown to be related to race/ethnicity, income, marital status, a positive attitude toward taking a physician's advice, knowledge about the relationship between folic acid and birth defects, planning for the pregnancy, earlier pregnancies and earlier discussion between the women and her physician about vitamins (Ahluwalia et al, 2007; Carmichael et al, 2006; Cleves et al, 2004; French et al, 2003; Rosenberg et al, 2003). Studies also found that younger age is related to a lower intake of folic acid supplements (Morin et al, 2002; CDC, 2008; Timmermans et al, 2008).

Studies in the USA showed that African-American and Hispanic women were less likely to use folic acid supplements than Caucasian women (Ahluwalia et al, 2007; Carmichael et al, 2006; Cleves et al, 2004). Half of Hispanic women, and one third of African-American women aged 18-24 years, as compared to Caucasian women were taking folic acid supplements. An Irish study showed that women from Asia/Middle East, Eastern Europe, Africa and South America were less likely to use folic acid supplements than those from Western Europe and that the highest intake was among women from North America, Australia and New Zealand (McGuire et al, 2010). Ethnicity was also a factor influencing the uptake of folic acid supplements in the Netherlands, where non-western women were less likely to use supplements than western women (Timmermans et al, 2008).

The relationship between low income and a lower intake of supplements has been highlighted in the literature. In their report published in 2008, Petrini and colleagues showed that the lowest prevalences of folic acid intake were seen in those with an annual household income of <$25,000 compared to those with >$50,000; these prevalences varied from 24% to 32% between the years 2003 and 2007 for women with the lowest income, and from 38% to 43% between 2003 and 2007 for women with the highest income (CDC, 2008). In Australia, a low income of less than 30,000$ was also associated with low levels of supplements intake (Forster et al, 2009). Lower socio-economical status was related to an inadequate behavior concerning folic acid supplements (no intake or less than recommended intake) in 2 studies conducted in Ireland and The Netherlands (McGuire et al, 2010; Timmermans et al, 2008). At the same time, high level of education in women of childbearing age was associated with a high level of folic acid intake (Nasr Hage et al, 2011; Nawapun and Phupong, 2007; CDC, 2008).

Being married was frequently identified as a factor of high folic acid intake. Cleves and colleagues found that married women were almost twice more likely than single women to take a daily supplement (Cleves et al, 2004). In the Netherlands, 42% of married women used folic acid supplement as compared to 10% of single women ($p<0.001$) (Timmermans et al, 2008). Another factor related to folic acid usage is the planning of pregnancy. Studies have shown that women who intended their pregnancies were 3 times more likely to use adequately folic acid supplements than women with unintended pregnancies (Rosenberg et al, 2003). In Europe, countries such as Norway and Ireland, studies have shown a higher chance of folic acid usage among women with planned pregnancies compared to unplanned pregnancies (McGuire et al, 2010; Nilsen et al, 2006). A planned pregnancy was also a factor related to supplements consumption in non-western countries such as Lebanon and Korea (Kim et al, 2009; Nasr Hage et al, 2011). The impact of this factor increases with the proximity of the planned conception, with women who indicate their desire to become pregnant at some time in the future but with no specific plan, being no more likely to take a daily folic acid supplement than women never wanting to become pregnant (Cleves et al, 2004). The number of pregnancies was also found as a determinant of folic acid intake with women having had anterior pregnancies more likely to take folic acid supplements than women with their first pregnancy (Carmichael et al, 2006; Nasr Hage et al, 2011; Nilsen et al, 2006). Only one study conducted in Australia by Forster and his colleagues showed that having had other pregnancies is correlated with lower levels of folic acid intake (Forster et al, 2009). National studies in the USA showed that the pregnancy status was also a factor influencing positively the chance of folic acid intake (CDC, 2008).

Age is a very important factor in relationship with folic acid for many reasons. In the USA, women in the age of 18-24 years account for one third of all births. At the same time, studies have shown that this age group had the least awareness and knowledge about folic acid and the lowest reported daily use of supplements (Morin et al, 2002; CDC, 2008; Timmermans et al, 2008). Furthermore, women in this age group have multiple risk factors for inadequate folic acid consumption. They have a high rate of unintended pregnancies, reaching 80% of all pregnancies in this age group (Finer and Henshaw, 2006) and they adopt risky sexual behaviors, not using systematically birth controls in about 1 in 5 women (Chandra et al, 2005). In this age group, women have also the lowest median annual household income (DeNavas-Walt et al, 2006) and often haven't completed college. They engage in unhealthy dietary behavior and often fail to meet dietary intake recommendations (Anding et al, 2001). All these behavioral, economical, educational and nutritional factors contribute to the low level of folic acid consumption in this age group and to the increased risk of pregnancies affected by NTDs. One study found that women aged 14-19 years were twice as likely to have a pregnancy with NTD as women 25-29 years of age (Reefhuis and Honein, 2004). It is of noteworthy to highlight the fact that all these studies in this age group were conducted in western countries where sexual activities and pregnancies in young, single women are socially accepted in opposition to more conservative societies where data on this subject is lacking.

An interesting study conducted by Ahluwalia and his collegues showed that certain psychosocial factors as well as advice from a health care provider help women to make decisions about folic acid use (Ahluwalia et al, 2007). In this study, regular use of multivitamins was positively associated with perceived benefits and negatively associated with perceived barriers.

### 5.2 Strategies to improve folic acid use

In the years following the folic acid recommendations, many educational and promotional campaigns using different means of communication have been used to promote folic acid intake during the periconceptional period with variable results. A systematic review of the literature on interventions designed to improve knowledge, awareness and consumption concerning folic acid was conducted in 2007 (Chivu et al, 2007). Among consumers, the interventions studied were printed and audio-visual media (radio, TV, internet) and printed media with other channels such as counseling, free distribution of folic acid pills, advertisements, magnetized reminders, food labels (folate logo and messages from nutritionists on food packs), slide presentations and reminder phone calls. Among health professionals, the interventions studied consisted of printed materials, training, professional publications, letters, personal communication, incentives (coffee mugs, note pads) and reminder in the patient history form. The review showed that health professionals increased their knowledge about folic acid advised dose from 13 to 58% before intervention to 51% to 70% after intervention and about the recommended period for folic acid usage from 57% to 80% before intervention to 79% to 85% after intervention ($p<0.0001$). Also, 19% to 62% of health professionals were recommending folic acid to women after the intervention, as compared to 13% to 45% before the intervention. As for women, awareness concerning folic acid increased on average from 60% to 72%, knowledge increased from 21% to 45% and consumption increased from 14% to 23%. Even though variable interventions increased women's knowledge and awareness of folic acid, there were still wide discrepancies between awareness/knowledge and consumption. Studies have shown that, according to social marketing theory, mass media positively influences people's awareness and knowledge, whereas behavior is more influenced by things such as health professionals' counseling and interpersonal communication (Roger, 2003).

Many European countries have launched official educational campaigns on folic acid and its role in the prevention of NTDs. In Belgium, the ONE (Office Of Birth and Childhood) in association with ASBBF (Association Spina Bifida Belge Francophone) ran a campaign including leaflets, a website, information on radio and television and letters to gynecologists and family physicians about the benefits of periconceptional folic acid . After the campaign, a study was conducted in 2006 on 195 women in the first week after delivery. It showed a percentage of folic acid consumption before and during pregnancy of only 12% (EUROCAT, 2009). In Denmark, the Danish Veterinary and Food Administration published leaflets addressing women planning pregnancy and distributed them to clinics, hospitals, pharmacies and drugstores in 1999 and again in 2001.At the same time, a study on compliance with folic acid guidelines was launched in 2000 until 2002 and was able to evaluate the impact of the health education campaign on folic acid usage. This study showed an increase in the proportion of women complying with the recommendation after the campaign. However, even at the end of the period, only 22% of the women with planned pregnancies were following the recommendations on folic acid supplementation (Knudsen et al, 2004). In Germany, there are no official governmental guidelines on periconceptional folic acid and no official health education campaigns. However, in Munich, a non official campaign on folic acid took place from 1996 to 1998. The impact of this campaign was evaluated by measuring periconceptional folic acid intake. This study showed an increase of intake from 2% in 1996 to 5% in 1998. Still, the percentages reached for folic acid consumption were excessively low (Egen, 1999 as cited in EUROCAT, 2009). In Ireland, since the recommendations on the consumption of folic acid tablets were issued in 1993, many promotional campaigns were undertaken at the national level through periodic media campaigns. At a more local level, health promotion units and public health departments promoted folic acid through a variety of channels, usually on an on-going basis. Studies evaluating the impact of these campaigns showed that even though women's awareness and knowledge concerning the role of folic acid in NTD prevention have reached high levels (95% and 77% respectively in 2002), the consumption of periconceptional folic acid was very low and not improving , being 21% in 1998 and reaching only 23% in 2002 (Ward et al, 2004). In Sweden, since 2007, the Board of the National Food Administration is sending annual letters to all women 18-45 years of age with information on the link between folic acid and the risk of NTDs, in addition to an offer of free folic acid tablets. No Study was conducted in Sweden to evaluate the efficacy of this campaign (EUROCAT, 2009).

## 6. Health professionals' knowledge and behavior concerning folic acid

Some studies found that health professionals play a major role in folic acid usage by women of childbearing age. The survey conducted by the March of the Dimes Foundation showed that 42% of women, aware of folic acid but not consuming it, would take a multivitamin if advised to do so by a health professional (March of the Dimes, 2004). In the 2004 Health Styles Survey, 91% of women 18-45 years of age agreed to take a multivitamin daily to prevent NTDs if their doctor encouraged them (Williams et al, 2006). In order to evaluate health professionals' knowledge and practice, the CDC initiated a national study in USA in 2001 among obstetricians/gynecologists, family/general physicians, nurse practitioners, certified nurse midwives, physician assistants and registered nurses (Williams et al, 2006). The study showed that more than 85% of the health care professionals knew about the adequate time to use folic acid supplements and that these supplements were necessary beyond what is available in diet. At the same time, 42% of the health professionals surveyed did not know the correct folic acid dosage. Nurse practitioners were most likely and family/general doctors were least likely to recommend supplements. The strongest predictor for recommending supplements was the personal intake of multivitamins by the health professional. Since incorporating messages about folic acid into preventive health care messages is critical to increasing folic acid consumption, health professionals were asked if they addressed folic acid intake during well-women visits. More obstetricians/gynecologists than family/general practitioners said they mentioned folic acid regularly to women (65% v/s 50% respectively). The conclusion of this study was that even though knowledge among health professionals concerning folic acid was good, this knowledge did not necessarily translate into counseling patients about its benefits.

Consistent with these results, 2 other studies conducted in the USA showed that even though health care providers were aware of the importance of folic acid in the prevention of NTDs, only half of them discussed folic acid on a regular basis with women of childbearing age (Hauser et al,2004; Power et al, 2000). A pilot study conducted in Ontario, Canada showed that 43% of family physicians did not mention folic acid supplementation as a topic for discussion with women of childbearing age, with women actually planning pregnancies or with women in the first trimester of pregnancy (Pereleman et al, 1996). The same study showed that up to 40% recommended folic acid to an already pregnant woman, and 10%

recommend it only to pregnant women. Only 14% of physicians in this study had correct knowledge of the appropriate dosages and timing for folate supplements and only 17% of all contacted physicians recommended folate to any women of childbearing age. In Puerto Rico, 88% of primary care physicians demonstrated an inadequate knowledge about folic acid supplements with older physicians and women physicians demonstrating greater knowledge than other physicians in the study (Mirinda et al, 2003). In Israel, 2 studies evaluated physicians' knowledge and practice concerning folic acid. The first study showed that 94% of physicians recommended folic acid to their patients but knowledge in this study was insufficient since only 2% correctly estimated the efficacy of folic acid in decreasing NTDs, 12% knew about the adequate timing and 47% about the correct dosage of folic acid supplements (Abu-Hamad et al, 2008). Another study conducted among women and physicians in Israel showed that 87% of gynecologists recommended preconception folic acid compared to 60% of family physicians ($p<0.05$) (Auriel et al, 2011). In Germany, a study done in 1996 showed that only 38% of gynecologists in Munich recommended preconceptional folic acid, 8% recommended folic acid at the beginning of pregnancy, 17% recommended folic acid only in cases with family history of NTDS and 37% did not give any recommendation at all. Following an interventional campaign in 1998, 74% of gynecologists recommended preconceptional folic acid. However, there were still 15% of gynecologists who recommended folic acid with the beginning of pregnancy and 11% only in case of a family history (Egen, 2000 as in EUROCAT, 2009).

## 7. Conclusion

There is strong evidence that most NTDs are preventable by increasing folate status before conception. Responses to this evidence have been variable around the world. Many governments have issued recommendations regarding the necessity for women to take folic acid, from at least 1 month before conception and during the first 3 months of pregnancy. Up to 53 countries around the world issued regulations for mandatory folic acid fortification of staple food. These countries had the most reduction in NTD prevalence according to registries. Even though this was a success story, it was considered as a partial success since the reduction seen with fortification was less than the reduction seen in studies using folic acid supplements. This was the reason behind the recommendations for folic acid supplements during the periconceptional period, at the dose of 400-500µg/day for women with no history of NTDs and at the dose of 4-5 mg/day in case of family history or previous personal pregnancies with NTDs. Health education campaigns on local and national were launched in many countries with variable results. These campaigns have been mainly effective on increasing the knowledge and awareness of women concerning folic acid. Still, the actual intake of folic acid is quiet low during the periconceptional period. All these facts show that women's behavior is complex and influenced by many determinants. A package of different measures including actions targeting women and health professionals are needed in order to improve intake of folic acid by women of childbearing age.

## 8. References

Abu-Hammad, T., Dreiher, J., Vardy, D.A. and Cohen, A.D. (2008). Physicians' knowledge and attitudes regarding periconceptional folic acid supplementation: a survey in Southern Israel. *Med Sci Monit*; 14 95): CR262-7.

Ahluwalia, I.B., Lawrence, J.M. and Balluz, L. (2007). Psychosocial factors associated with use of multivitamins by women of childbearing age. *Journal of Community Health*; 32 (1): 57-69.

Almeida, L.C. and Cardoso, M.A. (2010). Recommendations for folate intake in women: implications for public health strategies. *Cad, Saude Publica* [serial on the internet]. Nov; 26 911): 2011-2026.

Anding, J., Suminski, R. and Boss, L. (2001). Dietary intake, body mass index, exercise and alcohol: Are college women following the dietary guidelines for Americans? *Journal of American College Health*; 49 (4): 167-71.

Auriel, E., Biderman, A., Belmaker, I., Freud, T. and Peleg, R. (2011). Knowledge, attitudes, and practice among women and doctors concerning the use of folic acid. *ISRN Obstet Gynecol*; 946041.

Beaudin, A.E. and Stover P.J. (2009). Insights into metabolic mechanisms underlying folate-responsive neural tube defects: a minireview. *Birth Defects Res A Clin Mol Teratol*; 85: 274-84.

Blencowe, H., Cousens, S., Modell, B. and lawn, J. (2010). Folic acid to reduce neonatal mortality from neural tube disorders. *International Journal of epidemiology*; 39 Suppl 1:110-21.

Blom, H.J., Shaw, G.M., Den Heijer, M. and Finnell, R.H. (2006) Neural tube defects and folate: case far from closed. *National Review of Neuroscience*; 7: 724-31.

Boulet, S.L., Yang, Q., Mai, C., Kirby, R.S., Collins, J.S., Robbins, J.M., Meyer, R., Canfield, M.A. and Mulinare, J.(2008)Trend sin the postfortification prevalence of spina bifida and anencephaly in the United states. *Birth Defects Res. A Clin. Mol. Teratol.*; 82: 527-32.

Bower, C. and Stanley, F.J. (1989). Dietary folate as a risk factor for neural tube defects: evidence from a case-control study in Western Australia. *Medical Journal of Australia*; 150(11): 613-9.

Boyles, A.L., Hammock, P. and Speer, M.C. (2005). Candidate gene analysis in human neural tube defects. *American Journal of Medical Genetics Part C: Seminars in Medical Genetics*, 135C:9-23.

Briefel, R.R. and Johnson, C.L. (2004). Secular trends in dietary intake in the United States. *Annual Review of Nutrition*; 24: 401-31.

Carmichael, S.L., Shaw, G.M., Yang, W.W., Laurent, C.C., Herring, A.A., Royle, M.H., Marjorie, H. and Canfield, M.M. (2006). Correlates of Intake of folic acid-containing supplements among pregnant women. *American Journal of Obstetrics and Gynecology*; 194 (1): 203-10.

Centers for Disease Control. (1989). Economic burden of spina bifida -- United States, 1980-1990. *Morbidity and Mortality Weekly Report* 38:264-7.

Centers for Disease Control. (1992). Recommendations for the use of folic acid to reduce the number of cases of spina bifida and other neural tube defects. *Morbidity and Mortality Weekly Report* 41(RR-14): 1-7.

Centers for Disease Control and Prevention. (2004). Spina bifida and anencephaly before and after folic acid mandate--United States, 1995-1996 and 1999-2000. *Morbidity and mortality weekly report* 53 (17):362-5.

Centers for Disease Control and Prevention. (2008). Use of supplements containing folic acid among women of childbearing age---United States, 2007. *Morbidity and mortality weekly report;* 57 (01):5-8.

Centers for Disease Control and Prevention. (2010). CDC grand rounds: additional opportunities to prevent neural tube defects with folic acid fortification. *Morbidity and mortality weekly report;* 59 (31): 973-9.

Chandra, A., Martinez, G.M., Mosher, W.D., Abma, J.C. and Jones, J. (2005). Fertility, family planning, and reproductive health of U.S. women: Data from the 2002 National survey of family growth. National Center for Health Statistics. *Vital Health Statistics;* 23 (25).

Chen, L.T. and Rivera, M.A. (2004). The Costa Rican experience: reduction of neural tube defects following food fortification programs. *Nutr. Rev.;* 62: S40-43.

Chivu C.M., Tulchinsky T.H., Soares-Weiser K., Braunstein R. and Brezis M. (2008). A systematic review of interventions to increase awareness, knowledge, and folic acid consumption before and during pregnancy. *American Journal of Health Promotion* Mar-Apr; 22 (4):237-45.

Cleves, M.A., Hobbs, C.A., Collins, B., Andrews, N., Smith, L.N. and Robbins, J. (2004). Folic acid use by women receiving routine gynecologic care. *Obstet Gynecol;* 103 (4): 746-53.

Crider, K.S., Bailey, L.B. and Berry, R.J. (2011). Folic acid food fortification-its history, effect, concerns and future directions. *Nutrients;* 3: 370-84.

Cuskelly, G.J., McNulty, H. and Scott, J.M. Effect of increasing dietary folate on red-cell folate: implications for prevention of neural tube defects. *Lancet;* 347:657-9.

Czeizel, A.E. and Dudas, I. (1992). Prevention of the first occurrence of neural-tube defects by periconceptional multivitamin supplementation. *BMJ;* 306 (6893): 1645-1648.

De Marco, P., Merello, E., Calevo, M.G., Mascelli, S., Raso, A., Carna, A., et al. (2006). Evaluation of a methylenetetrahydrofolate-dehydrogenase 1958 G>A polymorphism for neural tube defectrisk. *Journal Human Genetics;* 51:98-103.

DeNavas-walt, C., Proctor, B.D. and Lee, C.H. (2006). U.S. Census Bureau, Current Population Reports, P60-231, Income, Poverty, and Health Insurance Coverage in the United States: 2005, U.S. government printing Office, Washington, DC.

De Wals, P., Tairou, F., Van Allen, M.I., Uh, S.H., Lowry, R.B., Sibbald, B., Evans, J.A., Van den Hof, M.C., Zimmer, P., Crowley, M., Fernandez, B., Lee, N.S. and Niyonsenga, T. (2007) Reduction in neural tube defects after folic acid fortification in Canada. *N. Engl. J. Med.;* 357: 135-42.

De Wals, P., Tairou, F., Van Allen, M.I., Lowry, R.B., Evans, J.A., Van der Hof, M.C., Crowley, M., Uh, S.H., Zimmer, P., Sibbald, B., Fernandez, B., Lee, N.S. and Niyonsenga, T.(2008). Spina bifida before and after folic acid fortification in Canada. *Birth Defects Res A Clin Mol Teratol;* 82 (9): 622-6.

Eichholzer, M., tonz, O. and Zimmermann, R. (20060. Folic acid: a public-health challenge. *Lancet;* 367 (9519): 1352-61.

EUROCAT. (2009). Special report: prevention of neural tube defects by periconceptional folic acid supplementation in Europe. EUROCAT Central Registry, University of Ulster.

French, A.E., Grant, R., Weitzman, S., Ray, J.G., Vermeulen, M.J., Sung, L., Greenberg, M. and Koren, G. (2003). Folic acid food fortification is associated with a decline in neuroblastoma. *Clin Phamacol Ther;* 74 (3): 288-94.

Finer, L.B. and Henshaw, S.K. (2006). Disparities in rates of unintended pregnancy in the United states, 1994 and 2001. *Perspectives on Sexual and Reproductive Health*; 38: 90-96.

Food and Drug Administration. (1996). Food standards: amendment of standards of identity for enriched grain products to require addition of folic acid. *Federal Register*; 61: 8781-97.

Gregory, J.F. III, Bhandari, S.D., Bailey, L.B., Toth, J.P., Bumagartner, T.G. and Cedra, J.J. (1990). Stable-isotope methods for assessment of folate bioavailability. *American Journal of Clinical nutrition*; 51:212-5.

Green, L.W., and Kreuter, M.W. (1991). Health promotion planning: An educational and environmental approach. *Mountain View, CA: Mayfield Publishing Company.*

Godwin, K.A., Sibbald, B., Bedard, T., Kuzeljevic, B., Lowry, R.B. and Arbour, L. (2008). Changes in frequencies of select congenital anomalies since the onset of folic acid fortification in a canadian birth defect registry. *Canadian Journal of Public Health*; 99: 271-5.

Hertrampf, E., Cortes, F., Erickson, J.D., Cayazzo, M., Freire, W., Bailey, L.B., Howson, C., Kauwell, G.P. and Pfeiffer, C. (2003). Consumption of folic acid-fortified bread improves folate status in women of reproductive age in Chile. *Journal of Nutrition*; 133 (10): 3166-9.

Hertrampf, E. and Cortes, F. (2004). Folic acid fortification of wheat flour: Chile. *Nutr. Rev.*; 62: S44-9.

Hibbard, E.D. and Smithells, R.W. (1965). Folic acid metabolism and embryopathy. *Lancet*; 1 (7398), 1254.

Hauser, K.W. and Lilly, C.M. (2004). Florida health care providers' knowledge of folic acid for the prevention of neural tube defects. Southern Medical Journal; 97 (5): 437-9.

Honein, M.A., Paulozzi, L.J., Mathews, T.J., Erickson, J.D. and Wong, L.Y. (2001). Impact of folic acid fortification of the US food supply on the occurrence of neural tube defects. *JAMA*; 285:2981-6.

Institute of Medicine. (1998). *Report of the Institute of Medicine Food and Nutrition Board, Standing Committee on the Scientific Evaluations and Dietary Reference Intakes.* Washington, D.C.: National Academy Press.

Kim, M.H., Han, J.Y., Cho, Y.J., Ahn, H.K., Kim, J.O., Ryu, H.M., Kim, M.Y., Yang, J.H. and Nava-Ocampo, A.A. (2009). Factors associated with a positive intake of folic acid in the periconceptional period among Korean women. *Public Health Nutrition*; 12 (4): 468-71.

Knox, E.G. (1972). Anencephalus and dietary intake. *British Journal of preventive Social Medicine*; 26: 219-23.

Knudsen, V.K., Mikkelsen, T.B., Michaelsen, K.F. and Olsen, S.F. (2004). Low compliance with recommendations on folic acid in relation to pregnancy: is there a need for fortification? *Public Health Nutrition*; 7: 843-50.

Kumanyika, S.K., Bowen, D., Rolls, B.J., Van Horn, L., Perri, M.G., Czajkowsky, S.M. and Schron, E. (2000). Maintenance of dietary behavior change. *Health Psychology*; 19 (1): 42-56.

Laurence, K. M., N. James, M. H. Miller, G. B. Tennant, and H. Campbell. (1981).Double-blind randomised controlled trial of folate treatment before conception to prevent recurrence of neural-tube defects. *British Medical Journal* 282 (6275):1509-11.

Lopez-Camelo, J.S., Castilla, E.E. and Orioli. (2010). Folic acid flour fortification: Impact on the frequencies of 52 congenital anomaly types in three South American countries. *American Journal of Medical Genetics Part A*; 152: 2444-58.

March of Dimes (2005). Folic acid and the prevention of birth defects: A national survey of pre-pregnancy awareness and behavior among women of childbearing age 1995-2005.

Medical Research Council (MRC) Vitamin Study Research Group. (1991). Prevention of neural tube defects: results of the Medical Research Council Vitamin Study. *Lancet*. 338:131-7.

Mathews, T.J. (2008). Trends in spina bifida and anencephalus in the United States, 1991-2005. http://www.cdc.gov/nchs/products/pubs/pubd/hestats/spine_anen.htm

McGuire, M., Cleary, B., Sahm, L. and Murphy, D.J. (2010). Prevalence and predictors of periconceptional folic acid uptake-prospective cohort study in an irish urban obstetric population. *Human Reproduction*; 25: 535-43.

Meijer, W.M. and de Walle, H.E. (2005). Differences in folic acid policy and the prevalence of neural tube defects in Europe: Recommendations for food fortification in a EUROCAT report. *Ned Tijdschr Geneeeskunde*; 149 (46): 2426-2430.

Milunsky, A., Jick, H., Jick, S.S., Bruell, C.L., McLaughlin, D.S.Rothman, K.J. and Willett, w. (1989). Multivitamin/folic acid supplementation in early pregnancy reduces the prevalence of neural tube defects. *JAMA*; 262 9200: 2847-52.

Mills J.L., McPartlin J.M., Kirke P.N., Lee Y.J., Conley M.R., Weir D.G. and Scott J.M. (1995). Homocystein metabolism in pregnancies complicated by neural tube defects. *Lancet* 345: 149-151.

Mirinda, A., Davila Torres, R.R., Gorrin Peralta, J.J. and Montes De Longo, I. (2003). Puerto Rican primary physicians' knowledge about folic acid supplementation for the preservation of neural tube defects. *Birth Defects research Part A: Clinical and Molecular Teratology*; 67 (12): 971-3. Morin P. (2002). Pregnancy planning: a determinant of folic acid supplements use for the primary prevention of neural tube defects. *Canadian Journal of public Health*; 93 (4):259-263.

MRC Vitamin Study Research Group. (1991). Prevention of neural tube defects: results of the Medical Research Council Vitamin Study. *Lancet*; 338 (8760): 131-7.

Mulinare, J., Corderao, J.F., Erickson, J.D. and Berry, R.J. (1988). Periconceptional use of multivitamins and the occurence of neural tube defects. *JAMA*; 260 (21): 3141-5. Nasr Hage C., Jalloul M., Sabbah M. and Adib S. (2011). Awareness and intake of folic acid for the prevention of neural tube defects among Lebanese women of childbearing age. *Maternal child and health journal* Jan 6.

Nawapun, K. and Phupong, V. (2007). Awareness of the benefits of folic acid and prevalence of the use of folic acid supplements to prevent neural tube defects among Thai women. *Archives of Gynecology and Obstetrics*; 276 (1): 53-7.

Nazer, H.J., Cifuentes, O.L., Aguila, R.A., Juarez, H.ME., Cid, R.MP., Godoy, V. ML.,Garcia, A.K. and Melibosky, R.F. (2007). Effects of folic acid fortification in the rates of malformations at birth in Chile. *Rev Med Chil*; 135 (2): 198-204.

Nilsen, R.M., Vollset, S.E., Gjessing, H.K., Magnus, P., Meltzer, H.M., Haugen, M. and Ueland, P.M. (2006). Patterns and predictors of folic acid supplement use among pregnant women: the Norwegian Mother and Child Cohort Study. *American journal of Clinical Nutrition*; 84 (5): 1134-41.

North Carolina Folic Acid Council (2009). www.getfolic.com.

Pereleman, V., Singal, N., Einarson, A., Kennedy, D. and Koren, G. (1996). Knowledge and practice by Canadian family physicians regarding peri-conceptional folic acid supplementation for the prevention of neural tube defects. *Canadian Journal of clinical Pharmacology*; 3:145-8.

Posey D.L., KhouryM.J., Mulinare J., Adams M.J. Jr and Ou C.Y. (1996). Is mutated MTHFR a risk factor for neural tube defects? *Lancet*; 347:686-7.

Power, M.L., holzman, G.B. and Schulkin, J. (2000). Knowledge and clinical practice regarding folic acid among obstetrician-gynecologists. *Obstetrics and Gynecology*; 95: 895-908.

Ray, J., Meier, C., Vermeulen, M., Boss, S., Wyatt, P. and Cole, D. (2002). Association of neural tube defects and folic acid fortification in Canada. *Lancet*; 360: 2047-8.

Ray, J.G., Singh, G. and Burrows, R.F. (2004). Evidence for suboptimal use of periconceptional folic acid supplements globally. *BJOG: An International Journal of Obstetrics & Gynaecology*; 111: 399-408.

Reefhuis, J. and Honein, M.A. (2004). Maternal age and non-chromosomal birth defects, Atlanta-1968-2000: Teenager or thirty-something, who is at risk? *Birth Defects Research part A: Clinical and Molecular Teratology*; 70 (9): 572-9.

Roger, E.M. (2003). Diffusion of innovations. *Free Press.*

Rosenberg, K.D., Gelow, J.M. and Sandoval, A.P. (2003). Pregnancy intendedness and the use of periconceptional folic acid. *Pediatrics*; 1111: 1142-5.

Rosenblatt, D.S. (1995). Inherited disorders of folate transport and metabolism. In Scriver, C.R., Beaudet, A.L., Sly, W.S. et al. (eds), *The Metabolic And Molecular Bases of Inherited Disease.* McGraw-Hill, New York, USA, pp.3111-3128.

Sayed, A.R., Bourne, D., Pattison, R., Nixon, J. and Henderson, B. (2008). Decline in the prevalence of neural tube defects following folic acid foertification and its cost-benefit in South Africa. Birth Defects Res. A Clin. Mol. Teratol.; 82: 2011-6. Smithells, R.W., Sheppard, S. and Schorah, C.J. (1976). Vitamin deficiencies and neural tube defect. *Arch Dis Child*; 51: 944-9.

Subar, A.F., Block, G. and James, L.D. (1989). Folate intake and food sources in the US population. *American Journal of Clinical Nutrition*; 50: 508-16.

Timmermans, S., Jaddoe, V., Mackenbach, J., Hofman A., Steegers-Theunissen, R. and Steegers, E. (2008). Determinants of folic acid use in early pregnancy in a multi-ethnic urban population in the Netherlands: the Generation R study. *Preventive Medicine*; 47 (7): 427-32.

Turgul, O., anli, N., mandiracioglu, A., Bati, H. and Akkol, S. (2009). The regional campaign for women on awareness of neural tube defects and folic acid in Narlidere, Izmir: a community-based intervention. (2009). *Eur J of Contracept and Reprod Health Care*; 14 (1): 69-74.

Van Allen, M.I., Fraser, F.C., Dallaire, L. et al. (1993).recommendations on the use of folic acid supplementation to prevent the recurrence of neural tube defects. *Canadian Medical association Journal*; 149: 1239-43.

Ward, M. (2004). Folic acid supplements to prevent neural tube defects: trends in East of Ireland 1996-2002. *Irish Medical Journal*; 97: 274.

Williams, L.J., Mai, C.T., Edmonds, L.D., Shaw, G.M., Kirby, R.S., Hobbs, C.A., Sever, L.E., Miller, L.A., Meany, F.J. and Levitt, M. (2002). Prevalence of spina bifida and anencephaly during the transition to mandatory folic acid fortification in the United States. *Teratology*; 66: 33-9.

Williams, J.L., Abelman, S.M., Fassett, E.M., Stone, C.E., Petrini, J.R., Damus, K. and Mulinare, J. (2006). Health care provider knowledge and practices regarding folic acid, United States, 2002-2003. *Maternal and Child Health Journal*; 10 (5 suppl): S67-72.

World Health Organization. (2002). *Prevention of Neural Tube Defects: Integrated Management of Pregnancy and Childbirth.* Standards for Maternal and Neonatal Care. Available from: http://www.who.int/making_pregnancy_safer/publications/Standards1.5N.pdf Yang, Q. H., H. K. Carter, J., Mulinare, R. J. Berry, J. M. Friedman, and J. D. Erickson.(2007). Race-ethnicity differences in folic acid intake in women of childbearing age in the United States after folic acid fortification: findings from the National Health and Nutrition Examination Survey, 2001-2002. *The American journal of clinical nutrition* 85 (5): 1409-16. Zeisel, S.H. (2009). Epigenetic mechanisms for nutrition determinants of later health

# 4

# Prevention of NTDs – Proposal of a New Concept

Prinz-Langenohl Reinhild[1], Pietrzik Klaus[1] and Holzgreve Wolfgang[2]
[1]*Department of Nutrition and Food Science, University of Bonn,*
[2]*Institute of Advanced Research, Berlin,*
*Germany*

## 1. Introduction

Neural tube defects (NTDs) are a heterogeneous group of serious congenital structural abnormalities of the brain and spine due to inadequate formation and/or closure of the developing brain and lower spine in the first month of pregnancy. Anencephalus, spina bifida, and encephalocele are the main manifestations of NTDs. The most serious form of NTDs is an anencephalus incompatible with life. Although NTDs can be detected by increased levels of alpha-fetoprotein and especially by ultrasound investigations early in pregnancy (Holzgreve et al., 1994), the prenatal diagnosis is often missed. After prenatal detection of NTDs, careful and comprehensive counseling of the parents is needed. Some parents select to carry the affected child to term, others decide to have a termination of pregnancy within the legal frameworks of their countries. If an anencephaly is recognized only late in gestation or even only at birth, the psychologic shock for the parents is usually prominent, and in their desperation to have at least some positive aspect in an otherwise hopeless situation parents have even requested in these rare situations to have organs transplanted from anencephalic donors (Holzgreve et al. 1987). NTDs have multiple etiologies and the role of folate, other vitamins and various micronutrients as factors in their etiology has been investigated from different angles for a long time now (Holzgreve et al., 1991, Simpson et al., 2010, 2011) A number of observational and interventional studies have demonstrated that folic acid (FA) supplementation before and in early pregnancy reduces the risk of having a NTD-affected offspring (Laurence et al., 1981; Milunsky et al. 1989; Smithells et al., 1980; Vergel et al., 1990).

Two intervention trials examining the effect of FA supplementation on NTD occurrence and recurrence, published twenty years ago, supported the evidence of the protective role of FA in NTD prevention (Czeizel et al., 1992; Medical Research Council [MRC], 1991). In these two trials, daily FA supplementation, alone, or in combination with other micronutrients, had started before conception and continued throughout the first trimester of pregnancy. Both studies reported a considerable reduction in NTD prevalence. These results were later confirmed in a public health campaign trial in China. Berry et al. (1999) observed a risk reduction between 40% and 85% in China among women who supplemented 400 µg/day FA. The wide range of decrease depends on the different baseline rates of NTD prevalence in the geographic areas included in the study (Northern region of China with high NTD prevalence, Southern region of China with low NTD prevalence).

Periconceptional supplementation with FA is internationally recognized as an effective measure for prevention of NTD-affected pregnancies. Although not all forms of NTD will be avoidable by additional FA, it is estimated that 70% of NTDs can be circumvented by adequate folate status prior to conception. Health authorities worldwide recommend that all women capable of becoming pregnant should improve their folate status to reduce the likelihood of having an NTD-affected child. Means to achieve this aim include modification of eating habits by choosing more food naturally rich in folate, increasing consumption of FA-fortified food and/or taking FA-containing supplements. Recommendations of the various governmental and non-governmental organizations are nearly identical, advising women of reproductive age to have about 400 – 500 µg FA daily from supplements, fortified foods, or both in addition to a varied diet in order to reduce occurrence of NTD. Women should follow this counsel at least four weeks prior conception and during the first three months of pregnancy (Australian Government, Department of Health and Ageing, National Health and Medical Research Council, 2006; Centers for Disease Control [CDC], 1992; Commission of the European Communities, 1993; German Nutrition Society, Austrian Nutrition Society, Swiss Society for Nutrition Research, Swiss Nutrition Association, 2002; Health Council of the Netherlands, 2008; Institute of Medicine [IOM], 1998; Scientific Advisory Committee on Nutrition [SACN] UK, 2006; US Preventive Task Force [USPTF], 2009; World Health Organization [WHO], 2002).

The U.S. Food and Drug Administration [FDA] had directed that all enriched cereal grain products were to be fortified with FA by January 1, 1998 with the objective to raise FA intake in the population (FDA, 1996). Meanwhile, more than fifty countries in North and South America, the Caribbean, the Middle East, North and Sub Saharan Africa and Oceania followed this strategy of public health policy and have regulations for food fortification programs including FA (Berry et al., 2010). Member states of the European Union have not chosen this policy, partly due to health risks possibly associated with high intake of FA and to the consumer's choice among fortified and non-fortified food (Osterhues et al., 2009).

Concentrations of plasma folate, red blood cell [RBC] folate and total homocysteine [tHcy] are biomarkers for evaluating folate status. Plasma folate concentration depends mainly on actual folate intake whereas RBC folate concentration is an indicator of long-term folate status as erythrocytes accumulate folate only during erythropoiesis. Taken into account the average life span of erythrocytes in the human body (about 120 days), folate concentration in erythrocytes changes slowly. As shown by Daly et al. (1995) in a large Irish cohort study, a woman's risk of having an NTD-affected offspring is inversely associated with maternal RBC folate concentration in early pregnancy. Although the precise optimal effective RBC folate concentration cannot be calculated from the study, the data allow associating RBC folate concentration above 906 nmol/L with the lowest risk for a NTD-affected pregnancy.

The objective of this chapter is to give a short overview of the effect of recommendations on folate status and FA intake and the consequences for NTD prevalence. In countries with mandatory FA food fortification a concomitant decline in NTD prevalence is observed. In countries without this measure only a marginal decrease in NTD prevalence can be recognized. A reason might be futile educational work. An alternative concept to improve folate status is therefore needed and presented in this chapter. Combining FA supplementation with oral contraceptives [OC] would be a good policy in this context. The rationale behind this concept is based on steady state conditions and elimination kinetics of folate, on the rapid conception among prior OC users who want to become pregnant, and on the high percentage of unplanned pregnancies. Although the majority of studies showed that FA, the synthetic form of the B-vitamin folate, was effective in preventing NTDs, there is evidence to suppose that natural folate like 5-methyltetrahydrofolate [5-MTHF] might have the same effect. Replacement of FA by the natural folate form [6S]-5-methyltetrahydrofolate in supplementation should therefore be considered, too.

## 2. Folate status and folic acid intake in the post-recommendation era

Numerous studies have been published in the last decade to document variation in folate status and folic acid intake in the post-recommendation period. As mandatory fortification is not yet implemented in all countries worldwide, data for some selected countries both with and without mandatory fortification are presented.

### 2.1 Data representative of countries with national fortification programmes

The United States were the first to implement mandatory food fortification with FA. In 1996, the U.S. FDA included FA in the pre-existing list of vitamins and minerals which have to be added to grain products in order to restore the micronutrient content of processed food. This regulation became active in 1998, directing that enriched grain has to be fortified with 140 µg FA per 100 g (FDA, 1996). A subsequent increase of daily FA intake by about 100 µg was predicted.

Jacques et al. (1999) and Choumenkovitch et al. (2001) analyzed the effect of this regulation on folate status in the Framingham Offspring Cohort. An increase in plasma folate concentration after fortification was seen in individuals who did not use B-vitamin supplements (117% increase) as well as in those taking B-vitamin supplements (61% increase) (Jacques et al., 1999). Mean RBC folate concentration was also significantly higher after fortification compared to the pre-fortification value in supplement user (+38%) and no-user (+24%) (Choumenkovitch et al., 2001).

Data from three National Health and Nutrition Surveys (NHANES) 1988-2005 show that FA fortification significantly raised folate status in the U.S. population compared to the pre-fortification period (Ganji & Kafai, 2006). Geometric mean RBC folate concentrations were higher in the post-fortification period than in the pre-fortification period (1999-2000: +58.2%; 2001-2002: +56.5%). Similar results were obtained for the geometric mean serum folate concentrations (1999-2000: +149%; 2001-2002: +129.8%). A small decline in serum folate was observed between NHANES 1999-2000 and NHANES 2001-2002. This finding might be explained by a reduced FA content in fortified food in NHANES 2001-2002 compared to NHANES 1999-2000. At the beginning of the fortification period products might had more overage of FA compared to later years (Ganji & Kafai, 2006).

The data of NHANES 2003-2004 and 2005-2006 were used to calculate FA consumption of non-pregnant U.S. women of childbearing age (15-44 years) in the post-fortification period.

The total daily FA intake was estimated by adding the FA value from foods reported in 24-h dietary recalls and the FA content of supplements taken by the subjects. The median intake of FA was 245 µg/day. Less than a quarter of the total group (n=2617) achieved the recommended amount of ≥ 400 µg/day FA. The strongest determinant of realizing the recommended FA level was the use of supplements containing FA. The lowest proportion of supplement user was found among young women aged 15-24 years. The median intake of FA in supplement user (n=647) was 502 µg/day, and more than two thirds (72%) of this group were able to fulfill the recommended intake. Median FA consumption and percentage achieving recommendation was significantly lower in the non-user group (n=1,970; 163 µg/day FA; 1.4% of the subjects with recommended intake) (Tinker et al., 2010). The marginal intake of FA supplements by young women was reported before by CDC on the basis of national, random-digit-dialed telephone surveys of a proportionate stratified sample of women of childbearing age (CDC, 2008).

Data from other countries support the benefit of fortification on folate status (and NTD prevalence, see 3.1). In Canada, fortification became mandatory at the end of 1998. An increase in RBC folate concentration in women of reproductive age (18-42 years) was observed shortly after the implementation of this regulation (Ray et al., 2002). In Iran, FA fortification became active in 2008. Abdollahi et al. (2011) evaluated the effect of fortification on folate status in postpartum women recruited from hospitals. While intake of dietary folate was stable over time (2006: 198.3 µg/day; 2008: 200.8 µg/day), a significant increase in total folate intake was observed after fortification (2006: 198.3 µg/day; 2008: 413.7 µg/day). Mean serum folate concentration was higher in the post-fortification era than in the pre-fortification era (2006: 13.6 nmol/L; 2008; 18.1 nmol/L). In Australia, fortification with FA was mandated in September 2009. Between April 2009 and April 2010, a significant 31% rise in mean serum folate concentration (17.7. nmol/L vs. 23.1 nmol/L) and a significant 22% increase in mean RBC folate concentration (881 nmol/L vs. 1071 nmol/L) was observed in a sample of inpatients and outpatients living in South Australia, Victoria and Western Australia (Brown et al., 2011).

Worldwide, the number of countries with mandatory FA fortification is rising. Fortification results in an improvement of folate status and folic acid intake in the populations from these countries including women of childbearing age. Nevertheless, as shown by the U.S. data, the major part of the targeted group is not compliant with the recommended intake of FA (400 µg/day) by fortified food alone. This supports the need to take supplements containing FA additionally to fortified food. However, the proportion of women supplementing FA is still low.

### 2.2 Data representative of countries without national fortification programmes

Up to now, mandatory fortification is not introduced in any European country, although products fortified with FA on voluntary basis are available in some of these countries. Data of folate status and folic acid intake will be presented for some, but not all European countries.

In Germany, a wide range of FA fortified foods is available. In the German National Health Interview and Examination Survey 1998 (Bundesgesundheitssurvey [BGS]), RBC folate and serum folate concentration were analyzed in 1,244 women of childbearing age (18 and 40 years). Median RBC folate was 266.3 nmol/L and median serum folate was 7.6 nmol/L without significant difference between the age groups. A high proportion of the participants showed suboptimal RBC folate concentrations and only 13% of the women had RBC folate concentrations above the cut-off value for NTD prevention (906 nmol/L) according to Daly et al. (1995) (Thamm et al., 2002). Data of the German National Nutrition Survey II showed a mean folate equivalent intake of 318 µg/day in women aged 19-24 years, 311 µg/day of women aged 25-34 years, and 285 µg/day for women aged 35-50 years (Max-Rubner-Institute [MRI], 2009). Periconceptional use of FA supplements is low in Germany, ranging between 4% and 6% (Egen, 1999; Heinz, 2001). Information campaigns had only a small effect on supplementation. The intake of FA was monitored in two small cross-sectional studies before and after such a campaign. 9.3% of the women interviewed in childbed used FA supplements after the campaign compared with 3.8% before (Egen & Hasford, 2003).

Two recent published studies investigated the folate status and FA supplement use in Irish women. In a large population-based cohort (n= 61,252), data on FA supplementation were available for 61,056 women. 85% of these women reported FA intake at any time during the periconceptional period. However, less than a third (28%) used FA according to the recommendation. Noteworthy is the increase in the proportion of women with correct FA supplementation over the years (2000: 17%; 2006: 36%) (McGuire et al., 2010). McNulty et al. (2011) investigated the association between FA intake and RBC folate concentrations in pregnant Irish women at 14 wk gestation (n=296) in a hospital-based trial. 84% of the participants stated FA supplement use at any time in the first three months of pregnancy. But only 19% of the total sample followed the recommendation correctly, using FA prior to conception and during the first trimester of pregnancy. Serum folate and RBC folate concentration was higher in subjects who started supplementation before or during the first six weeks of pregnancy compared to those who started later in pregnancy. RBC folate concentrations above 906 nmol/L were achieved by 73% of the women using FA already prior to conception, by 62% of the women starting in the first 6 weeks of pregnancy, and by 47% beginning supplementation after the sixth week of gestation.

Inskip et al. (2009) also noticed a poor compliance with recommendation in British Women recruited for the Southampton Women's Survey. Among those women who became pregnant, 2.9% reported to follow the recommendations taking ≥ 400 µg/day FA compared to 0.66% in those women who did not conceive.

To sum up, in countries without mandatory fortification folate status of pregnant women or women of childbearing age is suboptimal and use of FA supplements prior to and during early pregnancy is still very low. On average, less than 10% of the women of reproductive age take FA according to the recommendation although health education initiatives were conducted in most countries. Best compliance with the recommendation in European countries is noticed for the north of the Netherlands and a Danish area where about 30% of the women obey the recommendation (EUROCAT, 2009b; EUROCAT 2009c).

## 3. Prevalence of NTD in countries with and without national food fortification programmes

The rate of NTDs varies widely depending on the geographic region considered. Worldwide, about 300,000 babies are estimated to be born with a NTD every year (Botto et al., 1999). In Europe, at least 4,500 NTD-affected pregnancies happen per year (EUROCAT, 2009a).

Current data on NTD prevalence will be given separated between countries with national FA fortification programmes and without such programmes.

### 3.1 Data representative of countries with national fortification programmes

In the United States, the numbers of annual NTD-affected birth in a pre-fortification period (1995-1996) were compared with those in a post-fortification period (1999-2000). The data indicate a 26% decline in spina bifida and anencephaly affected live births and stillbirths in the post-fortification period (CDC, 2004). Racial and ethnic disparities were observed. Hispanic women had the highest rate of NTDs. Updated data were presented in the course of the CDC's Public Health Grand Rounds in February 2010 and verified the previous calculations of the CDC. According to the new data, the prevalence of NTDs dropped by 37% in a 2-year post-fortification period (2005-2006) compared to a 2-year pre-fortification period (1995-1996), at least partially attributed to the FA fortification programme as a public health strategy (CDC, February 2010).

López-Camelo et al. (2010) reported the variation in birth prevalence of NTDs in 77 hospitals in Chile, Argentina, and Brazil associated with FA fortification programmes in these countries. This paper is a publication of the Latin American Collaborative Study of Congenital Malformations (Éstudio Colaborativo Latino Americano de Malformaciones Congénitas [ECLAMC]). ECLAMC investigates the risk factors and the occurrence of congenital anomalies in South American hospitals since the late 1960s and early 1970s, using a case-control approach. Pre- and post-fortification rates of NTDs within each hospital were used to calculate prevalence rates by country. In Chile, FA fortification policy was implemented in January 2000, in Argentina in November 2003, and in Brazil in June 2004. A statistically significant decrease in birth prevalence estimates for NTDs after fortification was documented in all the three countries. A summary of the results is shown in table 1.

| | Chile | | | | Argentina | | | | Brazil | | | |
|---|---|---|---|---|---|---|---|---|---|---|---|---|
| | before fortification | | after fortification | | before fortification | | after fortification | | before fortification | | after fortification | |
| | 1998-2000 | | 2001-2007 | | 2002-2004 | | 2005-2007 | | 2003-2006/2005 | | 2007/2005-2007 | |
| | isolated | total | isolated | total | isolated | total | isolated | total | isolated | total | isolated | total |
| Anencephaly | 0.52 | 0.63 | 0.26 | 0.37 | 0.69 | 0.86 | 0.29 | 0.37 | 0.90 | 1.12 | 0.45 | 0.69 |
| Spina bifida-total | 0.73 | 1.02 | 0.24 | 0.46 | 0.82 | 1.27 | 0.33 | 0.66 | 0.86 | 1.45 | 0.69 | 1.42 |

Table 1. Birth prevalence estimates for NTDs (isolated and total) before and after implementation of FA food fortification in three Latin American countries, live born babies/1,000 births (modified according to Lopèz-Camelo et al., 2010)

These findings were confirmed by a study recently published by Orioli et al. (2011) in a cross-sectional study of Brazilian live births. Spina bifida birth prevalence in each state of Brazil was estimated from the Live Births Information System (Sistema de Informações sobre Nascidos Vivos [SINASC]) for both a pre-fortification and a post-fortification period (2004 and 2006). The authors observed a significant 39% decline in spina bifida birth prevalence in 2006 compared to 2004.

In Iran, flour fortification with FA started in 2008. In a hospital-based study, Abdollahi et al. (2011) noticed a 31% reduction in NTD birth prevalence in a post-fortification period (December 2007 to December 2008; 2.19 cases per 1,000 births) compared to a pre-fortification period (September 2006 to July 2007; 3.16 cases per 1,000 births) in the north of Iran. Jordan has initiated national food fortification programmes including wheat flour fortification with FA in April 2002. Amarin & Obeidat (2010) conducted a hospital-based study to evaluate the effect of FA fortified foods on the incidence on NTD in live born babies. Fortification has led to a concomitant significant fall in the number of NTDs in the north of Jordan (pre-fortification period 2000-2001: 1.85 cases per 1,000 births; post-fortification period 2005-2006: 0.95 cases per 1,000 births). A similar downward trend could be seen in Oman, where flour fortification with FA started in 1996 (Alasfoor et al., 2010). Spina bifida incidence varied from 2.34 to 4.03 per 1,000 births between 1991 and 1996 and dropped to 0.29 per 1,000 births in 2006.

In summary, national fortification programmes are associated with a notable fall in NTD prevalence. But the reduction in NTD is not completely attributed to FA fortification as there was a declining trend in some countries before fortification. In addition, one has to bear in mind whether total prevalence or live birth prevalence is reported. Live birth prevalence published by Lopez-Camelo et al. (2010), Abdollahi et al. (2011), or Amarin & Obeidat (2010) is not the best variable to deduce progress in prevention of NTD from FA fortification. Other factors than FA may be responsible for the decline like high-quality prenatal screening and medical termination of pregnancy following diagnosis of NTD. It may be that reporting the live birth prevalence therefore underestimates the total prevalence of NTD and in consequence overestimates the effect of FA fortification on NTD prevention.

### 3.2 Data representative of countries without national fortification programmes

Prevalence of NTDs over time across Europe is monitored by the European Surveillance Registry for Congenital Anomalies and Twins [EUROCAT]. EUROCAT is a European network of population-based registries for the epidemiologic surveillance of congenital anomalies started in 1979. EUROCAT is also a WHO-collaborating center for the epidemiological surveillance of congenital anomalies. Nowadays, 21 countries[1] contribute data to EUROCAT. None of these countries has implemented regulation for mandatory FA food fortification. About 31% of the births in the European Union are covered by EUROCAT (Boyd et al., 2011). Both terminations of pregnancy and births are registered. Total prevalence rates are calculated, including all cases affected by NTD (live births, stillbirths, fetal deaths from 20 weeks of gestation, and terminated pregnancies of any gestational age)

[1]Austria, Belgium, Croatia, Denmark, Finland, France, Germany, Hungary, Ireland, Italy, Malta, Netherlands, Norway, Poland, Portugal, Slovenia, Spain, Sweden, Switzerland, Ukraine, United Kingdom (EUROCAT, 2009a)

divided by the number of all births, still and live, in the registry population. Live birth prevalence includes live born cases only.

In Europe (2004-2008), the total prevalence of NTDs was 0.96 per 1,000 births. The live birth prevalence in the same period was 0.24 per 1,000 births. The lowest live birth prevalence is observed in Spain (0.08/1,000 births), the highest in Malta (0.96/1,000 births). Portugal has the lowest total NTD prevalence (0.20/1,000 births) and France the highest (1.46/1,000 births). As an estimated 72% of NTD-affected pregnancies are interrupted, discrepancies between live birth and total NTD prevalence are primarily attributed to the termination of an NTD-affected pregnancy following prenatal diagnosis (EUROCAT, 2009d).

Data on the trend in prevalence of NTDs are extracted from the EUROCAT Central Registry database 1980-2007 (EUROCAT, 2009a). According to the EUROCAT report (EUROCAT, 2009a) a declining trend in NTD prevalence was observed in the years 1992-2007. This tendency is attributed to a slightly, but significantly decreasing trend for anencephaly whereas there is no significant reduction trend for spina bifida. However, changes in NTD rates in the period considered vary among the European countries, partly due to differences in collecting and reporting data. A significant fall in NTD since 1992 has been found in Ireland. No variation has been observed in the UK. In the Continental Europe, represented by France, Belgium, Switzerland, Northern Netherlands, Denmark, Germany, Austria, Norway, Poland, Hungary, Ukraine and Finland, a significant reduction in NTD prevalence has only been observed in the Northern Netherlands. In South Europe, exemplified by Italy, Croatia, Portugal, Malta, and Spain, NTD prevalence dropped significantly since 1992.

In Europe, there are geographical discrepancies in the prevalence and trend in prevalence in NTD. The decline in Ireland can not only be explained by FA supplementation as reduction has started already before the implementation of a national policy, but rather by an improvement of the general diet. Similar downward trends were observed in other non-European countries without or prior to mandatory fortification. For example, data from South Australia, Victoria and Western Australia show a fall in total prevalence years before onset of mandatory fortification in 2009. Abeywardana et al. (2010) reported a decreasing prevalence for NTDs in these states from 1992 to 2005 with the main reduction already occurring between 1992 and 1998.

## 4. Natural folate like [6S]-5-methyltetrahydrofolate as an alternative to folic acid in NTD prevention

### 4.1 Background information

The term folate refers to a group of biologically active metabolites of this water-soluble B-vitamin. Folates occur naturally in biological systems in different chemical forms (mono- and polyglutamate forms, different one-carbon units bound). Folate, in the form of tetrahydrofolate (THF), acts as a coenzyme required for the transfer and processing of one-carbon units. The vitamin is thereby involved in numerous metabolic reactions including nucleotide synthesis, aminoacid metabolism, methylation reactions, and gene expression. FA is a synthetic form of the vitamin that does not occur in nature. It is commonly used in pharmaceuticals, supplements and fortified food products because of its high stability (Pietrzik et al. 2010).

As folates are absorbed in the monoglutamate form, polyglutamates have to be hydrolyzed to monoglutamates in the gut by the mucosal brush border conjugase prior to absorption. Most folate monoglutamates are taken up by a saturable carrier-mediated active mechanism. Only a small percentage is absorbed by a non-saturable diffusion-mediated process. In the mucosal cell, the monoglutamates are converted to 5-methyltetrahydrofolate (5-MTHF). This form can be taken up by the liver where it is retained or released to the systematic circulation or bile. Before being stored in tissue or acting as a coenzyme, monoglutamates has to be converted to the polyglutamates. Release from tissue into circulation depends on previous hydrolyzation to the monoglutamate form (Pietrzik et al. 2010).

FA is absorbed by passive diffusion. It is reduced via dihydrofolate to THF by the enzyme dihydrofolate reductase in order to become metabolically active. THF is then metabolized to 5-MTHF in the human mucosal cell and/or liver. As the capacity of conversion is limited, unmetabolized FA can appear in the systemic circulation, even after low-dose application (Pietrzik et al., 2010). A physiological function of FA itself is not known and is not to be expected as FA does not occur in nature. The underlying mechanism by which FA reduces the risk of NTD is unknown. Obviously, the beneficial role of FA in NTD prevention bases on upgrading the pool of active folate forms.

### 4.2 Potential health risk associated with FA

There is evidence that harmful effects might be associated with intake of FA. High intake of FA may delay the diagnosis of vitamin B12 deficiency by masking the hematological manifestation of this deficit. Megaloblastic anemia is one symptom of a severe vitamin B12 deficiency due to secondary folate deficiency. High doses of FA can result in the recovery of hematological symptoms, thereby complicating the diagnosis of vitamin B12 deficiency and allowing neurological complications in these patients to progress. This problem is specially addressed to the elderly. The IOM therefore sets a tolerable upper intake level of 1,000 µg/day of FA from supplements or fortified food for adults (19 years and older) (IOM, 1998). Furthermore, concerns have been raised that FA blunts antifolate therapy, i.e. reducing seizure control by phenytoin and affecting the efficacy of methotrexate. In addition, high folate status may trigger the promotion of malignant and premalignant lesions. Unmetabolized FA in the human systemic circulation, observed even after application of low-dose FA, is discussed to interfere with the transport, metabolism und functions of natural folates and may have a negative effect on natural killer cell toxicity. Twinning, miscarriage and epigenetic hypermethylation are further possible side effects which are put up for discussion (Kelly et al., 1997; Pietrzik et al., 2010; Smith et al., 2008; Troen et al., 2006).

### 4.3 Folate status and NTD risk associated with dietary folate

Observational studies indicate that the risk of an NTD-affected pregnancy is inversely associated with the intake of food folate in unsupplemented women (Shaw et al., 1995; Werler et al., 1993). As reviewed in detail by Eskes (2002), several, but not all studies showed lower serum folate or RBC folate concentrations in early pregnancy in women with NTD-affected pregnancy compared to controls.

Brouwer et al. (1999) investigated the effect of additional dietary folate from vegetables and citrus fruits on folate status. In a placebo-controlled, parallel group nutrition intervention trial in 66 healthy male and female subjects three treatments were used: 1) a high folate diet (total folate intake: 560 µg/day) plus a placebo, 2) a low folate diet (total folate content: 210 µg/day) plus supplemental FA and placebo on alternate days (FA intake: 250 µg/day), and 3) a low folate diet (total folate intake: 210 µg/day) plus placebo. Baseline folate status was measured by plasma folate, RBC folate and homocysteine [tHcy] concentrations. These parameters did not differ significantly among these three groups. After four weeks of intervention, plasma folate and RBC folate increased and tHcy decreased in both the high folate diet and the FA groups. Changes in folate indices assumed the same proportions in the high folate diet and the FA group. However, achieving a high folate diet as used by Brouwer et al. (1999) in their study requires major modifications in dietary behavior. This is unlikely to be realized by most subjects in everyday life over a longer period of time.

### 4.4 Studies with the natural folate form [6S]-5-methyltetrayhdrofolate

Most dietary folate and FA are metabolized to 5-MTHF as described before (see 4.1). Since some years, 5-MTHF has been available commercially, both in the natural form [6S]-5-MTHF and as the racemic mixture [6RS]-5-MTHF. However, the [6R]-isomer of the racemic mixture is presumed to be biologically inactive and therefore without nutritional significance. In addition, adverse effects of the [6R]-isomer on storage are under discussion (Mader et al., 1995; Willems et al., 2004). Thus, interventional trials with the racemic mixture of 5-MTHF as conducted by Fohr et al. (2002), Litynski et al. (2002), and Willems et al. (2004) are not considered in this chapter.

[6S]-5-MTHF is the biologically active diastereoisomer, also known as L-5-MTHF. It is available as a calcium salt, and in this form used in some vitamin supplements and pharmaceuticals. Only studies with [6S]-5-MTHF administered to healthy adults in physiological doses will be reviewed in the following sections.

#### 4.4.1 Bioavailability studies with [6S]-5-methytetrahydrofolate in physiological doses in healthy adults

Prinz-Langenohl et al. (2009) compared the bioavailability of [6S]-5-MTHF and FA in a short-term study, using a methodological approach which is standard in pharmacology for testing the pharmacokinetics of active drug ingredients. Twenty-four healthy females of childbearing age received a single oral dose of FA (400 µg) as reference and equimolar amount of [6S]-5-MTHF (416 µg as calcium salt) as test in a randomized, double-blind, crossover design. Plasma folate was monitored at various time points up to 8 h after application. Parameters to compare the bioavailability of both treatments included the concentration time-profile (area under the curve of the plasma folate concentration versus time [AUC]), the maximal plasma folate concentration [$C_{max}$] and the time to reach the maximum. Plasma folate concentration peaked significantly higher and within a shorter period of time with [6S]-5-MTHF than with FA. These findings confirm the result of a previous trial conducted by Prinz-Langenohl et al. (2003). In that randomized, double-blind, four period cross-over study, 21 healthy young females received a single oral dose of 400 µg FA and 416 µg [6S]-5-MTHF (as calcium salt) either without or with FA pre-saturation (1 mg/10 days prior to the study day). The volunteers were pre-saturated with FA in order to minimize difference in volunteers' baseline plasma folate concentrations. Plasma responses were measured up to 8 h after vitamin intake. With respect to the primary variables of bioavailability, AUC and $C_{max}$, the authors concluded that [6S]-5-MTHF is more effective in increasing plasma folate in comparison to FA depending on the procedure of FA pre-loading. This finding is in line with the results of Pentieva et al. (2004). Pentieva et al. (2004) compared the bioavailability of [6S]-5-MTHF with that of FA by monitoring plasma folate responses for a 10-h period after administration of the two vitamin forms. Both interventions were given in an oral single dose (500 µg) to 13 males pre-saturated with FA in a randomized, double-blind, placebo-controlled, crossover trial. No differences in the bioavailability endpoints AUC and $C_{max}$ were observed between [6S]-5-MTHF and FA.

### 4.4.2 Intervention studies with [6S]-5-methytetrahydrofolate in physiological doses in healthy adults

Several studies suggest that long-term intervention with [6S]-5-MTHF in a physiological low dose has at least the same effect on folate indices in healthy subjects as has FA. A long-term study in New Zealand compared the changes in blood folate in women of childbearing age (n=104) supplemented with either [6S]-5-MTHF (113 µg/day, calcium salt), FA (100 µg/day), or placebo for 24 wk (Venn et al., 2002). In this randomized, double-blind, parallel-group trial, RBC folate and plasma folate concentrations increased to a similar extent under both vitamin treatments. A second study with a similar design was published one year later by this working group (Venn et al., 2003). Venn et al. (2003) confirmed in a group of middle-aged volunteers of both genders (n=167) that the increase in RBC folate and plasma folate concentrations did not differ significantly between the FA (100 µg/day) and the [6S]-5-MTHF (113 µg/day) groups supplemented for 24 wk. In addition, they were able to show that [6S]-5-MTHF was significantly more effective than FA in lowering plasma tHcy. Lamers et al. (2004) compared the tHcy-lowering and plasma folate rising effect of [6S]-5-MTHF and FA during 24 wk of supplementation. Female subjects (n=144) were randomly allocated to one of the four intervention groups: 400 µg/day FA, 416 µg/day [6S]-5-MTHF, 208 µg/day [6S]-5-MTHF, or placebo. In comparison to the placebo group, tHcy decreased by 15%, 19%, and 19% in the three vitamin groups. The differences between the groups were not significant. The increase in plasma folate was significant compared to placebo (151%, 164%, and 101%). However, supplementation with the low-dose [6S]-5-MTHF resulted in a significant lower increase relative to the two other folate groups. A second long-term study with the same treatment regime and identical duration (24 wk) was performed by Lamers et al. (2006). The primary objective was to investigate the effect of treatment on RBC folate and plasma folate concentration in healthy females (n=144). The increase in RBC and plasma folate was significantly higher in the group receiving 416 µg [6S]-5-MTHF than in the two other folate groups. Whereas plasma folate reached a plateau after 12 wk supplementation in all groups, a steady state for RBC folate was not observed. The authors concluded that [6S]-5-MTHF is more effective in increasing RBC folate when given in doses equimolar to FA. In addition, they recommended to extent the preconceptional period of supplementation to 12 weeks or more; consequently one would make sure to reach the most preventive RBC folate concentration according to Daly et al. (1995). Houghton et al. (2006) conducted a randomized, placebo-controlled study with healthy women (n=72) to assess the effectiveness of [6S]-5-MTHF, FA, and placebo in upholding RBC folate concentration during lactation. After delivery, the lactating women were assigned to receive [6*S*]-5-MTHF (416 µg/day), folic acid (400 µg/day), or placebo for 16 wk. At the end of the treatment period, RBC folate concentration in the [6S]-5-MTHF group was higher than in the two other groups after adjustment for baseline concentrations at 36 wk gestation. In conclusion, the authors classified [6S]-5-MTHF to be as effective as, or even more than FA in maintaining RBC folate concentrations during lactation.

The main characteristics of the studies described are summarized in Table 2.

| Authors (year) | Design | Subjects | Intervention | Outcome variable | Main result |
|---|---|---|---|---|---|
| | ***Short-term bioavailability studies*** | | | | |
| Prinz-Langenohl et al. (2003) | randomized, double-blind, crossover | young females (n=21) | single dose: 400 µg FA and 416 µg [6S]-5-MTHF with /without FA preload | plasma folate | [6S]-5-MTHF as effective as FA in increasing plasma folate |
| Pentieva et al. (2004) | randomized, double-blind, crossover, placebo-controlled | young males (n=13) | single dose: 500 µg FA and 500 µg [6S]-5-MTHF with FA preload | plasma folate | [6S]-5-MTHF as effective as FA in increasing plasma folate |
| Prinz-Langenohl et al. (2009) | randomized, double-blind, crossover | young females (n=24) | single dose: 400 µg FA and 416 µg [6S]-5-MTHF without FA preload | plasma folate | [6S]-5-MTHF as effective as FA in increasing plasma folate |
| | ***Long-term intervention studies*** | | | | |
| Venn et al. (2002) | randomized, double-blind, parallel-group, placebo-controlled | young females (n=104) | 24 wk: 100 µg FA/d or 113 µg [6S]-5-MTHF/d or placebo | plasma folate, RBC folate | similar increase in plasma folate and RBC folate in the folate groups; no plateau in plasma or RBC folate reached after 24 wk |
| Venn et al. (2003) | randomized, double-blind, parallel-group, placebo-controlled | middle-aged males and females (n=167) | 24 wk: 100 µg FA/d or 113 µg [6S]-5-MTHF/d or placebo | plasma folate, RBC folate, tHcy | similar increase in plasma folate and RBC folate in the folate groups; [6S]-5-MTHF more effective in lowering tHcy than FA |
| Lamers et al. (2004) | randomized, double-blind, parallel-group, placebo-controlled | young females (n=144) | 24 wk: 400 µg FA/d or 416 µg [6S]-5-MTHF/d or 208 µg [6S]-5-MTHF/d or placebo | tHcy, plasma folate | both doses of [6S]-5-MTHF effective as FA in lowering tHcy; plasma folate increase in all groups, but lower in low-dose [6S]-5-MTHF than in the two other folate groups |

| Authors (year) | Design | Subjects | Intervention | Outcome variable | Main result |
|---|---|---|---|---|---|
| Lamers et al. (2006) | randomized, double-blind, parallel-group, placebo-controlled | young females (n=144) | 24 wk: 400 µg FA/d or 416 µg [6S]-5-MTHF/d or 208 µg [6S]-5-MTHF/d or placebo | RBC folate, plasma folate | increase in RBC folate higher in high-dose [6S]-5-MTHF than in the two other folate groups, no plateau in RBC folate reached in the three folate groups after 24 wk; increase in plasma folate higher in high-dose [6S]-5-MTHF than in the two other folate groups, plateau in plasma folate reached after 12 wk |
| Houghton et al. (2006) | randomized, double-blind, parallel-group, placebo-controlled | lactating healthy women (n=72) | 16 wk: 400 µg FA/d or 416 µg [6S]-5-MTHF/d or placebo | RBC folate | [6S]-5-MTHF at least as effective as FA in maintaining RBC folate |

FA, folic acid; tHcy, total plasma homocysteine; [6S]-5-MTHF, [6S]-5-methyltetrahydrofolate; RBC, red blood cell

Table 2. Interventional studies: effect of [6S]-5-MTHF supplementation in physiological doses on folate parameters in healthy adults.

In conclusion, short-term and long-term studies with healthy adults and women of childbearing age have shown that the natural folate form [6S]-5-MTHF administered in doses equimolar to FA is at least as effective as FA in improving folate status indices. A placebo-controlled trial to explore the effect of [6S]-5-MTHF given in the periconceptional period on the occurrence of NTDs as primary endpoint would be unethical. However, the inverse relation between RBC folate concentration as a surrogate endpoint and the risk of NTD has been calculated by Daly et al. (1995). Based on this observation [6S]-5-MTHF is considered to be an adequate alternative to FA supplementation in prevention of NTDs. In contrast to FA, the natural form of folate has never been linked to adverse effects as discussed for FA (Pietrzik et al., 2010).

## 5. Rationale for a new prevention concept – combining oral contraceptives with folic acid or folates

Although public is informed about the advantages mentioned above since more than two decades, the recommendations on NTD prevention by FA are marginally translated into practice in the majority of the European countries. Impact on NTD prevalence in Europe is small in contrast to countries with mandated FA food fortification. Therefore, an additional concept is needed to raise folate status in European women, taking into account both the steady state conditions of blood folate, the problem of unplanned pregnancies, and faster conception as expected.

### 5.1 Steady state conditions and elimination kinetics of red blood cell folate

Improvement of folate status should begin already in the preconceptional period to start pregnancy in an optimal folate status. Several intervention trials have investigated the time-effect of long-term supplementation on folate status indices in healthy adults. Bakker et al. (2009) studied RBC folate, plasma folate, and tHcy concentration in 27 healthy women in a 8-wk period of supplementation with 500 µg/day FA followed by a 12-wk period without supplementation. Serum folate and RBC folate concentrations significantly increased by supplementation compared to the control group (no supplementation). The authors assumed that a steady state was not reached in the 12-wk intervention period. In addition, Bakker et al. (2009) observed that serum folate and plasma tHcy returned to baseline after a 12-wk wash-out period following FA discontinuation. In contrast, RBC folate concentration remained significantly higher in the prior vitamin intervention group compared with the control group at the end of the wash-out phase. Other studies showed that low dose FA or [6S]-5-MTHF supplementation over 24 wk resulted in plasma folate steady state, but not in RBC folate steady state (Lamers et al., 2006; Venn et al., 2002). RBC folate seems to cumulate slower than plasma folate as erythrocytes take up folate only during erythropoiesis and have an average life span of 120 days.

Pietrzik et al. (2007) published a working model for appearance and elimination kinetics of RBC folate, assuming that steady state conditions of RBC folate can be calculated based on linear pharmacokinetics and the biological half-life of RBC folate (8 wk). This model predicts that a mean steady state of RBC folate would be achieved after 5 half-life periods (40 wk) after starting low-dose folate supplementation. In addition, Pietrzik et al. (2007) hypothesized that the period of time for the elimination of RBC folate after supplementation cessation is equal to the period of time needed to reach steady state in RBC folate by supplementation.

The latter assumption was partly confirmed by a study which assessed the pharmacokinetic effect on plasma folate and RBC folate during 24 wk of daily treatment with 451 µg [6S]-5-MTHF (as calcium salt) or with 400 µg FA, both in combination with an OC followed by 20 wk elimination phase with OC mono-application. Healthy women (n=172) between 18 to 40 years of age were randomly assigned to one of the treatments. Subjects were not allowed to consume FA-fortified food and vitamin supplements. Plasma and RBC folate increased by supplementation over 24 wk and decreased in the elimination phase reaching nearly baseline values after 20 wk in the MTHF group (FDA, 2010a).

Hao et al. (2008) evaluated the changes in RBC folate and plasma folate concentrations in young Chinese women (n=1108) treated with different doses and dosing schedules of FA for six months (100 µg/day FA, 4 x 25 µg/ day FA, 400 µg/day FA, 4 x 100 µg/d FA, 4000 µg/day FA, 4000 µg/wk FA) in a randomized, double-blind, parallel group trial. Folate status was measured at baseline, three times during the intervention, and after a wash-out period of three months following the discontinuation of FA supplementation. Plasma folate plateaued between three and six months in all intervention groups. Three months after cessation of FA administration, plasma folate remained higher than baseline. A plateau in RBC folate was not observed over the treatment period. The concentrations of RBC folate at the end of the wash-out period were significantly higher than those at baseline only in the groups who had received ≥ 400 µg/day FA. However, the practical aspect of the high dose group is missing as women would not be exposed to 4000 µg of FA with respect to NTD occurrence reduction.

Houghton et al. (2011) conducted a study to evaluate the long-term effect of FA supplementation on RBC folate in healthy female subjects of fertile age. 144 women were randomly assigned to receive 140 µg FA/day, or 400 µg FA/day, or placebo for 40 wk. RBC folate concentration as primary endpoint of the trial was measured at different time points during the study (baseline, 6, 12, 29, and 40 wk after start of supplementation). The statistical analysis of the data was restricted to subjects with a supplement compliance of ≥ 70%. RBC folate concentration increased in both FA groups throughout the intervention period, but RBC folate did not stabilize in neither of the two groups. The authors concluded that the time required to reach steady state is even longer than assumed by Pietrzik et al. (2007).

To substantiate the different hypothetical assumptions, a study is needed with FA supplementation as recommended, an intervention period of sufficient duration to achieve RBC folate steady state, and a wash-out period monitoring RBC folate concentration till return to baseline values.

### 5.2 Planned and unplanned pregnancy

Recommendations and health education campaigns to raise folate status with respect to NTD prevention address fertile women. Success depends on the fact that pregnancies are planned. However, pregnancies are often unplanned, subsuming that they are unintended, untimed and/ or unwanted. Blumenthal et al. (2011) and Finer & Henshaw (2006) identified a number of risk factors for an unplanned pregnancy including young age of the women, poor education of women, low-income, racial origin, domestic violence, poor access to contraceptive supplies, lack of knowledge about contraception, and being unmarried. Failure of OC and other contraceptive methods also contributes to unplanned pregnancy. According to Finer and Henshaw (2006) nearly half of the unintended conceptions occur during a month when contraceptive methods were used. Typical failure rates for oral formulations of hormonal contraceptives range from <3% to 5% mainly due to failures in compliance followed by vomiting and diarrhea (Barjot et al., 2006; Frye, 2006).

Data on the proportion of planned or unplanned pregnancies have a high variability between the countries. Moreover, evidence is limited because data are often based upon small-scale, non-representative surveys with different design.

Ray et al. (2004) published a systematic overview of 52 survey studies worldwide regarding the pre- and periconceptional use of folic acid supplements. In 19 of these studies, information about the proportion of unplanned pregnancies was available which ranged from 10 to 78%. Data from the National Survey of Family Growth (NSFG) 2002 combined with birth, abortion and population data from other sources indicate that nearly half (49%) of the pregnancies in the United States are unintended (Finer & Henshaw, 2006). In a Chinese study, about 72% of the women had not planned their pregnancy (Gong et al., 2010).

In Europe, more than half of the pregnancies are unplanned (EUROCAT, 2009a). The data of the country specific reports (EUROCAT, 2009b, 2009c) can be summarized as follows:

No information is available for Austria, Belgium, France, Malta, Slovenia, Ukraine, and Portugal. The percentage of pregnancies that are planned in Switzerland and Poland is thought to be very low. In Denmark, the compliance with contraception is rather high. Therefore, the rate of planned pregnancies is assumed to be somewhat higher than in the United States where about half of the pregnancies are planned. In one regional study in Denmark pregnant women attending a university hospital (n=3516) were recruited in the period 1994 to 1996. In this study 68% of the women confirmed that the pregnancy was planned. The study population was judged to be a representative subsample of the Danish population. In a small study in Finland, 547 women were interviewed during their first prenatal care visit in the year 2000. About 36% to 86% of the women had planned the pregnancy. The wide range depends on the different interpretation of the concept of a planned pregnancy. In Ireland, studies have shown that the percentage of women planning their pregnancy has been stable from 1996-2002 at 40-45%. There is little knowledge in Croatia about the rate of planned pregnancies, but 75% of pregnancies are assumed to be planned. Proportion of Italian planned pregnancies ranges between 61% and 64%. The proportion of Norwegian pregnancies that are planned is supposed to be between 50% and 75%. The situation in Sweden is assumed to be comparable to that in Norway. Basing on the data of one survey conducted from 1994 to 2006 in Barcelona, 50-75% of the Spanish pregnancies seem to be planned. Studies in the UK indicate that 60-75% of the pregnancies are planned. In the Netherlands, the proportion of planned pregnancies is high (85%) and not related to the socio-economic status of the women. In Hungary, 67.4% of pregnancies were found to be planned. In Germany, four studies were conducted in which women were asked after delivery whether or not their pregnancy was planned. According to these studies 66-72% of the women confirmed their pregnancy to be planned.

The data of planned and unplanned pregnancies in European countries according to EUROCAT (2009b, 2009c) are presented in table 3.

A study recently published, but not included in the EUROCAT report, indicate that in Germany 47% of the pregnancies in the Eastern federal states (newly formed German states, formerly GDR) and 29% in the Western federal states (old German states, BRD) are unplanned. Especially young women (16-19 years) in Germany have a high percentage of unplanned pregnancies (75%) (Rieback & Kreyenfeld, 2009).

The data indicate that a major percentage of pregnancies are unplanned. This fact is relevant for prevention of NTD because women, not planning a pregnancy, may be uninterested in prenatal instructions or will not receive preconceptional health information by their gynecologist, i.e. advice and information about NTD prevention by improving folate status preconceptionally. As shown by Gong et al. (2010) the proportion of Chinese women who took FA prior to conception was higher for those who had planned their pregnancy. Similar results are reported for Irish women. Less than recommended or no FA supplementation was associated with unplanned pregnancy (McGuire et al., 2010). As indicated in the systematic reviews of Ray et al. (2004) and Stockley & Lund (2008), unintended pregnancy is the most important factor for lack of compliance with the recommendations.

| Country | Percentage estimates of planned pregnancies | Percentage estimates of unplanned pregnancies |
|---|---|---|
| Austria | No data available | No data available |
| Belgium | No data available | No data available |
| Croatia | 75% | 25% |
| Denmark | 50%-68% | 32%-50% |
| Finland | 36%-86% | 14%-64% |
| France | No data available | No data available |
| Germany | 66%-72% | 28%-34% |
| Ireland | 40%-45% | 55%-60% |
| Italy | 61%-64% | 36%-39% |
| Malta | No data available | No data available |
| Netherlands | 85% | 15% |
| Norway | 50%-75% | 25%-50% |
| Poland | Thought to be very low | Thought to be very high |
| Portugal | No data available | No data available |
| Spain | 50%-75% | 25%-50% |
| Slovenia | No data available | No data available |
| Sweden | 50-75% | 25%-50% |
| Switzerland | Thought to be very low | Thought to be very high |
| UK | 60%-75% | 25%-40% |
| Ukraine | No data available | No data available |

Table 3. Planned and unplanned pregnancies in Europe (EUROCAT, 2009b, 2009c)

### 5.3 Pregnancy after discontinuation of an oral contraceptive

Oral contraceptives represent a commonly used method of reversible conception control in industrialized countries. In the German BGS 1998, for example, 30% of the women between 18 and 45 years of age in the Western federal states and 47% in the Eastern federal states reported use of OC (Knopf & Melchert, 1999). Ovulation returns rapidly after stopping OC as shown by Cronin et al. (2009). In a prospective, non-interventional cohort study of 59,510 users of OC in seven European countries the rate of pregnancy over time was monitored in those participants who stopped use of OC because of a planned pregnancy (n=2,064). 21.1% of the prior OC users became pregnant one cycle after OC cessation. The rate of pregnancy increased to 45.7% after three cycles, and 79.4% after 13 cycles. Nearly half of the women who did not become pregnant in the first 13 cycles after OC cessation did so in the second year. 26 cycles after OC cessation, overall pregnancy rate was 88.3%. The age of the women only had a minor influence on the rate of pregnancy up to the age of 35 years.

The findings of this study have important consequences with respect to the periconceptional improvement of folate status. First of all, a considerable part of the prior OC users may become pregnant before being able to transfer the recommendations of NTD prevention in practice. Moreover, achieving the preventive level of RBC folate is nearly impossible when becoming pregnant sooner than expected (≤ 3 months after stopping OC), assuming that the women are counseled by the gynecologist before stopping OC and act according to the recommendation already while using OC.

## 6. Conclusion

Optimization of folate status by consumption of food naturally rich in folate and/or fortified with FA, and FA supplementation is possible. A daily intake of 400 µg/day FA is recommended to women of childbearing age and/or women planning to get pregnant. However, as reviewed in this chapter compliance with recommendations is poor even in countries with mandatory food fortification. Impact on total NTD prevalence is marginal in countries without mandatory FA food fortification. Regarding this unsatisfactory development in prevention of NTD, an additional concept is needed.

Combing OC with folate could be such an alternative. At first glance, this concept does not make sense as women, using OC, will prevent conception and therefore do not represent the target group of the recommendation. However, referring to the information given in section 4 and 5 of this chapter several advantages of this approach are obvious.

Firstly, fortifying OC with FA will minimize the risk of a NTD-affected baby if pregnancy will happen due to failure of this contraceptive method. As shown by Barjot et al. (2006) and Frye (2006) the failure rate of OC is up to 5% mainly due to inconsistencies or mistakes in taking the OC, vomiting and diarrhea. Failure of contraceptive methods is one reason for an unplanned pregnancy. Secondly, unplanned pregnancy is one predictor of low compliance to the FA recommendation as reviewed by Ray et al. (2004) and Stockley & Lund (2008). Combining OC with folate would result in a protective maternal folate status for OC users being advantageous to those conceiving under OC therapy. Thirdly, as shown by Cronin et al. (2009) conception may happen in a short period after cessation of OC use: more than a 20% of prior OC users got pregnant one cycle after discontinuation in this study, and 50% were pregnant 3 cycles after stopping use of OC. There is reasonable doubt that women transfer the recommendations into practice directly after discontinuation of OC, provided that knowledge about NTD prevention by FA exists. But the timing of FA supplementation is critical because the neural tube closes within 28 days after conception. Even if the women starts with FA supplementation directly after discontinuation of OC, the supplementation period might be too short to achieve protectable serum folate and RBC folate concentrations. At least 12 wk of supplementation are needed to get a steady state in plasma folate concentrations (Hao et al., 2008; Lamers et al., 2006), the medium by which the fetus is supplied with nutrients. A more extensive supplementation period is necessary to reach the plateau in RBC folate concentrations (Hao et al., 2008, Houghton et al., 2010; Lamers et al., 2006; Venn et al., 2002). A combined FA/OC would guarantee a good folate status for a certain period of time (3 months or more) after cessation of OC as RBC folate concentration decreases slowly (Bakker et al., 2009; Hao et al., 2008; Houghton et al., 2010). Fourthly, use of OC is the most common method of contraception worldwide. By combining OC with folate, the majority of the targeted group will be set into a good folate status. Fifthly, only the targeted group, women of childbearing age, will receive the product under medical care. Discussion on potential risks of high FA exposure for the whole population by mandatory fortification is therefore less relevant. In addition, there is evidence from several studies that [6S]-5-MTHF has the same beneficial effect on NTD compared with FA, but is less likely to have health risks as discussed for FA. Therefore [6S]-5-MTHF should be preferred to FA for combining with OC.

Thus, combining OC with [6S]-5-MTHF or FA is a reasonable und promising approach to minimize NTD prevalence. In 2010, the U.S. FDA approved two OC products combined with [6S]-5-MTHF (FDA, 2010a, 2010b) which have been introduced in the U.S. market in 2011. These OCs are not only approved for the primary indications of an OC, but also secondarily for improving folate status to reduce the risk of a NTD-affected pregnancy in those women who conceive while using the product or shortly after discontinuation. The concept of a combined OC-folate product would be ingenious and useful in European and other countries, too.

## 7. References

Abdollahi, Z.; Elmadfa, I.; Djazayery, A.; Golalipour, M.J.; Sadighi, J.; Salehi, F. & Sadeghian Sharif, S. (2011). Efficacy of flour fortification with folic acid in women of childbearing age in Iran. *Annals of Nutrition & Metabolism*, Vol.58, No.3, pp. 1988-196, ISSN 0250-6807

Abeywardana, S.; Bower, C.; Halliday, J.; Chan, A. & Sullivan, E.A. (2010). Prevalence of neural tube defects in Australia prior to mandatory fortification of bread-making flour with folic acid. *Australian and New Zealand Journal of Public Health*, Vol.34, No.4, pp. 351-355, ISSN 1326-0200

Alasfoor, D.; Elsayed, M.K. & Mohammed, A.J. (2010). Spina bifida and birth outcome before and after fortification of flour with iron and folic acid in Oman. *East Mediterranean Health Journal*, Vol. 16, No.5, pp. 533-538, ISSN 1020-3397

Amarin, ZO. & Obeid, A.Z. (2010). Effect of folic acid fortification on the incidence of neural tube defects. *Paediatric and perinatal Epidemiology*, Vol. 24, No.4, pp. 349-451, ISSN 1365-3016

Australian Government, Department of Health and Ageing, National Health and Medical Research Council (2006). Folate, In: *Nutrient reference values for Australia and New Zealand including recommended dietary intakes.* Australian Government, Department of Health and Ageing, National Health and Medical Research Council (Ed.), 98-104, ISBN 1864962372, Canberra, Australia

Bakker, D.J.; de Jong-van den Berg, L.T.W. & Fokkema, R.M.(2009). Controlled study on folate status following folic acid supplementation and discontinuation in women of child-bearing age. *Annals of Clinical Biochemistry*, Vol.46, No.Pt3, pp. 231–234, ISSN 0004-5632

Barjot, P.; Graesslin, O.; Cohen, D.; Vaillant, P.; Clerson, P. & Hoffet, M. (2006). Pregnancies occurring during oral contraception: lessons from the GRECO study. *Gynécologie, Obstétrique & Fertilité*, Vo.34, No.2, pp.120-6, ISSN 1297-9589

Berry, R.J.; Li, Z.; Erickson,J.D.; Li, S.; Moore, C.A.; Wang, H.; Mulinare, J.; Zhao,P.; Wong, L.Y.; Gindler, J.; Hong, S.X. & Correa, A. (1999). Prevention of neural-tube defects with folic acid in China. China-U.S. Collaborative Project for Neural Tube Defect Prevention. *New England Journal of Medicine*, Vol. 341, No.20, pp. 1485–1490, ISSN 0028-4793

Berry, R.J.; Bailey, L.; Mulinare, J. & Bower, C. (2010). Folic Acid Working Group. Fortification of flour with folic acid. *Food and Nutrition Bulletin,* Vol.31, No. 1, pp. S22-35, ISSN 0379-5721

Botto, L.D.; Moore, C.A.; Khoury, M.J. & Erickson, J.D. (1999). Neural-tube defects. *The New England Journal of Medicine*. Vol. 341, No.20, pp. 1509-1519, ISSN 0028-4793

Botto L.D.; Lisi A.; Robert-Gnansia, E.; Erickson, J.D.; Vollset, S.E.; Mastroiacovo, P.; Botting, B.; Cocchi, G.; de Vigan, C.; de Walle, H.; Feijoo, M.; Irgens, L.M.; McDonnell, B.; Merlob, P.; Ritvanen, A.; Scarano, G.; Siffel, C.; Metneki, J.; Stoll, C.; Smithells, R. & Goujard, J. (2005). International retrospective cohort study of neural tube defects in relation to folic acid recommendations: are the recommendations working? *British Journal of Medicine*, Vol.330, No.7491, p. 571, ISSN 0959-8138

Boyd, P.A.; Haeusler, M.; Barisic, I.; Loane, M.; Garne, E. & Dolk, H. (2011). Paper 1: The EUROCAT Network—Organization and Processes. *Birth Defects Research. Part A, Clinical and molecular teratology*, Vol. 91, Suppl.1, pp. S2–S15, ISSN 1542-0752

Brown, R.D.; Langshaw, M.R.; Uhr, E.J.; Gibson, J.N. & Joshua, D.E. (2011). The impact of mandatory fortification of flour with folic acid on the blood levels of an Autralian population. *Medical Journal of Australia*, Vol.194, No.2, pp. 65-67, ISSN 0025-729X

Brouwer, I.A.; van Dusseldorp, M.; West, C.E.; Meyboom, S.; Thomas, C.M.G.; Duran, M.; van het Hof, K.H.; Eskes T.K.A.B.; Hautvast, .J.G.A.J. & Steegers-Theunissen, R.P.M. (1999). Dietary folate from vegetables and citrus fruit decreases plasma homocysteine concentrations in humans in a dietary controlled trial. *Journal of Nutrition*, Vol.129, No.6, pp. 1135–1139, ISSN 0022-3166

Centers for Disease Control and Prevention (CDC )(1992). Recommendations for the use of folic acid to reduce the number of cases of spina bifida and neural tube defects. *Morbidity and Mortality Weekly Report* , Vol.41, No.1, pp. 2-8, ISSN 1057-5987

Centers for Disease Control and Prevention (CDC) (2004). Spina bifida and anencephaly after folic acid mandate - United States, 1995-1996 and 1999-2000. *Morbidity and Mortality Weekly Report, Vol.* 53, No.17, pp. 362-365, ISSN 0149-2195

Centers for Disease Control and Prevention (CDC) (2008). Use of supplements containing folic acid among women of childbearing age - United States, 2007. *Morbidity and Mortality Weekly Report, Vol.* 57, No.1, pp. 5-8, ISSN 0149-2195

Centers for Disease Control and Prevention (CDC) (February 2010). Public Health Grands Rounds. Presentation. Folic acid in the prevention of birth defects. 07-07-2011, Available from: http://www.cdc.gov/about/grand-rounds/archives/ 2010/02-February.htm

Choumenkowitch, S.F.; Jacques, P.F.; Nadeau, M.R.; Wilson, P.W.F.; Rosenberg, I.H. & Selhub, J. (2001). Folic acid fortification increases red blood cell folate concentrations in the Framingham study. *Journal of Nutrition*, Vol.131, No.12, pp.3277-3280, ISSN 0022-3166

Commission of the European Communities (1993). Folate. In: *Reports of the Scientific Committee for Food: 31st Series - Nutrient and energy intakes for the European Community*. Commission of the European Communities, Office for Official Publications of the European Communities, 99-106, ISBN 92-826-6409-0, Luxembourg, Luxembourg,

Cronin M.; Schellschmidt, I. & Dinger J. (2009). Rate of pregnancy after using drospirenone and other progestin-containing oral contraceptives. *Obstetrics & Gynecology*, Vol.114, No.3. pp. 616-622, ISSN 0029-7844

Czeizel, A.E & Dudás, I. (1992). Prevention of the first occurrence of neural-tube defects by periconceptional vitamin supplementation. *New England Journal of Medicine*, Vol.327, No.26, pp. 1832-1835, ISSN 0028-4793

Daly, L.E.; Kirke, P.N.; Molloy, A.; Weir, D.G. & Scott, J.M. (1995). Folate levels and neural tube defects. Implications for prevention. *Journal of the American Medical Association*, Vol.274, No.21, pp. 1698-1702, ISSN 0098-7484

Egen V. (1999). Die Prophylaxe von Neuralrohrdefekten durch Folsäure: Umsetzung eines medizinischen Forschungsergebnisses in der Praxis. Dissertation an der Medizinischen Fakultät der Ludwig-Maximilians-Universität München

Egen, V. & Hasford, J. (2003). Prevention of neural tube defects: effect of an intervention aimed at implementing the official recommendations. *Sozial- und Präventivmedizin*, Vol. 48, No.1, pp.24-32, ISSN 0303-8408

Eskes, T.K.A.B (2002). Folate, homocysteine, and neural tube defects. In: *Folate and Human Development*, E.J. Massaro & J.M. (Ed.), 137-164, ISBN 0-89603-936-6, Humana Press Totowa, New Jersey, USA

EUROCAT (2009a). Folic Acid Special Reports. Special Report: Prevention of Neural tube defects by periconceptional folic acid supplementation in Europe - December 2009. Part I - Overview. 08-07-2011, Available from: http://www.eurocat-network.eu/PREVENTIONandRISKFACTORS/FolicAcid/FolicAcidSpecialReports

EUROCAT (2009b). Folic Acid Special Reports. Special Report: Prevention of Neural tube defects by periconceptional folic acid supplementation in Europe - December 2009. Part IIa - Country Specific Chapters (Austria to Ireland). 08-07-2011, Available from: http://www.eurocat-network.eu//PREVENTIONandRISKFACTORS/FolicAcid/FolicAcidSpecialReports

EUROCAT (2009c). Folic Acid Special Reports. Special Report: Prevention of Neural tube defects by periconceptional folic acid supplementation in Europe - December 2009. Part IIb - Country Specific Chapters (Italy to UK). 08-07-2011, Available from: http://www.eurocat-network.eu/PREVENTIONandRISKFACTORS/FolicAcid/FolicAcidSpecialReports

EUROCAT (2009d). Prevalence Tables. 08-07-2011, Available from: http://www.eurocat-network.eu/ACCESSPREVALENCEDATA/PrevalenceTables

Finer, L.B. & Henshaw, S.K. (2006). Disparities in rates of unintended pregnancy in the U.S., 1994 and 2001. *Perspectives on Sexual and Reproductive Health*, Vol.38, No.2, pp. 90-96, ISSN 1538-6341

Flynn, M.A.T.; Anderson, W.A.; Burke, S.J. & Reilly A. (2008). Session 1: Public health nutrition Folic acid food fortification: the Irish experience. *Proceedings of the Nutrition Society*, Vol. 67, No.4, pp. 381–389, ISSN 0029-6651

Fohr, I.; Prinz-Langenohl, R.; Brönstrup, A.; Bohlmann, A.M.; Nau, H.; Berthold, H.K. & Pietrzik, K. (2002). 5,10-methylenetetrahydrofolate reductase genotype determines the plasma homocysteine-lowering effect of supplementation with 5-methyltetrahydrofolate or folic acid in healthy young women. *American Journal of Clinical Nutrition*, Vol.75, No.2, pp. 275–282, ISSN 0002-9165

Food and Drug Administration (FDA) (1996). Food standards. Amendment of standards of identity of enriched grain products to require addition of folic acid. *Federal Register*, Vol. 61, No.44, pp. 8781-8797, ISSN 0097-6326

Food and Drug Administration (FDA) (2010a). FDA Approved Drug Products. Safyral. 08-07-2011, Available from: http://www.accessdata.fda.gov/scripts/cder/drugsatfda/index.cfm?fuseaction=Search.DrugDetails

Food and Drug Administration (FDA) (2010b). FDA Approved Drug Products. Beyaz. 08-07-2011, Available from: http://www.accessdata.fda.gov/scripts/cder/drugsatfda/index.cfm?fuseaction=Search.DrugDetails

Frye, C.A. (2006). An overview of oral contraceptives: mechanism of action and clinical use. *Neurology,* Vol.66, No.6 (Suppl 3), pp. S29-36, ISSN 0028-3878

Ganji, V. & Kafai, M.R. (2006). Trends in serum folate, RBC folate, and circulating total homocysteine concentrations in the United States: Analysis of data from National Health and Nutrition Examination Surveys, 1988–1994, 1999–2000, and 2001–2002. *Journal of Nutrition,* Vol.136, No.1 ,pp.153– 158, ISSN 0022-3166

German Nutrition Society, Austrian Nutrition Society, Swiss Society of Nutrition Research, Swiss Nutrition Association (2002). Folate. In: *Reference values for nutrient intake.* German Nutrition Society (Ed.), 117-122, Umschau Braus GmbH, Frankfurt, ISBN 3-8295-7114-5

Gong R.; Wang, Z.P.; Gao, L.J.; Lu Q.B.; Sun, X.H. & Zhao, Z.T. (2010). A case-control study of the effect of pregnancy planning on neural tube defects and its primary prevention. *Birth Defects Research Part A. Clinical and Molecular Teratology.* Vol.88, No.9, pp. 737-742, ISSN 1542-0752

Hao, L.; Yang, Q.-H.; Zhu, Y.; Bailey, L.B.; Zhu, J.-H.; Hu, D.J.; Zhang, B.-L.; Erickson J.D., Zhang, L.; Gindler, J.; Li, S. &Berry R.J. (2008). Folate status and homocysteine response to folic acid doses and withdrawal among young Chinese women in a large -scale randomized double-blind trial. *American Journal of Clinical Nutrition,* Vol.88, No.2, pp. 448-457, ISSN 0002-9165

Health Council of the Netherlands. Towards an optimal use of folic acid. The Hague (The Netherlands): Health Council of the Netherlands. 2008. Publication No 2008/02E.

Holzgreve, W.; Wagner H. & Rempen , A. (1984). Möglichkeiten der pränatalen Beurteilung von normaler und gestörter Neuralrohrentwicklung durch Ultraschall. *Medizinische Welt,* Vol.35, pp. 1344-1347, ISSN 0025-8512

Holzgreve, W.; Buchholz, B. & Beller, F.K. (1987). Kidney transplantation from anencephalic donors. *New England Journal of Medicine,* Vol.316, No.17, pp. 1069-1070, ISSN 0028-4793

Holzgreve, W.; Tercanli, S. & Pietrzik, K. (1991). Vitamins to prevent neural tube defects. *Lancet,* Vol. 338, pp.639-640, ISSN 0140-6736

Houghton, L.A.; Sherwood, K.L.; Pawlosky, R.; Ito, S. & O'Connor, D.L. (2006). [6S]-5-methyltetrahydrofolate is at least effective as folic acid in preventing a decline in blood folate concentrations during lactation. *American Journal of Clinical Nutrition,* Vol.83, No.4, pp. 842–850, ISSN 0002-9165

Houghton, L.A.; Gray, A.R.; Rose, M.C.; Miller, J.C.; Hurthouse, N.A. & Gregory III, J.F. (2011). Long-term effect of low-dose folic acid intake: potential effect of mandatory fortification on the prevention of neural tube defects. *American Journal of Clinical Nutrition,* Vol.94, No.1, pp. 136-141, ISSN 0002-9165

Inskip, H.M.; Crozier, S.H.; Godfrey, K.M.; Borland S.E.; Cooper, C. & Robinson S.M. (2009). Women's compliance with nutrition and lifestyle recommendations before pregnancy: general population cohort study. *British Medical Journal,* Vol. 338, No.2 pp.481-486, ISSN 0959-8138

Institute of Medicine (IOM) (1998). Folate. In: *Dietary reference intake for thiamin, riboflavin, niacin, vitamin B6, folate, vitamin B12, pantothenic acid, biotin, and choline*. pp. 196-305, National Academy Press, Washington D.C., ISBN 0-309—06554-2

Jacques, P. F.; Selhub, J.; Bostom, A. G.; Wilson, P. W. & Rosenberg, I. H. (1999). The effect of folic acid fortification on plasma folate and total homocysteine concentrations. *New England Journal of Medicine*, Vol. 340, No.19, pp. 1449–1454, ISSN 0028-4793

Kelly, P.; McPartlin, J.; Goggins, M.; Weir, D.G. & Scott, J. (1997). Unmtabolized folic acid in serm: acute studies in subjects consuming fortified food an supplements. *American Journal of Clinical Nutrition*, Vol. 65, No.6, pp.1790-1795, ISSN 0002-9165

Knopf H. & Melchert, H.-U. (1999). Subjektive Angaben zur täglichen Anwendung ausgewählter Arzneimittelgruppen - Erste Ergebnisse des Bundesgesundheitssurveys 1998. *Gesundheitswesen*, Vol.61, Sonderheft 2, pp. 151-157, ISSN 0941-3790

Lamers, Y.; Prinz-Langenohl, R.; Moser, R. & Pietrzik, K. (2004). Supplementation with [6S]-5-methyltetrahydrofolate or folic acid equally reduces plasma total homocysteine concentrations in healthy women. *American Journal of Clinical Nutrition*, Vol.79, No.3, pp. 473–478, ISSN 0002-9165

Lamers, Y.; Prinz-Langenohl, R.; Brämswig, S. & Pietrzik, K. (2006). Red blood cell folate concentrations increase more after supplementation with [6S]-5-methyltetra-hydrofolate than with folic acid in women of childbearing age. *American Journal of Clinical Nutrition*, Vol.84, No.1, pp. 156–161, ISSN 0002-9165

Laurence, K.M. ; James, N. ; Miller, M.H. et al. (1981). Double-blind randomised controlled trial of folate treatment before conception to prevent recurrence of neural-tube defects. *British Medical Journal (Clinical Research Ed)*, Vol. 282, No.6275, pp.1509–1511, ISSN 1468-5833

Litynski, P.; Loehrer, F.; Linder, L.; Todesco, L. & Fowler, B. (2002). Effect of low dose of 5-methyltetrahydrofolate and folic acid on plasma homocysteine in healthy subjects with or without the 677C→T polymorphism of methylenetetrahydrofolate reductase. *European Journal of Clinical Investigation, Vol.*32, No.9, pp. 662–668, ISSN 1365-2362

López-Camelo, J.S.; Castilla, E.E. & Orioli, I.M.( 2010). Folic acid flour fortification: Impact on the frequencies of 52 congenital anomaly types in three South American countries. *American Journal of Medical Genetics* Part A, Vol.152, No.19, pp. 2444–2458, ISSN 1552-4825

Mader, R.M.; Steger, G.G.; Rizovski, B.; Djavanmard, M.P.; Scheithauer, W.; Jakesz, R. *et al.* (1995). Stereospecific pharmacokinetics of rac-5-methyltetrahydrofolic acid in patients with advanced colorectal cancer. *British Journal of Clinical Pharmacology*, Vol.40, No.4, pp. 209–215, ISSN 1365-2125

McGuire, M.; Cleary, B; Sahm, L. & Murphy, D.J. (2010). Prevalence and predictors of periconceptional folic acid uptake - prospective cohort study in an Irish urban obstetric population. *Human Reproduction*, Vol. 25, No.2, pp. 535-543, ISSN 0268-1161

McNulty B.; Pentieva, K.; Marshal, B.; Ward, M.; Molloy A.M.; Scott J.M. & McNulty, H. (2011). Women's compliance with current folic acid recommendations and achievement of optimal vitamin status for preventing neural tube defects. *Human Reproduction*, Vol. 26, No.6, pp.1530-1536, ISSN 0268-1161

Medical Research Council (1991). Vitamin prevention of neural tube defects: results of the Medical Research Council Vitamin Study. MRC Vitamin Study Research Group. *Lancet* 1991, Vol.338, No.8760, pp.131-137, ISSN 0140-6736

Max-Rubner-Institut (MRI) (2008). Nationale Verzehrsstudie II, Ergebnisbericht, Teil 2. Max-Rubner-Institut (ed.), Karlsruhe, Germany

Mulinare, J.; Cordero, J.F.; Erickson, J.D. & Berry, R.J. (1988). Periconceptional use of multivitamins and the occurrence of neural tube defects. *Journal of the American Medical Association*, Vol.260, No.21, pp. 3141–3145, ISSN 0098-7484

Milunsky, A.; Jick, H.; Jick, S.S., et al. (1989).Multivitamin/folic acid supplementation in early pregnancy reduces the prevalence of neural tube defects. *Journal of the American Medical Assocation*, Vol. 262, No.20, pp. 2847–52, ISSN

Orioli, I. M.; Lima do Nascimento, R.; López-Camelo, J. S. & Castilla, E. E. (2011). Effects of folic acid fortification on spina bifida prevalence in Brazil. *Birth Defects Research Part A: Clinical and Molecular Teratology*, May 31. doi: 10.1002/bdra.20830, ISSN 1542-0752

Osterhues, A.; Holzgreve, W. & Michels, K.B. (2009). Shall we put the world on folate? *Lancet*, Vol.374, No.969,. pp.959-961, ISSN 0140-6736

Pentieva, K;: McNulty, H.; Reichert, R.; Ward, M.; Strain, J.J.; McKillop, D.; McPartlin, J.M.; Connolly, E.; Molloy, A.; Kramer, K. & Scott, J.M. (2004). The short-term bioavailabilities of [6S]-5-methyltetrahydrofolate and folic acid are equivalent in men. *Journal of Nutrition*, Vol. 134, No.3, pp. 580–585, ISSN 0022-3166

Pietrzik, K.; Bailey, L.; Shane, B. (2010) Folic acid and L-5-methytetrahydrofolate. *Clinical Pharmacokinetics*, Vol.49, No.8, pp 535-548, ISSN 0312-5963

Pietrzik, K.; Lamers, Y.; Brämswig, S. & Prinz-Langenohl R. (2007). Calculation of red blood cell folate steady state conditions and elimination kinetics after daily supplementation with various folate forms and doses in women of childbearing age. *American Journal of Clinical Nutrition*, Vol.86, No.5, pp. 1414-1419, ISSN 0002-9165

Prinz-Langenohl, R.; Lamers, Y.; Moser, R. et al. (2003). Effect of folic acid preload on the bioequivalence of [6S]-5-methyltetrahydrofolate and folic acid in healthy volunteers. *Journal of Inherited Metabolic Disease*, Vol.26, Suppl. 1, p. 124, ISSN 0141-8955

Prinz-Langenohl, R.; Brämswig, S.; Tobolski, O.; Smulders, Y.M.; Smith, D.E.C.; Finglas, P.M. & Pietrzik, K. (2009). [6S]-5-methyltetrahydrofolate increases plasma folate more effectively than folic acid in women with the homozygous or wild-type 677C,T polymorphism of methylenetetrahydrofolate reductase. *British Journal of Pharmacology*, Vol.158, No.8, pp. 2014–2021, ISSN 0007-1188

Ray, J.G.; Vermeulen, M.J.; Boss, S.C. & Cole, D.E. (2002). Increased red cell folate concentrations in women of reproductive age after Canadian folic acid food fortification. *Epidemiology*, Vol.13, No.2, pp.238-240, ISSN 1044-3983

Ray, J. G.; Singh, G. & Burrows, R. F. (2004). Evidence for suboptimal use of periconceptional folic acid supplements globally. *BJOG: An International Journal of Obstetrics & Gynaecology*, Vol.111, No.5, pp. 399–408, ISSN 1470-0328

Rieback, M. & Kreyenfeld, M. (2009). Ungeplantes Glück. *Deutsche Hebammenzeitschrift*, Vol.9, pp. 72-74, ISSN 0012-026X

Scholl, T.O. & Johnson, W.G. (2000). Folic acid: influence on the outcome of pregnancy. *American Journal of Clinical Nutrition*, Vol.71, No.5, pp.1295S–1303S, ISSN 0002-9165

Schwarz, E.B.; Sobota, M.; Gonzales, R. & Gerbert, B. (2008). Computerized counseling for folate knowledge and use: a randomized controlled trial. *American Journal of Preventive Medicine*, Vol.35, No.6, pp. 568-571, ISSN 0749-3797

Scientific Advisory Committee on Nutrition (2006). Folate and Disease Prevention. Food Standard Agency and the Department of Health, UK, ISBN 9780112431114

Shaw, G.M.; Schaffer, D.; Velie, E.M., et al. (1995). Periconceptional vitamin use, dietary folate, and the occurrence of neural tube defects. *Epidemiology*, Vol. 6, No.3, pp. 219–226, ISSN 1044-3983

Simpson, J.L.; Bailey, L.B.; Pietrzik, K.; Shane, B. & Holzgreve, W. ( 2010). Micronutrients and women of reproductive potential: required dietary intake and consequences of dietary deficiency or excess. Part I- folate, vitamin B12, vitamin B6. *Journal of Maternal-Fetal and Neonatal Medicine*, Vol.23, No.12, pp. 1323-43, ISSN 1476-7058

Simpson, J.L.; Bailey, L.B.; Pietrzik, K.; Shane, B. & Holzgreve, W. (2011). Micronutirients and women of reproductive potential: required dietary intake and consequences of dietary deficiency or excess. Part II- Vitamin D, Vitamin A, Iron, Zinc, Iodine, Essential Fatty Acids. *Journal of Maternal-Fetal and Neonatal Medicine*, Vol.24, No.1, pp.1-24, ISSN 1476-7058

Smith, A.D.; Kim, Y.I. & Refsum, H. (2008). Is folic acid good for everyone? *American Journal of Clinical Nutrition*, Vol. 87, No. 3, pp. 517–533, ISSN 1044-3983

Smithells, R.W.; Sheppard, S.; Schorah, C.J. et al. (1980). Possible prevention of neural-tube defects by periconceptional vitamin supplementation. *Lancet*, Vol. 1, No.8164, pp. 339–40, ISSN 0140-6736

Stockley L. & Lund, V. (2008). Use of folic acid supplements, particularly by low-income and young women: a series of systematic reviews to inform public health policy in the UK. *Public Health Nutrition*, Vol. 11, No.8, pp. 807-821, ISSN 1368-9800

Thamm, M.; Mensink, G.B. M. & Thierfelder, W. (2002). Folsäureversorgung von Frauen im gebärfähigen Alter. *Gesundheitswesen*, Vol. 61, Sonderheft 2, pp. 207–S212, ISSN 0941-3790

Tinker, S.C.; Cogswell, M.E.; Devine, O. & Berry, R.J. (2010). Folic acid intake among U.S. women aged 15-44 years, National Health and Nutrition Survey, 2003-2006. *American Journal of Preventive Medicine*, Vol.38, No.5, pp. 534-542, ISSN 0749-3797

Troen, A.M.; Mitchell, B.; Sorensen B.; Werner, M.H.; Johnston, A.; Wood B. et al. (2006). Unmetabolized folic acid in plasma is associated with reduced natural killer cell cytotoxicity among postmenopausal women. *Journal of Nutrition*, Vol. 136, No.1, pp.189-194, ISSN 0022-3166

US Preventive Services Task Force (2009). Folic acid for the prevention of neural tube defects: US preventive services task force recommendation statement. *Annals of Internal Medicine*, Vol.150, No.9, pp. 626-631, ISSN 0003-4819

Venn, B.J.; Green, T.J.; Moser, R.; McKenzie, J.E.; Skeaff, C.M. & Mann, J. (2002). Increases in blood folate indices are similar in women of childbearing age supplemented with [6S]-5-methyltetrahydrofolate and folic acid. *Journal of Nutrition*, Vol.132, No.11, pp. 3353–3355, ISSN 0022-3166

Venn B.J., Green T.J., Moser R. & Mann J.I. (2003) Comparison of the effect of low-dose supplementation with L-5-methyl-tetrahydrofolate or folic acid on plasma homocysteine: a randomized placebo-controlled study. *American Journal of Clinical Nutrition,* Vol. 77, No.3, pp. 658–662, ISSN, 0002-9165

Vergel, R.G.; Sanchez, L.R.; Heredero, B.L., et al. (1990). Primary prevention of neural tube defects with folic acid supplementation: Cuban experience. *Prenatal Diagnostic,* Vol.10, No.3, pp. 149–52, ISSN 0197-3851

Werler, M.M.; Shapiro, S. & Mitchell, A.A. (1993). Periconceptional folic acid exposure and risk of occurrent neural tube defects. *Journal of the Medical Association*, Vol.269, No. 10, pp. 1257-1261, ISSN 0098-7484

Willems, F.F.; Boers, G.H.J.; Blom, H.J.; Aengevaeren, W.R.M. & Verheugt, F.W.A. (2004). Pharmacokinetic study on the utilisation of 5-methyltetrahydrofolate and folic acid in patients with coronary artery disease. *British Journal of Pharmacology,* Vol. 141, No.5, pp. 825–830, ISSN 0007-1188

5

# Antenatal Prevention of Neural Tube Defects

Naomi Burke, Tom Walsh and Michael Geary
*Rotunda Hospital, Parnell Square, Dublin, Ireland*

## 1. Introduction

Neural tube defects (NTDs) are complex congenital anomalies. Spina bifida and anencephaly which arise from failure of closure of the neural tube during embryogenesis are the most common forms of NTDs. While anencephaly is a letal malformation, spina bifida is a common birth defect in which patients can suffer from a multitude of potential medical and surgical morbidities and increased risk of mortality throughout their life. The incidence and prevalence of NTDs varies in different parts of the world [1]. This is attributable to many factors including; geographic region, maternal age, obesity, ethnicity and socioeconomic status of the parents. However a declining trend has been seen in many countries. This in part may be explained by the availability of prenatal diagnosis, folic acid supplementation recommendations, folic acid food fortification initiatives and selective termination. Prevention of NTDs presents a complex problem as the underlying aetiologies of NTDs are an interplay of genetic, environmental and nutritional factors. Folate deficiency explains approximately 72% of NTDs cases and this chapter will primarily address the role of folic acid supplementation for the prevention of NTDs [2]. However, it is necessary to briefly review the metabolism of folate to understand how these prevention strategies were developed.

## 2. An overview of folate metabolism

Dietary folate polyglutamates need to be converted to monoglutamates before they can be absorbed. In the jejunum, polyglutamates are converted to monoglutamates by the enzyme γ -glutamyl hydrolyase prior to their absorption in the intestine. During absorption in the jejunum, the different monoglutamyl folates are converted to 5-methyltetrahydrofolate (5-MeTHF). 5-MeTHF is the principal circulating folate and is transported across the plasma membranes of cells and thus the principal form by which tissues are supplied with folate. Within cells, folate is involved in methylation reactions where it can either donate one carbon units for purine and thymidine synthesis or accept one carbon units from amino acids. There are three principal enzymes involved in these methylation reactions. Methylenetetrahydrofolate reductase (MTHFR) competes with thymidylate reductase (TS) and methylenetetrahydrofolate dehydrogenase (MTHFD) for one carbon units. MTHFR is controlled by S-adenosylmethinione. 5-MeTHF donates a methyl group via methionine synthase to homocysteine using Vitamin B12 as a co-factor to produce S - adenosylmethinione [3]. Homocysteine will accumulate when there are depleted amounts of folate or vitamin B12. S-adenosylmethinione is a key donor in the methylation of DNA, proteins and lipids. It is also essential in the metabolism of certain neurotransmitters. This outlines the importance of folate metabolism in cellular function especially in rapidly dividing cells i.e. periods of rapid growth. It is here we see the importance of folate metabolism in the aetiology of NTDs.

## 3. Genetics: Variations in folate metabolism

Normal folate levels with high homocysteine levels have been observed in women who have delivered children with NTDs [4]. This is an indicator that there must be other factors contributing to the aetiology of NTDs. Several genes coding for folate dependent enzymes have been examined for mutations that could account for NTDs. One gene that codes for a folate dependent enzyme is C677T polymorphism of 5,10 methylenetetrahydrofolate reductase (MTHFR). The function of MTHFR is to regulate production of 5-MeTHF, the main plasma form of the vitamin. This thermolabile variant is associated with decreased enzyme activity [5]. The C667T thermolabile variant gene was observed in 18% of spina bifida patients versus 6% of a controlled group in a study carried out by Shields et al in Ireland [6]. Several other studies confirmed the increased risk of NTDs in the offspring of women with this variant gene. The major implication of this finding is that these are a subset of women who may have increased folate requirements [7]. Although other mutations of the MTHFR gene have been identified, along with mutations in other key genes encoding for enzymes used in folate metabolism none have been implicated yet as contributing to cases of NTDs [8].

## 4. Environmental

As described earlier the incidence of NTDs can vary with geography, socioeconomic status of the parents and there is a seasonal variation. Discordance in monozygotic twinning has also been reported in NTDs. This suggests that environmental factors may contribute to the aetiology of NTDs. A whole host of physical, chemical and infectious agents have been suggested as possible teratogens including; solvents, anaesthetics agents, X-radiation, viruses and paints [9]. One physical agent, hyperthermia has been investigated as a possible teratogen and a meta-analysis by Moretti et al in 2005 showed that maternal hyperthermia during critical periods of neural tube development is associated with an increased incidence of NTDs (OR 1.95) [10]. Of course one cannot forget the possibility of susceptible gene-environment interactions which could help explain the geographical and seasonal variations seen in the incidence of NTDs.

## 5. Nutritional

Folic Acid supplementation had been shown to prevent NTDs. There had been an explosion of scientific and clinical data since the first seminal work by Smithsells et al more than thirty years ago[11]. The United Kingdom Medical Research Council Trial and the Hungarian Periconceptional folic acid supplementation randomised control trial in the early nineties outlined how folic acid supplementation could decrease the occurrence of NTD by 50-70% [2, 12]. This led to universal recommendations of periconceptional folic acid supplementation. A recent meta-analysis by the Cochrane collaboration identified five trials which examined the prevalence of NTDs in women receiving folic acid supplementation, those receiving folic acid had a significantly reduced risk of having baby with a NTDs (risk ratio 0.28 95% confidence intervals (CI) 0.15 to 0.52) [13]. Indeed the evidence from these five trials is so overwhelmingly in favour of folic acid supplementation there has been a paucity of supporting trials since the year 2000. The recommendations are to take 400µg of folic acid daily (either from dietary sources or supplements) for at least one month before conception (World Health Organisation). This dosing regimen has been largely based on the association between maternal red cell folate (RCF) levels and the risk of NTDs.

## 6. Red cell folate and serum folate and its relationship to NTD

Irish researchers have made substantial contributions to the understanding of NTD epidemiology. In a large case-control study based on over 56,000 women attending the maternity hospitals in Dublin from 1986 to 1990, the folate and vitamin B12 levels of blood samples taken at the first ante-natal visit were noted as independent risk factors for neural tube defect [14]. Later, data representing the blood folate concentrations of NTDs cases (n = 84) and selected controls (n = 266) was used to calculate the degrees of risk of an NTDs birth [15]. Cases and controls were similar with regard to maternal age. All controls were representative of normal births. The red cell folate (RCF) level in early pregnancy emerged as a premier indicator of such risk. The overall NTDs rate was 1.9/1000 births in this study. They showed that the risk of NTDs is associated with RCF levels in a continuous dose-response relationship. The risk is reduced as RCF levels increase. With a RCF level of <150µg/l the risk of NTD is 6.6/1000 but if the RCF level is increased beyond 400µg/l the risk falls to 0.8/1000. The RCF levels can be increased over a 6 month period with doses of 400µg of folic acid which can reduce the risk of NTDs by 47% [15]. This dose is also considered safe. However, in the context of food fortification programmes it may be worth reviewing this recommendation. There is no consensus on the minimal effective dose of folic acid. Table 1 shows the distribution of RCF in cases and controls and NTDs risk in each category.

| RED CELL FOLATE ng/mL | RISK OF NTD PER 1000 BIRTHS |
|---|---|
| 0-149 | 6.6 |
| 150-199 | 3.2 |
| 200-299 | 2.3 |
| 300-399 | 1.6 |
| >400 | 0.8 |

Table 1. Overall risk of a neural tube defect pregnancy associated with low red cell folate status.

The largely European drive for improved periconceptional education and folic acid supplementation has not seen the reduction in NTDs predicted. A large international cohort study involving ten countries and covering more than 13 million births concluded that recommendations alone did not improve trends of incidence of NTDs[16]. Countries which had implemented food fortification programmes were excluded from this study. This underlines the entire problem with the prevention of NTDs. For folic acid to work it must be taken within the first four weeks of pregnancy, before the woman knows she is pregnant!

## 7. Food fortification

Many countries have identified new strategies to increase serum folate levels in women of reproductive age. In the US, Canada, South Africa and Chile they have adopted national floor fortification policies and have seen a substantial decrease in the numbers of new cases of NTDs. In March 1996, the U.S. Food and Drug Administration (FDA) issued a final rule, effective January 1998, that required all enriched cereal-grain products (flour, rice, breads, rolls and buns, pasta, corn grits, corn meal, farina, macaroni and noodle products) to be fortified with folic acid 0.14mg folic acid /100g flour and 0.24 mg/100g pasta in addition to the iron, thiamin, riboflavin and niacin already added to these enriched cereal-grain products. Mandatory food fortification has been the solution to NTDs in the USA, and has had a dramatic effect on the folate status there [17, 18]. Further evidence to support the process of food fortification has emerged. Jacques et al. looked at blood folate status in a control group before fortification and a group after fortification. They found that the mean plasma folate (for non-users of B-vitamin supplementation) increased from 4.6μg/L before fortification to 10μg/L after folic acid fortification. They also noted that with fortification there was a decrease in the prevalence of high homocyteine levels from 18.7 to 9.8% [19].The U.S. Centres for Disease Control and Prevention reported that there has been a three-fold increase in the serum folate status of women aged 15-44 years who did not use supplements[18]. Another report published in 2000 looked at data collected from the Framingham Offspring Cohort Study. It was found that among non-supplement users, folic acid intake increased by a mean of 190μg/day and total folate intake increased by a mean of 323μg/day dietary folate equivalents in the exposed participants[20]. In Canada a mandatory fortification policy was also adopted; specific cereal grain products had to be fortified with folic acid at a level of 0.15mg/100g by November 1st 1998. Persad et al looked to see if folic acid supplementation or fortification changed the annual incidence of open NTDs in Nova Scotia. The study looked at the total number of births and stillbirths with NTDs and the number of terminated pregnancies affected with NTDs from perinatal and fetal anomaly databases. They reported that the incidence of open NTDs (spina bifida, anencephaly, encephaloceles) decreased by 54% after the Canadian fortification program was implemented. In 1991 to 1997 the mean annual rate was 2.58 per 1000 births and from 1997 to 2000 was 1.17 per 1000 births [21]. De Wals et al demonstrated similar results, showing a decline in the prevalence of NTDs from 1.58 per 1000 pregnancies before fortification to 0.86 per 1000 pregnancies thereafter giving a 46% reduction (95% CI 40-51) [22]. Mandatory fortification has also been introduced in other countries in Central and South American and in the Middle East. In Chile, the addition of folic acid to wheat flour commenced in January 2000. A study looking at the prevalence rate of spina bifida and anencephaly there demonstrated a decrease in the years 2001 and 2002 [23]. The decrease was approximately 51% for spina bifida and 46% for anencephaly. These results showed an obvious benefit in folic acid fortification and do not significantly differ from those published from other folic acid fortified populations in Canada and the USA. The main strength of this paper is that termination of pregnancy is illegal in Chile and therefore the observed data is complete and not influenced by termination of pregnancy such as occurs in other countries. In the USA the level of folic acid fortification, at 140ug/gm of flour, was chosen to be sufficient to prevent NTDs and to provide less than 1mg/day additional folate, a limit set by the Institute of Medicine (IOM) in 1998. There is a concern that excessively high levels might delay the diagnosis of a haematological or neurological impairment due to vitamin B12 deficiency, which could potentially be masked by high serum folate. Food fortification policies in Europe have been delayed due to difficulty in determining the effective dose and concerns about safety. This helps explain the disparity in reduction of NTDs in Europe when compared to the USA and Canada [24]. An Irish study carried out in the late nineties indicated effectiveness and safety at a dose between 100µg and 200µg[25].

## 8. The cases for high dose folic acid

### 8.1 Epilepsy and Anti-Epileptic Drugs (AED)

The association of epilepsy and NTDs is well known. The risk of a woman with epilepsy on AEDs of having a child affected with a NTDs is 1-2% [26]. The known anti-folate mechanism of action of AEDs (especially valporate and carbamazepine) would intuitively indicate a recommendation of folic acid supplementation and is supported by a study in Hungary showing that the risk of congenital abnormalities could be reduced but not eliminated by folic acid supplementation[27]. However, the benefits have not been clearly demonstrated by a large prospective study in the United Kingdom [28]. A Cochrane review on the effectiveness of pre-conception counselling for women with epilepsy did not outline any consensus on the recommended dose, which varies in different countries from 0.4µg to 5mg[29].

## 9. Obesity

Many countries have seen a substantial rise in the prevalence of obesity in women of reproductive age in the last twenty years. It is an important observation and of critical value when interpreting the effects this may have on the observed rates of NTDs. Several studies have reported an increased risk of NTDs in the offspring of obese women. This risk can vary from no risk at all as demonstrated in one study[30] to a 3 fold increase in risk in a study by Shaw et al in 1996[31]. A recent meta-analysis by Rasmussen et al in 2008 identified 12 studies (4 cohort and 8 case controls) which investigated the relationship between maternal obesity and the risk of NTDs[32]. The odds ratio for a NTD-affected pregnancy was 1.22 (95% CI 0.99-1.49) for overweight women, 1.70 (95% CI 1.34-2.15) for obese women and 3.11 (95% CI 1.75-5.46) for severely obese women. This meta-analysis controlled for confounding factors such as date of publication, diabetes and folic acid intake. There are three main hypotheses for this increased risk of NTDs in obese women. Firstly, the association of NTDs and the teratogenic effects of hyperglycaemia may be a possible explanation [33]. Altered glucose metabolism in these women leads to hyperinsulinaemia, which has been shown to be associated with NTDs. This is similar to the mechanisms causing the increased NTD-affected pregnancies in diabetic patients. A second possible explanation for the association of obesity and NTDs is that obese women have a higher dietary requirement for folic acid. It is well established that higher plasma and red cell folate levels are associated with a lower risk of NTDs. A study carried out by Werler et al and published 1996 showed that obese women, specifically those greater than 70 kgs, were less responsive to the WHO recommended 400µg dose than women of a normal weight[34]. Further investigations of women with a higher BMI showed overall lower serum folate levels and advised that obese women should take 750µg of folic acid to reach satisfactory RCF levels[35]. The final hypothesis is that these findings simply reflect that prenatal diagnosis of NTDs in women who are obese is limited. Therefore more NTD-affected pregnancies would result in live births and this more likely to be identified in the birth defects surveillance systems which were used to identify the cases for the meta-analysis. This factor may have led to an over estimation of the risk associated with maternal obesity.

## 10. Conclusion

This chapter outlines the aetiologies and strategies for preventing neural tube defects. It is clear from international data that we should be striving for national policies for food fortification programmes to effectively reduce the incidence of neural tube defects. Future studies focus on identifying those who may have an increased folate requirement either due to a genetic predisposition or co-morbidities.

## 11. References

[1] Au, K.S., A. Ashley-Koch, and H. Northrup, *Epidemiologic and genetic aspects of spina bifida and other neural tube defects.* Developmental Disabilities Research Reviews, 2010. 16(1): p. 6-15.

[2] Group, M.V.S.R., *Prevention of neural tube defects: results of the Medical Research Council Vitamin Study. MRC Vitamin Study Research Group.* Lancet, 1991. 338(8760): p. 131-7.

[3] Blom, H.J., et al., *Neural tube defects and folate: case far from closed.* Nature Reviews Neuroscience, 2006. 7(9): p. 724-31.

[4] van der Put, N.M., et al., *Altered folate and vitamin B12 metabolism in families with spina bifida offspring.* Qjm, 1997. 90(8): p. 505-10.

[5] Weisberg, I., et al., *A second genetic polymorphism in methylenetetrahydrofolate reductase (MTHFR) associated with decreased enzyme activity.* Molecular Genetics & Metabolism, 1998. 64(3): p. 169-72.

[6] Shields, D.C., et al., *The "thermolabile" variant of methylenetetrahydrofolate reductase and neural tube defects: An evaluation of genetic risk and the relative importance of the genotypes of the embryo and the mother.* American Journal of Human Genetics, 1999. 64(4): p. 1045-55.

[7] Molloy, A.M., et al., *Thermolabile variant of 5,10-methylenetetrahydrofolate reductase associated with low red-cell folates: implications for folate intake recommendations.* Lancet, 1997. 349(9065): p. 1591-3.

[8] Parle-McDermott, A., et al., *Analysis of the MTHFR 1298A-->C and 677C-->T polymorphisms as risk factors for neural tube defects.* Journal of Human Genetics, 2003. 48(4): p. 190-3.

[9] Padmanabhan, R., *Etiology, pathogenesis and prevention of neural tube defects.* Congenital Anomalies, 2006. 46(2): p. 55-67.

[10] Moretti, M.E., et al., *Maternal hyperthermia and the risk for neural tube defects in offspring: systematic review and meta-analysis.* Epidemiology, 2005. 16(2): p. 216-9.

[11] Smithells, R.W., et al., *Apparent prevention of neural tube defects by periconceptional vitamin supplementation.* Archives of Disease in Childhood, 1981. 56(12): p. 911-8.

[12] Czeizel, A.E. and I. Dudas, *Prevention of the first occurrence of neural-tube defects by periconceptional vitamin supplementation.* New England Journal of Medicine, 1992. 327(26): p. 1832-5.

[13] De-Regil, L.M., et al., *Effects and safety of periconceptional folate supplementation for preventing birth defects.* Cochrane Database of Systematic Reviews, 2010(10): p. CD007950.

[14] Kirke, P.N., et al., *Maternal plasma folate and vitamin B12 are independent risk factors for neural tube defects.* Q J Med, 1993. 86(11): p. 703-8.

[15] Daly, L.E., et al., *Folate levels and neural tube defects. Implications for prevention.* JAMA, 1995. 274(21): p. 1698-702.

[16] BMJ, d.b., et al., *International Retrospective Cohort Study of Neural Tube Defects in Relation to Folic Acid Recommendations: Are the Recommendations Working? [Miscellaneous]*2005: Obstetrical & Gynecological Survey September 2005;60(9):563-565.

[17] Williams, L.J., et al., *Prevalence of spina bifida and anencephaly during the transition to mandatory folic acid fortification in the United States.* Teratology, 2002. 66(1): p. 33-9.

[18] Honein, M.A., et al., *Impact of folic acid fortification of the US food supply on the occurrence of neural tube defects.[Erratum appears in JAMA 2001 Nov 14;286(18):2236].* JAMA, 2001. 285(23): p. 2981-6.

[19] Jacques, P.F., et al., *The effect of folic acid fortification on plasma folate and total homocysteine concentrations.* New England Journal of Medicine, 1999. 340(19): p. 1449-54.

[20] Choumenkovitch, S.F., et al., *Folic acid fortification increases red blood cell folate concentrations in the Framingham study.* J Nutr, 2001. 131(12): p. 3277-80.

[21] Persad, V.L., et al., *Incidence of open neural tube defects in Nova Scotia after folic acid fortification.* CMAJ Canadian Medical Association Journal, 2002. 167(3): p. 241-5.

[22] De Wals, P., et al., *Reduction in neural-tube defects after folic acid fortification in Canada.* New England Journal of Medicine, 2007. 357(2): p. 135-42.

[23] Lopez-Camelo, J.S., et al., *Reduction of birth prevalence rates of neural tube defects after folic acid fortification in Chile.* American Journal of Medical Genetics. Part A, 2005. 135(2): p. 120-5.

[24] Busby, A., et al., *Preventing neural tube defects in Europe: a missed opportunity.[Erratum appears in Reprod Toxicol. 2006 Jan;21(1):116].* Reproductive Toxicology, 2005. 20(3): p. 393-402.

[25] Daly, S., et al., *Minimum effective dose of folic acid for food fortification to prevent neural-tube defects.* Lancet, 1997. 350(9092): p. 1666-9.

[26] Yerby, M.S., *Management issues for women with epilepsy: neural tube defects and folic acid supplementation.* Neurology, 2003. 61(6 Suppl 2): p. S23-6.

[27] Kjaer, D., et al., *Antiepileptic drug use, folic acid supplementation, and congenital abnormalities: a population-based case-control study.* BJOG: An International Journal of Obstetrics & Gynaecology, 2008. 115(1): p. 98-103.

[28] Morrow, J.I., et al., *Folic acid use and major congenital malformations in offspring of women with epilepsy: a prospective study from the UK Epilepsy and Pregnancy Register.* Journal of Neurology, Neurosurgery & Psychiatry, 2009. 80(5): p. 506-11.

[29] Winterbottom, J., et al., *The effectiveness of preconception counseling to reduce adverse pregnancy outcome in women with epilepsy: what's the evidence?* Epilepsy Behav, 2009. 14(2): p. 273-9.

[30] Moore, L.L., et al., *A prospective study of the risk of congenital defects associated with maternal obesity and diabetes mellitus.* Epidemiology, 2000. 11(6): p. 689-94.
[31] Shaw, G.M., E.M. Velie, and D. Schaffer, *Risk of neural tube defect-affected pregnancies among obese women.* JAMA, 1996. 275(14): p. 1093-6.
[32] Rasmussen, S.A.M.D.M.S.a., et al., *Maternal obesity and risk of neural tube defects: a metaanalysis. [Review].* American Journal of Obstetrics & Gynecology June, 2008. 198(6): p. 611-619.
[33] Loeken, M.R., *Current perspectives on the causes of neural tube defects resulting from diabetic pregnancy.* American Journal of Medical Genetics. Part C, Seminars in Medical Genetics, 2005. 135C(1): p. 77-87.
[34] Werler, M.M., et al., *Prepregnant weight in relation to risk of neural tube defects.* JAMA, 1996. 275(14): p. 1089-92.
[35] Mojtabai, R., *Body mass index and serum folate in childbearing age women.* Eur J Epidemiol, 2004. 19(11): p. 1029-36.

# 6

# Selective Abortion and Folic Acid Fortification as Contrasting Strategies for Prevention of Congenital Neural Tube Defect

John A. A. Nichols
*The Postgraduate Medical School,*
*The University of Surrey*
*UK*

## 1. Introduction

Prenatal diagnosis of severe disability and the option of termination of pregnancy (TOP) have been widely available to parents in most countries in the Western world for three decades. This has come to be known as selective abortion. The ethics of this procedure is a large subject that I will not attempt to address in this paper. Some countries have laws that forbid selective abortion unless the mother's life is at risk. Where neural tube defects (NTDs) are concerned, medical opinion might favour TOP in a mother carrying an anencephalic fetus. The anencephalic infant will not normally survive for more an hour after birth but the mother may have a difficult and even life threatening labour because the lack of a fetal head prevents normal labour from progressing. The pregnancy tends to go overdue and vaginal delivery is complicated by shoulder dystocia and can be very difficult and hazardous for the mother. However 60% of women in the world would not be able to access an early TOP for this type of pregnancy due to poverty, religious reasons or anti-abortion legislation. In the republic of Ireland, which has anti-abortion legislation, this situation has encouraged legislators to consider minimising the need for selective abortion by introducing mandatory fortification of flour with folic acid (FA).

### 1.1 Objections to folic acid fortification of bread, flour and grain

Scientists, oncologists and politicians have urged caution in implementing folic acid fortification of bread, flour and grain. Oncologists were amongst the first to point out that many cancer chemotherapy drugs work by inhibiting folate metabolism and subsequent research showed that giving folic acid can accelerate tumour growth in animal models (Hubner et al., 2007). The arguments for and against fortification depend on the interpretation of data from countries where fortification has already been implemented. In Chile, which has similar anti-abortion legislation to The Republic of Ireland, a ten year policy of fortification has reduced the incidence of NTD births by 40% - from 17/10,000 births to 10.1/10,000 births (Hertrampf et al., 2004). However the UK and Irish governments have held back on fortification and the following issues have caused pause for thought:

### 1.1.1 There has been a slight increase in colorectal and prostate cancer in middle life in the USA

Mandatory FA fortification has been in force for ten years in the USA and Canada and the incidence of NTD conceptions has dropped 20-40% varying between different regions of North America. However, a slight increase in the incidence of colorectal and prostate cancer was noticed which coincided with the introduction of fortification (Mason et al., 2007).The latest paper from the USA on colorectal cancer since fortification (n=535,000) showed that far from an increased risk, subjects with the highest folate intakes were 30% less likely to develop cancers (Gibson et al., 2011).

### 1.1.2 Supplementation trials and cancers risk

A trial comparing FA supplementation and low dose aspirin with placebo suggests that giving folic acid 1000 microgram daily increases the risk of middle life cancers, especially colorectal and prostate (Cole et al 2007). This is thought to occur in folate replete populations when an unnaturally high folate status accelerates cell proliferation in early cancers. However, supplementation with folic acid and other B vitamins in folate deficient populations and populations where there is a high incidence of the gene for slow folate metabolism (MTHFR C677T) may decrease the risk of these cancers (Le Marchand et al., 2002; Figueiredo et al., 2011).

### 1.1.3 Masking of vitamin B12 deficiency

Masking of B12 deficiency by giving folic acid for macrocytic anaemia was a problem in the last century but B12 deficiency is much less likely to go undiagnosed in a modern medical setting. However, there have been warnings that folic acid fortification might have an adverse effect on B12 status and cognitive function in older age groups (Clarke et al., 2004).

### 1.1.4 Folic acid in not a natural substance

Folates are the natural form of the vitamin and are present in fruit and vegetables whereas FA is a synthetic man made substance. However, folates are labile molecules that break down with storage and heat. Folic acid is a relatively stable synthetic molecule and is quickly metabolised into the folate pathways in small quantities but a high dose may not be metabolised so well. High intake of FA results in a measurable residue of circulating folic acid which could, theoretically, have adverse effects, on the development of the fetal central nervous system for instance (Smith et al., 2008). Research in Ireland has shown that fortification that delivers a dose of 100 microgram daily is safe, in this respect. There was no detectable unmetabolised serum folic acid at this dose (Sweeney et al, 2007).

### 1.1.5 30% of NTD conceptions will still occur

The precise reason for this is unknown but some genetic combinations may make the development of some NTDs inevitable. However, other B vitamins are involved in the folate-methionine-homocysteine cycle (Figure 1; McNulty et al., 2002). Instability of this cycle and build up of high levels of homocysteine are thought to play a key role in delaying neural tube closure (Rosenquist et al., 2002). Zinc deficiency might also be a factor in some NTDs (Srinivas et al., 2001).

### 1.2 Benefits from public health measures for prevention of NTDs

In terms of public health benefit, we should also concern ourselves with the efficacy of folic acid fortification compared with the policy in the United Kingdom and other European countries where women are encouraged to take folic acid 400 μg daily starting about six weeks before a planned conception and offered ultrasound screening and the option of TOP if a NTD fetus is diagnosed. Is prevention of NTD conceptions by folic acid fortification a valid alternative? It has the advantage that the 40% of conceptions that are unplanned but not unwanted (Botto et al., 2005; Gipson & Stanelli, 2011) will benefit from this policy whereas the UK policy will only achieve an intake of folic acid sufficient to reduce the risk of NTD conceptions in 60% of subjects at the very most. However, the concordance rate for starting folic acid before conception in planned pregnancies is poor and does not seem to make a significant impact on the incidence of NTD conceptions (Botto et al., 2005). The best concordance data shows only 10-20% of women with both planned pregnancies and starting a folic acid supplement before conception (Rezan et al., 2002).

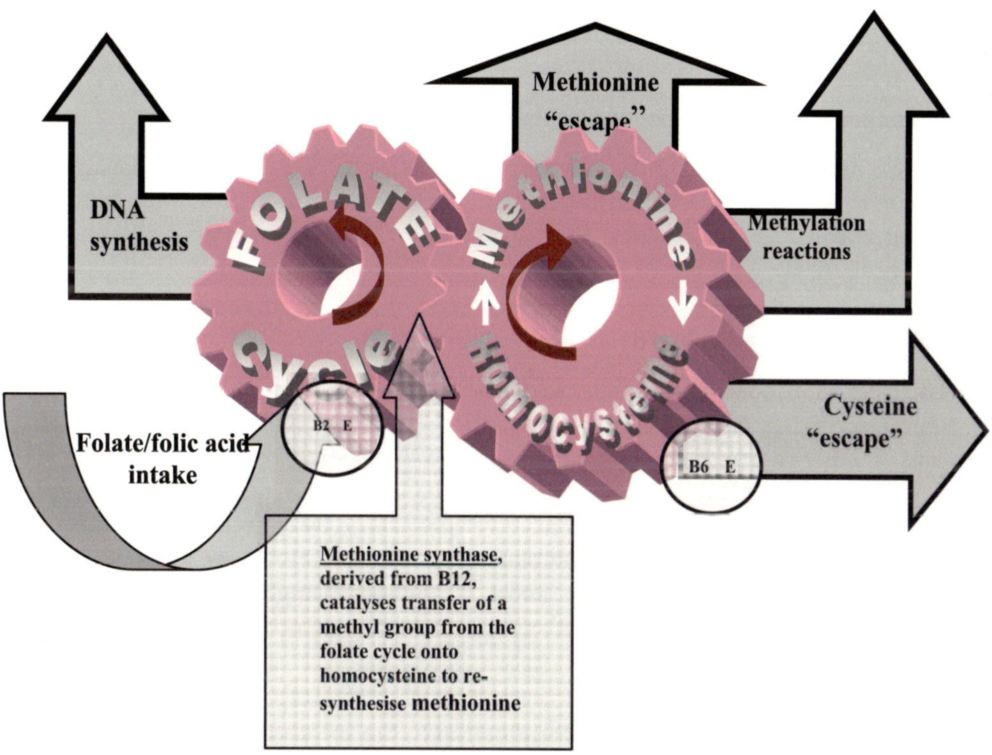


**B2 E denotes an enzyme pathway dependant on vitamin B2**
**B6 E denotes an enzyme pathway dependant on vitamin B6**

Fig. 1. Simplified version of the folate-methionine-homocysteine cycle illustrating the role of vitamins B2 (riboflavin), B6 (pyridoxine) and B12 (cobalamin) in modulating the cycle and directly or indirectly lowering homocysteine burden.

### 1.3 Objections to policy of pre-conception advice with option of selective abortion

Having listed the objections to fortification, we need to consider the reasons why a policy of advising pre-conception folic acid and ultrasound screening for NTDs in early pregnancy may be considered unsatisfactory. This will always involve a significant number of women being offered TOP as an option when screening shows a NTD fetus.

#### 1.3.1 Pre-conception folic acid concordance has failed

The level of success for starting folic acid before conception is too low to make a measurable impact on the rate of NTD conceptions. Since the neural tube develops before a woman knows she is pregnant, starting folic acid as soon as pregnancy is confirmed will never make a noticeable impact on the incidence of NTD conceptions. According to a survey based on data for England and Wales published by the UK Office for National Statistics (Morris & Wald, 2007) 969 NTD conceptions were recorded in 2004 (801 women had TOPs for NTD but 168 were recorded as going to term with NTD infants). The authors estimate that there are 1,100 NTD conceptions in the whole of the UK (if Scotland and Northern Ireland are included).

#### 1.3.2 Selective abortion is a psychological trauma

The distress to mothers who opt for selective abortion for a NTD conception is a significant issue. A review of the evidence on the impact of selective abortion concludes that women experience a bereavement reaction that is similar to that experienced with a stillbirth (Statham et al., 2000).

#### 1.3.3 Screening misses a significant proportion of NTDs

The data from Morris and Wald indicates that a significant minority of NTDs are missed on ultrasound screening (see 1.2.1) which is approximately 17% of all NTD conceptions. However, another source of error is the pregnancies that spontaneously abort due to NTDs which has been estimated at 600-1200 per year in the UK (UK Department of Health report 2000). In at least half of these aborted foetuses NTD is caused by chromosomal abnormalities so that folate status has no bearing on aetiology or prevention. However, some women with NTD conceptions who spontaneously abort in this way might have benefitted from increased intake of FA before conception and they certainly get no benefit from the policy of selective abortion.

### 1.4 Assessing the case for folic acid fortification in the UK and Ireland

The success of fortification in Chile and North America is encouraging and the recent data on cancers in these countries has reassured the public health experts that the apparent increased risk of cancers with fortification is either very small or just a statistical aberration. It is particularly significant that the USA and Canada have not wavered from the policy of FA fortification. Ultimately, the question of whether fortification is a cost-effective exercise has to be addressed. This can be estimated by comparing: A/ costs mandatory fortification reimbursed to UK millers by government = government reimbursement to millers for adding folic acid 140 µg/100mg + cost of government monitoring B/ government savings from mandatory fortification = cost of TOP x drop in number of TOPs done for NTD+ lifetime medical cost of treatment for NTD patients x drop in number of NTD births This can be estimated for the UK from Morris and Wald's data on selective abortion for NTDs and live NTD births who survive infancy and from research carried out in Surrey (Nichols et al 2008a) using data on total folate intake from a women attending local midwives' booking in clinics.

## 2. Estimation of benefits of UK adopting policy of mandatory folic acid fortification of flour and bread

The research carried out by the author and colleagues at The University of Surrey, UK was used, with data from other sources, to estimate the impact of fortification for the whole nation.

### 2.1 Two groups of women were investigated

a. Eighteen Surrey women were assessed for dietary folate intake as part of a larger research project (Nichols et al 2008b) which assessed dietary folate intake using weighed food diet diaries. Each subject was given a seven-day diet diary to complete and given the use of battery operated microtonic scales with detailed instructions. Research has demonstrated the weighed seven-day diet diary to be a reasonably accurate tool for measuring nutrient intake in free-living individuals (Day et al., 2001, Nelson et al 1998). The diet diary data was entered into "WinDiets Professional", a computerised database for analysis of nutritional intake (Wise, 1999). The output included an estimate of daily folate intake for each of the 18 subjects. Although this was a small sample, the mean folate intake at 267 µg/day was very similar to the UK national averages from the UK National Diet and Nutritional Survey 2002 (229 µg/day for women aged 19-24 yr, 234 µg/day for women aged 25-34 yr). Therefore the figure of 267 µg/day was assumed to be the approximate dietary intake for group B women and the basis for calculating total folate intake by adding together this presumed dietary folate and folic acid supplementation in the larger sample of Surrey Group B women attending the district midwife booking-in clinic.
b. 200 women were asked to complete questionnaires when they attended midwives' booking in clinics in the catchment area of The Royal Surrey Count Hospital. The response rate was 43.5%. The women were asked to complete the questionnaire and return it to the researchers in a stamped addressed envelope. The questions asked the following:

- whether the pregnancy was planned or unplanned
- whether the pregnancy was natural or an assisted pregnancy
- whether a supplement was started before or after conception
- if before conception, number of weeks taken
- exactly what brand(s) of supplement was used
- age, and age at completion of education

With a good response rate, this sample was thought to be adequate to calculate statistical significance for the different amounts of folic acid in the different over-the-counter supplements and for estimation of total folate intake (TFI).

### 2.2 Estimation of total folate intake

Owing to the poor availability of dietary folate resulting from loss of folate content in cooking and poor absorption of food folate compared with synthetic folic acid (McKillop et al., 2002; Standing committee on the Scientific Evaluation of Dietary Reference Intakes, Washington DC, 1998), various authorities have recommended a downward adjustment of approximately 50% for dietary folate (Eichholzer et al., 2006) when calculating a combined value for dietary folate/day + FA/day (FAD). Therefore, corrected total folate (TFI) was calculated using the estimated mean dietary intake for all Group B Surrey women (DM) using the formula:

$$\text{TFI} = [(\text{DM}) \div 2] + \text{FADmg / day}$$

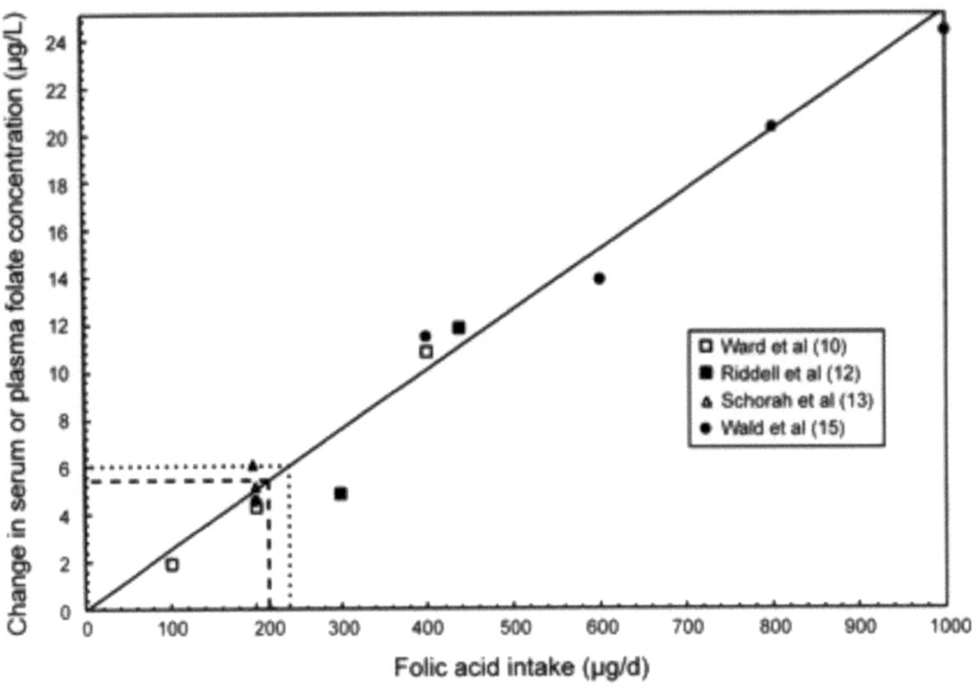


Fig. 2. Relation between controlled folic acid intake and the resulting change in median or adjusted mean serum or plasma folate concentration. Data were derived from intervention studies looking at the effect of longitudinal folic acid supplementation or fortification with known daily amounts of folic acid on median or adjusted mean serum or plasma folate concentrations. The broken and dotted lines represent the change in plasma or serum folate concentration observed by two research groups (Jacques et al., 2000; Lawrence et al, 1999) respectively, in 2 studies examining the effect of the current US folic acid fortification regimen on folate status. $y = 0.0254x + 0.0514$ ($r = 0.984$, $P < 0.0001$).

The predicted average uplift from FA fortification at the level of 140 µg/100gm of flour TFI is 220 µg/day (Eichholzer et al., 2006; Quinlivan & Gregory, 2003). Figure 2 was used to calculate the uplift of folate intake with fortification which was estimated for women in group B using the formula:

$$\text{Estimated TFI after fortification} = [(\text{DM}) \div 2] + \text{FAD} + 220\text{mg / day}$$

Since at least 70% of mothers will achieve a serum folate level that prevents the NTD malformation on an intake of >700 µg/day (Homocysteine Lowering Trialist's Collaboration, 2005; Rosenquist & Finnell 2001) (Figure 1), the data for estimated TFI after fortification was analysed using this standard. 24% (21/87) of women attending the DMCs had unplanned pregnancies and were younger (mean age 29.8 yr, compared with average 33 yr). Numerous surveys suggest that the national average for pregnancies that are unplanned, but not necessarily unwanted, is 40%. However, there were probably a higher proportion of women with unplanned pregnancies among the 113 women who had failed to return a completed questionnaire so that the true figure for Surrey women having unplanned pregnancies may be closer to the 40% national average. Using the above formula, the expected uplift of TFI was estimated for all pregnancies and separately for unplanned pregnancies (Table 1).

| | Mean TFI before fortification | Mean TFI after fortification | Increased to >700 µg/day before-after fortification | P values for uplift |
|---|---|---|---|---|
| All district midwife clinic | 497 µg/day (95% Cl 358-635) | 717 µg/day (95% Cl 579-855) | 21%-55%* | 0.01 |
| Unplanned pregnancies | 160 µg/day (95% Cl 81-240) | 380 µg/day (95% Cl 301-460) | 4.8%-4.8% | ns |

* 34% improvement in reaching >700 µg/day TFI

Table 1. Estimated total daily folate acid intake - dietary folate + folic acid (TFI) before and after fortification with folic acid 140 µg/100 g of flour as implemented in The USA. P values are given for the difference between number of subjects with an adequate intake of total folate (700 µg/day or more) before and after fortification (from Nichols et al., 2008a).

Only one woman with an unplanned pregnancy had been taking FA 400 µg/day (in a multivitamin tablet), compared with 75% of women with planned pregnancies.

### 2.3 Estimation of expected number of NTD malformations averted with folic acid fortification for the UK

The estimated number of UK NTD conceptions/year is 1100 (Morris & Wald, 2007). If fortification achieves a national 34% improvement in the number of women attaining the optimal level of daily TFI >700 µg/day for prevention of NTDs (Homocysteine Lowering Trialist's Collaboration), this would result in 374 of these 1100 women/year reaching this standard. In this "high risk" group, achieving optimal TFI should protect 62-94% (Berry et al, 1999) = 232-352 NTD malformations/year averted. Thus approximately 292 infants a year will be born normal and healthy after fortification that are currently either being diagnosed as NTD and aborted or born with a NTD malformation. An alternative calculation is based on expected rise in serum folate with fortification (Wald et al., 2003). The rise in serum folic acid in group B subjects was estimated from FA intake before and after fortification by reading off expected plasma folate values from Figure 2:

$$\text{Estimated plasma folic acid before fortification} = 12.6\text{mg} / \text{L}$$

$$\text{Estimated plasma folic acid after fortification} = 18.4\text{mg} / \text{L}$$

$$\text{Estimated change in plasma folic acid} = 5.4\text{mg} / \text{L}$$

$$\text{Percentage change} = (5.8 / 12.6)\text{x}100\% = 46\%$$

Doubling serum folate (100% rise) halves the risk of NTD (Berry et al., 1999), therefore a 46% increase would reduce the total number of UK NTD conceptions by 253/year (from 1100 to 847). Therefore from the two methods of calculation a mean value of 273 averted NTD conceptions is assumed, though this may be an underestimate as improving folate intake without reaching the 700 μg/day will prevent the NTD malformation in some cases.

### 2.4 Estimation of expected cost-benefit balance with folic acid fortification of flour in the UK

Calculations of cost-benefit expected from folic acid fortification will depend on the balance between:

a. The costs of mandatory fortification

= government reimbursement to millers for adding folic acid 140 μg/100mg

and

b. government savings from mandatory fortification

= cost of TOP x drop in number of TOPs done for NTD + average lifetime cost of treatment for NTD patients x drop in number of NTDs births

#### 2.4.1 Cost to the UK government of mandatory folic acid fortification

The national Association of British and Irish Millers estimated in March 2011 that 5600,000 tonnes of wheat are milled to make flour/year in the UK. The cost per ton for fortification in 2011 British Pounds Sterling, estimated from the experience of fortification and monitoring expenses in Chile (Llanos et al., 2007) is £0.13/ton. Therefore the expected cost of fortification for the UK is £728000/year

#### 2.4.2 Cost saving benefits from UK mandatory fortification

Of the 273 averted NTD conceptions averted, 17% (46) will, on past evidence, be NTD births which will be associated with a range of lifetime medical costs and 83% (227) of women will opt for selective abortion. Although I could not find a UK estimate for average lifetime costs of infants that survive birth with an NTD malformation, there were a range of costs from other countries ranging from £15,400 - 326,000. The median figure was £240,000 (Ouyang et al., 2007). However, this was an estimation of mean average costs for the USA and USA medical expenses are higher than UK prices (even the same drugs cost roughly twice as much) and average per capita health expenditure is 2.2 times higher (Kaiser Family Foundation 2008). I assume here that the same x2.2 difference will apply to lifetime NTD medical costs. Therefore an estimate of mean average lifetime NTD medical costs in the UK = £240,000÷2.2 = £109,091. The UK cost of a therapeutic TOP is £800. Therefore the annual saving from fortification in British pounds is:

$$109{,}091\text{x}46 + 800\text{x}227 = 5{,}018{,}181 + 181{,}600 = 5{,}199{,}781$$

### 2.4.3 Estimated cost benefit of UK mandatory fortification

Therefore the estimated annual cost saving of fortification in British pounds is:

$$4{,}471{,}781 - 728{,}000 = 5{,}126{,}981$$

This converts to approximately $7 million. A comparison with the estimated savings for Chile in 2001-2001 of only $2.3 million (Llanos et al., 2007) may be largely because their health services are less able to cope with complex medical problems that arise in children who survive with NTD malformations, early deaths will often occur and this will be associated with lower lifetime costs. The Centre for Disease Control and Prevention, USA gives a much higher estimate of $453 million/year. Apart from the higher US costs and larger population, this estimate includes the loss of earning for parents who stop work to care for a spina bifida child which is not included in my estimate for the UK.

## 3. Conclusions

The above figures are only an estimate of the cost-benefit of fortification and there are a number of factors that would have to be taken into consideration if fortification was implemented in the UK. It will never completely eliminate the need for selective abortion or the advisability of women who plan their pregnancies to start taking a FA supplement before conception. We estimated (Nichols et al., 2008a) that 45% of women in group B would still fail to achieve optimal total folate intake after fortification. When women attend to see a primary care doctor or nurse for contraceptive advice or review of ongoing contraception, there is an opportunity to raise the importance of pre-conception issues and boost FA concordance whenever there is a possibility of a future planned pregnancy. A comprehensive package of pre-conception care will be even more effective at reducing the risk of NTDs and other congenital malformations as described in section 3.3. The combined effect of fortification and adequate preconception advice, linked to contraceptive advice, could double the number of NTDs averted. This chapter has concentrated on the benefits of FA fortification with respect to averted NTD malformations, but there are other expected benefits and several remaining concerns (Table 2). In particular, there is growing evidence that other fetal malformations are prevented by fortification and FA supplementation has been shown to reduce the risk of intrauterine growth retardation. It is interesting to note that most of these benefits from improving folate status were predicted by Bryan Hibbard nearly 50 years ago (Hibbard, 1964) and now we have evidence that improving folate status may also prevent childhood cancers (Table 2). Added to this, there is growing evidence that FA fortification may deliver more benefits than side effects amongst elders (Table 2). It is too soon to claim this as a dependable measure of cost benefit from FA fortification but close monitoring of FA intake, blood folate levels and outcomes may help to clarify matters.

### 3.1 Remaining concerns

After fortification a monitoring protocol should include B12 status in view of the 25-43% incidence of borderline and moderate vitamin B12 deficiency found in three UK elder studies and the suspicion that high folate intake may exacerbate both B12 deficiency and associated cognitive decline (Green & Miller, 2005; Table 2) and the evidence for a role for borderline vitamin B12 deficiency in NTD (Ray JG et al., 2007; Molloy et al., 2009;), other fetal malformations and low birth weight (Table 2). The structure of the UK National Health Service (NHS) should make monitoring of B12 status an eminently achievable objective. Another concern is that high folate intake may reduce the efficacy of anti-folate drugs used in treatment of cancers, rheumatoid arthritis and psoriasis (Smith et al., 2008). This, however, is avoidable if these patients are advised to avoid the fortified bread and their folate status is monitored by blood tests, when appropriate. The issue of unmetabolised FA is unresolved but the North American experience of fortification has been encouraging. The predicted problems relating to unmetabolised FA have failed to materialise in the post-fortification decade. One prediction is that high levels of unmetabolised FA may have an adverse effect on immune function in elders by inhibiting the action of NK cells. This has only been described in one study (Pfeiffer at al., 2004) and there are no reports to suggest that fortification has caused NK cell problems. Lastly, the possibility that high intake of FA may influence gene expression by modifying epigenetic imprinting (Smith et al., 2008) and this has been demonstrated in animal models but there is, as yet, no evidence that this is harmful to humans. Remaining concerns that have to be taken into consideration and answered are summarized in table 2.

| | **Remaining concerns** | **Answers to concerns** |
|---|---|---|
| FA fortification and infant health | 15% of group B had predicted TFA above 1000 μg/day which might increase unmetabolised FA in circulation and there are purely hypothetical suggestions that this could have adverse affects on fetal development. However, the USA have set this safe upper limit due to relatively slender evidence that masking of vitamin B12 deficiency may start at this level (Standing Committee on the Scientific Evaluation 1998) which is unlikely to apply to pregnant women. | Although the evidence linking TFI with NTDs is strongest, there is also evidence that FA prevents several other major congenital malformations, including congenital heart defects, limb defects, and orofacial clefts (Eichholzer et al., 2006) and fetal trisomy (Eskes et al., 2006), and that inadequate maternal TFI plays a role in intrauterine growth retardation (Relton et al., 2005a; Relton et al., 2005b) and lymphoblastic leukaemia in childhood (Thompson et al., 2001). |

| | Remaining concerns | Answers to concerns |
|---|---|---|
| FA fortification and cancers | Research already mentioned has raised the possibility that fortification may increase the incidence of colorectal and prostate cancers. Recent trials failed to confirm this risk (Figueiredo et al., 2011,Gibson et al., 2011). The initial increase in these cancers observed in USA was either very small or a statistical aberration | FA fortification may have been responsible for a drop in the incidence of childhood cancers: neuroblastomas (French et al., 2003) and several other childhood cancers (Preston-Martin et al., 1998; Grupp SG et al., 2010) and even coloectal cancers may be averted in subjects with low folate status (Figueiredo et al., 2011). |
| Affects of fortification on elders | Although low folate status is known to be a factor in cognitive decline, FA intake greater than 1000 μg/day may exacerbate borderline vitamin B12 deficiency and exacerbate cognitive decline (Morris et al., 2004; Clarke et al., 2004; McCracken et al., 2006; Clarke et al., 2007). | Since fortification was introduced in North America a 5% reduction in stroke related mortality has been observed (Yang et al., 2006; Selhub et al., 2000). A well established association between folate status and cognitive decline was tested in The Netherlands using 800 μg/day, given to subjects with raised serum homocysteine. This showed a significantl slowing of the rate of cognitive decline (Durga et al 2007). |
| General inad-equacies of FA fortification | FA fortification does nothing for borderline deficiencies in the other B vitamins that are relevant to fetal development and elder health issues and the problem of unmetabolised FA at the suggested level of fortification has not been solved. In the Surrey research (Nichols et al., 2008a) 45% of women still had a sub-optimal FA intake and the USA experience shows that fortification has failed to reduce NTD conceptions in some ethnic groups (Yang et al., 2007). | The established benefits in terms of averting NTD malformations may outweigh any remaining concerns. However, any campaign associated with introduction of fortification should emphasize the need for women to continue to take a pre-conception B vitamin supplement. Public policy on voluntary fortification can be used to control the excessive levels of FA added to some products to minimise the risk of pushing FA intake above 1000 μg/day. |

Table 2. Remaining concerns about FA fortification compared with established benefits

### 3.2 Opportunistic linkage of advice on pre-conception FA to contraception appointments

First, consider if the patient is likely (or most unlikely) to become pregnant in the future. Second, if future pregnancy is a possibility, ask if they expect to "become pregnant" or "start a family" at some time in the near or distant future. Lastly, offer them the brochure (outlined below) that explains the importance of taking pre-conception FA and, where appropriate, advise them to tell their friends (an intelligent young woman will usually want to do this).

**Before pregnancy**

The government recommends that all women planning to become pregnant should start taking folic acid vitamin tablets from at least six weeks before the planned pregnancy and up to the twelfth week of pregnancy.

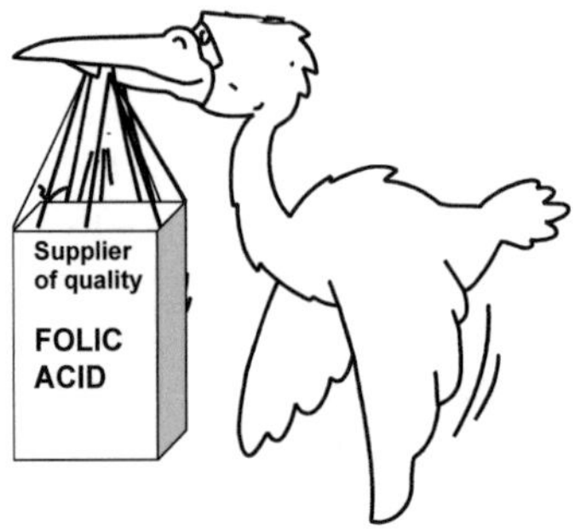


Folic acid plays an important role in the early development of the human embryo. For about 35 years medical scientists have claimed that lack of folic acid is a cause of miscarriage, congenital malformations and handicap but only after particularly convincing research in 1991, has the government recommended a daily tablet of folic acid for all women.Women who have had a previous baby with the rare but serious spinal cord defect "spina bifida" should take a relatively high dose of 5 milligrams, but these women are likely to be under the care of their doctor or a specialist for this treatment. All other women should ask at their chemist for the folic acid 0.4 mg tablet, which should be available at any chemist shop Other pre-pregnancy advice which you may or may not be aware of is listed below.

**Non-Smoking**

Children of smoking parents are more likely to be born with health problems such as baby asthma. Sometimes smoking may cause serious problems for the baby and when babies are born very underweight this will usually be partly due to smoking before pregnancy, not just during pregnancy. But the effects of smoking are unpredictable and most babies born to smoking mothers will appear to be quite normal. Research has shown, however, that these babies never do quite so well in later life as the children of non-smokers.

**Alcohol**

Both parents should cut back on alcohol before conception. Views differ as to what is a safe limit, but it is probably safest for both of you to cut it out completely

### Contraception and smear test

Women should discuss contraception with the family doctor or practice nurse when they start to plan for pregnancy. Some delay may be advisable if you have had a pregnancy in the last year or two, whatever the outcome. Statistics show that a minimum of 15-month gap between children is advisable. This gives the body time to recover fully. Most experts agree that it is best to switch from the contraceptive pill to another form of contraception two or three months before pregnancy. This allows normal hormone balance to be restored and pregnancy is less likely to be troublesome. There is even some evidence that there is an increased risk of miscarriage when women become pregnant immediately after stopping the pill. Normally, smear tests should be done every three years, but if you are planning to become pregnant, an earlier smear test is advisable - i.e. within the year before attempting to conceive.

### Diet

Although women need extra folic acid as already described, most of the other vitamins, micro nutrients and body building nutrients that are needed for fertility and good health can be obtained from a really healthy diet with plenty of fresh fruit and vegetables and unprocessed whole foods. Recent evidence suggests that eating fish is also beneficial to the outcome of pregnancy, especially in prevention of premature birth. How healthy is your diet? Everyone thinks his or her diet is "quite good" but most of us are in the "could do better" category. Some men and women will benefit from special help with their diet from a doctor or dietician. Pre-conception supplements (e.g. Pregnacare) are available which contain extra micronutrients, in addition to folic acid. This may be helpful if you feel run down and tired or if you have had problems with pregnancy in the past such as a miscarriage or postnatal depression.

Foods which are better avoided before and during pregnancy are:

- Liver and liver products (contain too much vitamin A)
- Swordfish and other large fish should not be eaten around the time of conception or during pregnancy due to traces of mercury
- Soft ripe cheese, pate and raw eggs can contain harmful bacteria that infect the placenta
- Raw meat including cured meat such as parma ham may be a source of toxoplasma parasite (see next section).
- Too much "junk" food such as sweets, biscuits cakes and fizzy drinks

Lastly, remember that you should build up your strength and bodily resources for pregnancy. If you are underweight you may have trouble conceiving and your baby may be underweight at birth, which is not a good start for a baby. Now is not the time to lose weight.

### Infection

Most women will have had a rubella jab at some time, but we now know that it is best to have a blood test to check immunity to rubella, even if you did have the jab at school. Another infection, which very occasionally causes miscarriage or abnormalities, is toxoplasmosis, which is caught mainly from uncooked meat but maybe also from cat faeces. You should, perhaps, avoid contact with sick cats or litter trays whilst you are pregnant. Chickenpox infection during pregnancy also carries a small but significant risk to both mother and baby but if you are sure you have had chickenpox there is nothing to worry about. Women who think they have never had chickenpox should discuss this with their doctor. Sexually transmitted diseases are a particular problem when you are planning to start a family. Both the man and woman should attend The Genitourinary Clinic if there is any suspicion of infection as lingering infection can cause infertility or miscarriage and can sometimes have a damaging effect on the baby.

**Medical problems**

If you or your partner has a medical problem such as diabetes or epilepsy you should see your doctor for advice before starting a pregnancy. If either of you are on any regular medication for any condition (including over the counter medications) you should discuss this with a doctor or nurse. If you have a family history of a hereditary disease such as Haemophilia or Muscular Dystrophy you should see your doctor about being referred to see a genetic counsellor at a hospital clinic.

### 3.3 Implications for future research

Future considerations include the further development of gene testing to determine which subjects need a higher dose of FA before a first conception rather than waiting for a NTD conception before offering such advice and further consideration of advice on preconception supplementation with the other B vitamins and nutrients such as zinc.

Future research therefore should include:

- Establishing a way of linking contraceptive advice to pre-conception advice on FA supplementation, diet and other aspects of preparation for a healthy pregnancy.
- Resolving the issue of a safe upper limit for total combined folate and folic acid intake, currently set at 1000 μg/day.
- Investigating the biochemistry of unmetabolised FA.
- Investigating interactions between folate status and B12 status by monitoring reliable biomarkers for both after fortification and monitoring outcome (NTDs and cognitive decline etc.).
- Further research into gene-nutrient interactions involving B vitamins and both well established genetic variants and candidate genes revealed by genome wide association studies.

A true and accurate cost-benefit analysis for FA fortification can only be completed when this research has been done.

## 4. Acknowledgements

I am indebted to my co-authors and research collaborators, Professor Margaret Rayman of The University of Surrey and Mr. Paul Curtis, consultant Gynaecologist at The Royal Surrey County Hospital, for allowing me to use data from our paper (Nichols et al., 2008). I would have been unable to collect this data without the co-operation of senior community midwife Catherine-Anne Wilkins and her district midwife team based on The Royal Surrey County Hospital. I am especially indebted to the 18 diet diary participants our and 87 supplementation respondents. Lastly, I am grateful for the guidance and help of Dr Andrew

Taylor of The University of Surrey who helped me to plan and complete the diet diary analysis of the 18 diet diary participants.

## 5. Glossary of acronyms

| | |
|---|---|
| DM | Mean daily dietary folate for group A women (used for group B calculations) |
| FA | Folic acid (also has chemical name pteroylmonoglutamate) |
| FAD | Daily FA intake from supplements |
| n | Number of participants in a research project |
| NTD | Neural tube defect (the developmental fault in the early embryo that causes spina bifida, hydrocephalus and anencephaly) |
| TFI | Total folate intake (a combined value for dietary folates and FA) |
| TOP | Termination of pregnancy |

## 6. References

Berry RJ, Li Z, Erickson JD, Li S et al (1999). Prevention of neural-tube defects with folic acid in China. *New Eng J Med*;341(20):1485-91.

Botto LD, Lisi A, Robert-Gnansia E, Erickson JD, Vollset SE, Mastroiacovo P, Botting B, Cocchi G, de Vigan C, de Walle H (2005). International retrospective cohort study of neural tube defects in relation to folic acid recommendations: are the recommendations working? *British Medical J ournal*;330:571.

Clarke R, Grimley Evans J (2004). Reply to NJ Wald et al: Folic acid fortification in the prevention of neural tube defects. *American Journal of Clinical Nutrition*;79:338–9.

Clarke R, Birks J, Nexo E, Ueland PM, Schneede J, Scott J, e Molloy A, Grimley Evans J (2007). Low vitamin B-12 status and risk of cognitive decline in older adults. *Am J Clinical Nutrition*;86:1384 - 1391.

Cole BH, Baron JA. Sandler RS, Haile RW, Ahnen DJ, Bresalier RS, McKeown-Eyssen G, Summers RW, Rothstein RI, Burke CA, Snover DC, Church TR, Allen JI, Robertson DJ, Beck GJ, Bond JH, Byers T, Mandel JS, Mott LA, Pearson LH, Barry EL, Rees JR, Marcon N, Saibil F, Ueland PM, Greenberg ER, Polyp Prevention Study Group (2007). Folic Acid for the Prevention of Colorectal Adenomas- A Randomized Clinical Trial. *JAMA*;297(21):2353-2359.

Day NE, McKeown N, Wong MY. Welch A, Bingham S (2001). Epidemiological assessment of diet: A comparison of a 7-day diary with a food frequency questionnaire using urinary markers of nitrogen, potassium and sodium. *International Journal of Epidemiology*;30(2):309-317.

Durga J. van Boxtel MP. Schouten EG. Kok FJ. Jolles J. Katan MB. Verhoef P (2007). Effect of 3-year folic acid supplementation on cognitive function in older adults in the FACIT trial: a randomised, double blind, controlled trial. *Lancet*;369(9557):208-16.

Eichholzer M, Tönz O, Zimmerman R (2006). Folic acid: a public health issue. *Lancet*;367:1352-1361.

Eskes TK, Eur J (2006). Abnormal folate metabolism in mothers with Down syndrome offspring: review of the literature. *Obstet Gynecol Reprod Biol*;124(2): 130-3.

Figueiredo JC, Mott LA, Giovannucci E, Wu K, Cole B, Grainge MJ, Logan RF,. Baron JA (2011). Folic acid and prevention of colorectal adenomas: a combined analysis of randomized clinical trials. *International Journal of Cancer*: 129, 192–203.

French AE, Grant R, Weitzman S, Ray JG. Vermeulen MJ. Sung L. Greenberg M. Koren G. (2003). Folic acid food fortification is associated with a decline in neuroblastoma. *Clinical Pharmacology and Therapetics*;74:288-94.

Gibson TM, Weinstein RM, Pfeiffer RM, Hollenbeck AR, Subar AF, Schatzkin A, Mayne ST, Stolzenburg-Soloman R (2011). Pre- and postfortification intake of folate and risk of colorectal cancer in a large prospective cohort study in the United States. *American J of Clinical Nutrition*;94(4):1053-1062.

Gipson JD, Stanelli JS (2011). Unplanned and assisted conceptions - high prevelance of unplanned pregnanacy warrants primary and secondary preventon efforts. *BMJ*;343:378-9

Green R. Miller JW (2005). Vitamin B12 deficiency is the dominant nutritional cause of hyperhomocysteinemia in a folic acid-fortified population. *Clinical Chemistry & Laboratory Medicine*;43(10):1048-51.

Grupp SG. Greenberg ML. Ray JG. Busto U. Lanctot KL. Nulman I. Koren G (2011). Pediatric cancer rates after universal folic acid flour fortification in Ontario. *Journal of Clinical Pharmacology*;51(1):60-5.

Hertrampf E, Corte´s F (2004). Folic Acid Fortification of Wheat Flour: Chile. *Nutrition Reviews*;62(6):S44–S48.

Hibbard BM (1964). The role of folic acid in pregnancy - with particular reference to anaemia, abruption and abortion. *British Jounal of Obstetrics and Gynaecology*;71(4):529-542

Homocysteine Lowering Trialist's Collaboration (2005). Dose-dependent effects of folic acid on blood concentrations of homocysteine: a meta-analysis of the randomised trials. *Am J Clin Nutr*; 82(4):806-12.

Houlston RD, Hubner RA, Muir KR (2007). Should folic acid fortification be mandatory? - No. *British medical Journal*;334:1253

Jacques PF, Selhub J, Bostom AG, Wilson PWF, Rosenberg IH (2000). The effect of folic acid fortification on plasma folate and total homocysteine concentrations. *N Engl J Med*;340:1449–54.

Kaiser Family Foundation (2008). Health Expenditure Per Capita (PPP; International $), In: *US Global Health Policy- and online gateway for the latest data and information on the US role in global health,* Available from: www.globalhealthfacts.org/data/topic/map.aspx?ind=66

Lawrence JM, Petitti DB,Watkins M, Umekubo MA (1999). Trends in serum folate after food fortification. *Lancet*;354:915-6.

Llanos A, Hertrampf E, Cortes F, Pardo A, Grosse SD, Uauy R (2007). Cost-effectiveness of a folic acid fortification program in Chile. *Health Policy*;83:295-30

Le Marchand L, Donlon T, Hankin JH, Kolonel LN et al (2002). B-vitamin intake, metabolic genes and colorectal cancer risk (United States). *Cancer Causes & Control*;13(3):239-8.

Mason JB, Dickstein A, Jacques PF, Haggarty P, Selhub J, Dallal G, Rosenberg IH (2007). A temporal association between folic acid fortification and an increase in colorectal cancer rates may be illuminating important biological principles: a hypothesis. *Cancer Epidemiology, Biomarkers & Prevention*;16(7):1325-9.

McCracken C, Hudson P, Ellis R, McCaddon A (2006). Methylmalonic acid and cognitive function in the Medical Research Council Cognitive Function and Ageing Study. *Am J Clin Nutr*;84:1406-1411.

McKillop DJ, Pentieva K, Daly D, McPartlin JM, Hughes J, Strain JJ, Scott JM, McNulty H (2002). The effect of different cooking methods on folate retention in various foods that are amongst the major contributors to folate intake in the UK diet. *British Journal of Nutrition*;88(6):681-8.

McNulty H, McKinley C, Wilson B, et al (2002). Impaired functioning of thermolabile methylenetetrahydrofolate reductase is dependent on riboflavin status: implications for riboflavin requirements. *American Journal of Clinical Nutrition*;76:436–41.

Molloy AM. Kirke PN. Troendle JF. Burke H. Sutton M, Brody LC, Scott JM. Mills JL (2009). Maternal vitamin B12 status and risk of neural tube defects in a population with high neural tube defect prevalence and no folic Acid fortification. *Pediatrics*;123(3):917-23.

Morris JK, Wald NJ (2007). Prevalence of neural tube defect pregnancies in England and Wales from 1964 to 2004. *Journal of Medical Screening*;14(2):55-9.

Morris MC, Evans DA, Bienias JL, Tangney CC, Hebert LE, Scherr PA, Schneider JA (2005). Dietary folate and vitamin B12 intake and cognitive decline among community-dwelling older persons. *Archives of Neurology*;62(4):641-5.

Nelson M, Bingham SA (1998). Assessment of food consumption and nutrient intake; In: *Design Concepts in nutritional epidemiology* by Margetts, Nelson M; Oxford University Press: 87-104

Nichols JAA, Curtis EPP, Rayman MP (2008). Survey of total folate intake at conception and assessment of impact of fortification. *Journal of Nutritional & Environmental Medicine*;17(1):44-55.

Nichols JAA, Curtis EPP, Rayman MP, Taylor A (2008). A survey to estimate total nutrient intake at conception – Dietary and supplementary. *Journal of Nutritional & Environmental Medicine*;17(1):12-43.

Pfeiffer CM, Fazili Z, McCoy L, Zhang M, Gunter EW (2004). Determination of folate vitamers in human serum by stable-isotope-dilution tandem mass spectrometry and comparison with radioassay and microbiologic assay. *Clin Chem*;50:423-32.

Ouyang L, Grosse SD, Armour BS, Waitzman N J (2007). Health Care Expenditures of Children and Adults with Spina Bifida in a Privately Insured U.S. Population. *Birth Defects Research (Part A)*; 79:552–558.

Ray JG. Wyatt PR. Thompson MD. Vermeulen MJ. Meier C. Wong PY. Farrell SA. Cole DE (2007). Vitamin B12 and the risk of neural tube defects in a folic-acid-fortified population. *Epidemiology*;18(3):362-6.

Rezan A, Kadir, Demetrios L, Economides (2002). Neural tube defects and periconceptional folic acid. *Canadiab Medical Association Journal*; 167 (3):255.

Relton CL, Pearce MS, Burn J, Parker L (2005) An investigation of folate-related genetic factors in the determination of birthweight. *Paediatric and Perinatal Epidemiology*;19(5):360-7.

Relton CL, Pearce MS, Parker L (2005). The influence of erythrocyte folate and serum vitamin B12 status on birth weight. *British Journal of Nutrition*;93(5):593-9.

Rosenquist TH, Finnell RH (2001). Genes, folate and homocysteine in embryonic development. *Proceedings of the Nutrition Society*; 60(1):53-61

Srinivas M, Gupta DK, Rathi SS, Gover JK, Vats V, Sharma JD, Mitra DK (2001). Association between lower hair zinc levels and neural tube defects. *Indian Journal of Pediatrics*;68(6):519–22.

Selhub J, Jacques PF, Bostom AG, Wilson PW, Rosenberg IH (2000). Relationship between plasma homocysteine and vitamin status in the Framingham study population. Impact of folic acid fortification. *Public Health Reviews*;28(1-4):117-45.

Smith AD, Youn-In K, Refsum H (2008). Is folic acid good for everyone? *American Journal of Clinical Nutrition*;87:517 - 33.

Standing committee on the Scientific Evaluation of Dietary Reference Intakes and its Panel on Folate, other B vitamins and Choline and Subcommittee on Upper Reference Levels of Nutriennts, Food and Nutrition Board, Institute of Medicine. Folate. In: Dietary reference intakes for thiamine, riboflavin, niacin, vitamin B6, folate, vitamin B12, pantothenic acid, biotin, and Choline. Washington DC: National Academy Press, 1998:196-305

Statham H, Solomou W, Chitty L (2000). Prenatal diagnosis of fetal abnormality: psychological effects on women in low-risk pregnancies. *Best Practice & Research in Clinical Obstetrics & Gynaecology*;14(4):731-47.

Standing committee on the Scientific Evaluation of Dietary Reference Intakes and its Panel on Folate, other B vitamins and Choline and Subcommittee on Upper Reference Levels of Nutriennts, Food and Nutrition Board, Institute of Medicine. Folate. In: Dietary reference intakes for thiamine, riboflavin, niacin, vitamin B6, folate, vitamin B12, pantothenic acid, biotin, and Choline. Washington DC: National Academy Press, 1998:196-305

Sweeney MR, McPartlin J, Scott J (2007). Folic acid fortification and public health: Report on threshold doses above which unmetabolised folic acid appear in serum. *BMC Public Health*;7:41-48.

Thompson JR, FitzGerald P, Willoughby MLN, Armstrong BK (2001). Maternal folate supplementation in pregnancy and protection against lymphoblastic leukaemia in childhood: a case control study. *Lancet*;358:1935-1940.

UK Department of health. Report on health and social subjects No. 50. *Folic Acid and Prevention of Disease*. Report of The Committee on medical aspects of Food and Nutrition Policy. ISBN 0 11.

Yang Q, Botto LD, Erickson JD, Berry RJ, Sambell C, Johansen H, Friedman JM (2006). Improvement in stroke mortality in Canada and the United States, 1990 to 2002. *Circulation*;113(10):1335-43.

Yang QH, Carter HK, Mulinare J, Berry RJ, Friedman JM, Erickson JD (2007). Race-ethnicity differences in folic acid intake in women of childbearing age in the United States after folic acid fortification: findings from the National Health and Nutrition Examination Survey, 2001-2002. *American Journal of Clinical Nutrition*;85(5):1409-16.

Wise A (1999). Appropriate uses for spreadsheets, databases and statistical software for the analysis of dietary data. *International Journal of Food Sciences & Nutrition*;50(2):111-5.

# 7

# Folate and Prevention of Neural Tube Disease

Ramya Iyer and S. K. Tomar
*National Dairy Research Institute, Karnal, India*

## 1. Introduction

A birth defect also referred to as "congenital anomalies" or "congenital abnormalities" is a health problem or a physical abnormality that a baby has at birth. It can be very mild or severe. Congenital malformations occur all over the world and are responsible for about 15% of the prenatal mortality in India (Merchant, 1989; Kulshteshtra et al., 1983; Swain et al., 1994; Datta & Chaturvedi, 2000). The relative importance of congenital malformations *per se* has snowballed as they manifest into a major public health concern owing to associated problems mortality, morbidity, social cost, and human suffering.

Among the various birth defects Neural Tube Defects (NTDs) are the most common malformations of the central nervous system that occur because of a defect in the neurulation process (Finnell et al., 2003; Sadler, 2005). Any woman of child-bearing age is potentially prone to give birth to a child suffering from an NTD. There are no means to predict the susceptibility of a woman to a NTD pregnancy as 95% of NTDs affect women without any history of such ailment in their families. Some affected pregnancies are spontaneously or electively aborted. Jaquier et al., 2006). Distinct variability has been reported in the occurrence rates for NTDs according to geographic area, socioeconomic status, and ethnic background (Frey & Hauser, 2003; Nazer et al., 2001; Pitkin, 2007; Benton, 2008).

The main cause of NTDs is yet to be known. They can be attributed to a combination of environmental and genetic factors (Sadler 2005). Among the various factors, nutrition has particularly been a significant factor effecting intrauterine development of fetus. Most of the attention has focused on folic acid as several research studies have shown that maternal folic acid supplementation reduce NTD incidence in humans ranging from 30-40% reduction in the general population to 70% for women given high levels of folic acid following a previous NTD pregnancy (MRC Vitamin Study Research Group,1991; de Wals et al., 2007). Folic Acid is a B group vitamin which plays an essential role in cellular division. Folate is required by human body to synthesize, repair and methylate DNA as well as to act as a cofactor in biological reactions involving folate (Goh & Koren, 2008). It s present ensures prolific cell division and growth, such as in infancy and pregnancy (Iyer & Tomar, 2009; Iyer et al., 2011) when the folic acid requirements are higher than usual. In consequence to the health benefits associated with increased folate intakes many countries now possess mandatory folate enrichment programs. The dose of folic acid, either alone or as part of a multivitamin preparation, varied between 400 to 5000 µg (0.4-5 mg) per day and was taken at least 1 month before conception and throughout the first trimester. In some countries, such as the

United States, Chile, Canada, and Israel, the food supply (usually flour) is fortified with folic acid as a way of bringing folic acid to women of childbearing age (Penchaszadeh, 2002).

Although folic acid supplementation is recognized to extend benefits for mothers-to-be, yet necessity of putting folic acid in the food supply is debatable (Iyer & Tomar, 2011). There has been discussion about the long-term effects of food fortification, as well as what effects folic acid may have on the general population, who would also be consuming the fortified foods (Yang et al., 2010). Lately, a number of studies have shown in comparison to natural folate, high intakes of folic acid, the chemically synthesized form (tolerable upper intake level, 1000 $\mu g\ d^{-1}$), can cause adverse health effects as highlighted by the Food and Drug Administration (FDA, 1996) such as the masking of the early hematological manifestations of vitamin B12 deficiency, leukemia, arthritis, bowel cancer and ectopic pregnancies. The Institute of Medicine (IOM, 1998) has established a tolerable upper intake level (UL) for folate from fortified foods or supplements (i.e. folic acid) for ages one and above. Intakes above this level increase the risk of adverse health effects. Therefore, naturally produced folates seem to be more rationale for fortification purposes. This article describes in the factors causing NTDs, role of folic acid, its side effects, advantage of natural folate over synthetic folic acid, need for novel food variants and further research needs.

## 2. Neural tube disease

NTD is a congenital malformation which takes place between the 20th and 28th day after conception (Sadler, 2005; Marco et al., 2011). It is an opening in the spinal cord or brain that occurs very early in human development. The cells of the neural plate make up the fetus' nervous system which during normal development folds back onto themselves to create the neural tube, which then becomes the back bone and the spinal cord and ultimately the brain. In the case of an NTD, the neural tube is unable to close completely and hence the brain and spinal cord remains exposed (Botto et al., 1999).

### 2.1 Types of NTDs

NTDs can be classified, based on embryological considerations and the presence or absence of exposed neural tissue, as open or closed types (Wald et al., 1991; Van Der Put et al., 2001; Greene et al., 2009a). Open NTDs are the most common which occurs due to a d defect in the skull or vertebrae and leads to exposed brain and/or spinal cord. Examples of open NTDs are spina bifida (myelomeningocele), anencephaly, and encephalocele. Closed NTDs are the rarer forms in which the spinal defect is covered by skin. Examples of closed NTDs are lipomyelomeningocele, lipomeningocele, and tethered cord. Anencephaly and spina bifida are the most common NTDs and occur with about equal frequency, whereas encephalocele is seen less frequently (Brody & Shane 2001).

Anencephaly is the cranial defect in which the cerebral cortex and overlying bony calvarium fail to develop. Infants with this disorder are born without a scalp or cerebellum. It is invariably lethal, with death either before or shortly after birth (Jaquier 2006). In spina bifida (about two-thirds of NTDs) there is a caudal defect in which the spinal cord is dysplastic and the overlying spinal column is absent. It is not usually fatal but can cause paraplegia, with paralysis of the lower extremities and impaired bladder and bowel function (Pitkin, 2007). Infants born with NTDs have increased risk of mortality within the first year of life, and survivors face life-long morbidities including neurologic, cognitive, urologic, and gastrointestinal complications (Marean et al., 2011). NTDs are devastating conditions as most of the lesions are always associated with neurological deficits producing varying degree of limb paresis/paralysis, bladder and anorectal incontinence (Digra, 2004).

NTDs are multifactorial as are believed to reflect a combination of genetic predisposition and environmental influences (Penchaszadeh, 2002). It may be the result of genetic abnormalities, the intrauterine environment, morphogenesis errors, or a chromosomal abnormality. The wide geographic variations in incidence suggest the prime role of importance of intra uterine environmental factors (Penchaszadeh, 2002). Neural tube defects indeed are particularly prevalent in China (Xiao et al., 1990), Mexico (Mutchinik, 1988), Central America (Saborio, 1992) and Chile (Nazer et al., 2001). Among intrauterine environmental factors, nutrition plays the most critical role in fetal growth and development (Belkacemi et al., 2010). Maternal under nutrition during gestation reduces placental and fetal growth of both domestic animals and humans (Barker & Clark, 1997; Redmer et al., 2004; Wu et al., 2006). Substantial evidence suggests that fetal growth is most susceptible to maternal dietary deficiencies of nutrients (protein and micronutrients) during the peri-implantation period and the period of rapid placental development (Sugden & Holness, 2002; Waterland & Jirtle, 2004; Wu et al., 2004). During pregnancy, when the woman's nutritional intake also provide for the growing foetus, a woman's requirement for numerous micronutrients mainly folate, Vitamin A, C, D, K, B12 is on the rise. Among these, folate is a B vitamin which women require in increased amounts during pregnancy - to assist with cell division in the baby. Intrauterine folic acid deficiency is a well known factor predisposing to neural tube defects and possibly other congenital anomalies (Czeizel & Dudás, 1992).

## 3. Folate versus folic acid

The generic term "folate" represents the complete group of all form of folate, a water soluble B vitamin, including synthesized fully-oxidized "folic acid" commonly used for food fortification and nutritional supplements.and the polylglutamates naturally present in foods (Iyer & Tomar, 2009). Folic acid or pteroyl glutamic acid (PGA) is comprised of *p*-aminobenzoic acid (PABA) linked at one end to a pteridine ring and at the other end to L-glutamic acid (Fig. 1a). The naturally occurring forms of folate differ in the extent of the reduction state of the pteroyl group, the nature of the substituents on the pteridine ring and the number of glutamyl residues attached to the pteroyl group (Fig. 1b).

Good dietary sources of folate include breakfast cereals; other cereals or cereal based foods (e.g. bread); yeast extract; beans and legumes etc. Natural food folates or pteroylpolyglutamates are conjugated to a polyglutamyl chain containing different numbers of glutamic acids which is removed in the brush border of the mucosal cells by the enzyme folate conjugase (Scott & Weir, 1994). Subsequently the polylglutamates are hydrolyzed to monoglutamate prior to absorption in the small intestine. The primary form of folate entering human circulation from the intestinal cells is 5-methyltetrahydrofolate monoglutamate. If enough folic acid is given orally, unaltered folic acid appears in the circulation (Kelly et al., 1997), is taken up by cells, and is reduced by dihydrofolate reductase to tetrahydrofolate.

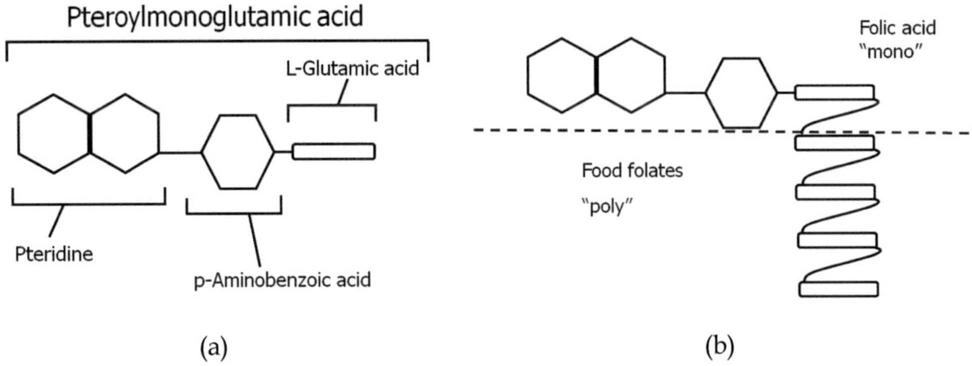


Fig. 1. Structure of a) folic acid (pteroyl-L-glutamic acid), and b) native food folates, e.g. reduced, one-carbonsubstituted forms of polyglutamates.

The bio-availability of natural folates is affected by the removal of the polyglutamate chain by the intestinal conjugase and therefore the monoglutamate forms, including folic acid, are easily transported across small intestine (Shils et al., 1994; Hendler & Rorvik, 2001). The absorption efficiency of natural folates is approximately half from that of synthetic folic acid. As folate requires hydrolysis to monomeric forms before it can be used thus relative bioavailability of dietary folates is estimated to be only 50% compared with synthetic folic acid (Sauberlich et al., 1987; Forssen et al., 2000; Fitzpatrick, 2003; Iyer & Tomar, 2009).

### 3.1 Folate deficiency

Folate is an essential nutrient component of normal human diet involved in numerous metabolic reactions as DNA and RNA biosynthesis and amino acid inter-conversions (Iyer & Tomar, 2009). Functional folates have one-carbon groups derived from several metabolic precursors (e.g., serine, *N*-formino-L-glutamate, folate, etc.). The DNA and methylation cycles both regenerate tetrahydrofolate (Fig.2.).

However, there is a considerable amount of catabolism of folate and hence there is always a need to replenish the body's folate content by uptake from the diet. If there is inadequate dietary folate, the activity of both DNA and methylation cycles will be reduced and thereby affects cell division and amino acid interconversion. Folate deficiency has been implicated in a wide variety of disorders from Alzheimer's to coronary heart diseases, neural tube defects, anemia, increased risk of breast and colorectal cancer (Verhoef et al., 1998; Verhaar et al., 2002; Le Blancet al., 2007; Tomar & Iyer, 2011). Although folate is found in a wide variety of foods, it is present in a relatively low density (Chanarin, 1979).

Though a normal human diet has sufficient amount of folate, still folate deficiencies occur frequently, even in well-developed countries (Konings et al., 2001; O'Brien et al., 2001). As activity of natural folates tend to rapidly diminish over periods of days or weeks hence a significant loss of biochemical activity is liable to occur during harvesting, storage, distribution, and cooking. Moreover owing to inability of the mammalian cells to synthesize this vital biomolecule; an external supply is essential to prevent nutritional deficiency.

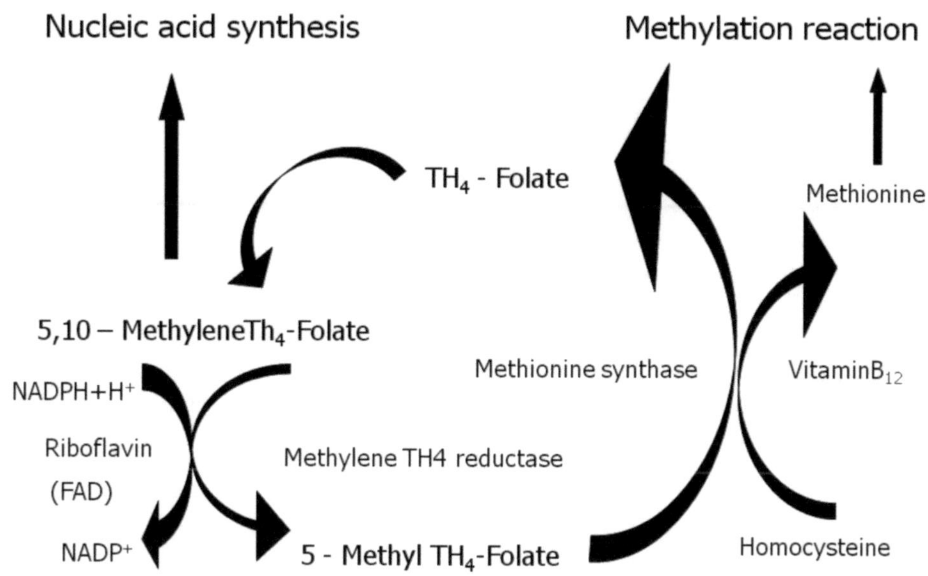


Fig. 2. Role of folate in metabolism

### 3.2 Role of folic acid in NTD pathophysiology

Besides the common reasons of malnutrition, malabsorption and low intake, increased requirement is also one of the important cause of folate deficiency. As folate plays an essential role in cellular division, pregnancy doubles the need of dietary folates (Forssen et al., 2000; Patterson et al., 2008). Pregnancy is associated with a marked acceleration in 1-carbon transfer reactions, including those required for nucleotide synthesis and thus cell division, which is the basis for the substantial increase in folate requirements during pregnancy. Low maternal folate status has been associated with premature birth, low birth-weight and increased risk of NTDs in the offspring (Iyer & Tomar, 2009; Kim et al., 2011).

The possibility that folic acid played a vital in NTD role was first reported by Hibbard (1964) and further scientists in 1976, observed that women who gave birth to NTD babies had low serum rates for folates and low vitamin levels in their red cells. Later Professor Smithhells in 1976, showed that an additional intake of 0.4 mgs of folic acid prior and at the initiation of a pregnancy caused significant drop in NTD rates. Several clinical trials subsequently demonstrated that the risk of recurrence and first occurrence of these abnormalities were declined by periconceptional folic acid supplementation prior to and during pregnancy (MRC vitamin study research group, 1991; Czeizel & Dudas, 1992; Werler et al., 1993; Czeizel et al., 1993). Several other studies have also shown that further related congenital anomalies can be prevented by folic acid intake (Czeizel 1993, Antony & Hansen, 2000). Besides, a good number of studies indicate that folic acid could potentially reduce the risk of miscarriage (George et al., 2002). Also reports are there which shows that folic acid supplementation before conception may potentially reduce the frequency of Down's syndrome (James et al., 1999; Barkai et al., 2003; Patterson, 2008).

Despite the importance of folate in NTD prevention, the mechanism by which folic acid exerts its preventive effect is unknown. Moreover folic acid also induces epigenetic changes during development and can conceivably affect the epigenetic regulation of gene expression (Lillycrop et al., 2005; Mathers et al., 2010; Li et al., 2011). Thus, the identification of genetic risk factors for human NTDs is complicated by the multiplicity of genes participating in neurulation, and the importance of gene–environment interactions (Greene et al., 2009a, b). Research on NTD pathophysology suggests several gene defects affecting enzymes and proteins involved in transport and metabolism of folate have been associated with NTDs (Carroll et al., 2009). Among them methionine synthase activity is one of the important factors involved. This enzyme transforms homocysteine into methionine for which folic acid acts as methyl group donor. Besides folate and vitamin B12 concentrations being the independent risk factors for NTDs, homocysteine concentrations also mildly get increased in maternal blood and amniotic fluid of NTD pregnancies (Kirke et al., 1993) which signifies the potential role of disregulated methionine synthase in NTDs development. Moreover, genetic association between the methionine synthase gene and NTDs in affected families remains ambiguous (De Marco et al., 2002; Pulikkunnel & Thomas, 2005; Doudney et al., 2009). Though the role of enzyme 5, 10-methylene tetrahydrofolate reductase (MTHFR) in the NTD etiology is well documented (Van der Put et al., 1995), but is still debatable (de Franchis et al., 1995; Koch et al., 1998). Thus, folic acid deficiency or an enzyme anomaly prevents the closure of the neural tube.

In humans, most genetic causes of NTDs remain unknown. Fleming & Copp, (1998) identified a mouse model of folate- preventable NTD using deoxyuridine suppression test so as to detect disturbance of folate metabolism in homozygous *splotch* (*Pax3*) mouse embryos developing NTDs *in vitro*. They observed that as folic acid and thymidine can prevent NTDs in *splotch* embryos, having abnormal pyrimidine biosynthesis which mainly leads to NTD,and hence suggested that thymidine therapy could serve as an adjunct to folic acid supplementation to prevent human NTDs. Till date mouse models of NTDs are beginning to provide insight into the genetic causes and developmental origins of NTDs in humans (Greene et al., 2009b) and over 240 genes are identified to be important in neural tube closure in mice (Harris & Juriloff, 2010). Moreover, mouse NTD models have the potential to aid in understanding the genetics underlying folic acid responsiveness or non-responsiveness in NTD prevention (Harris, 2009). Recently Marean et al., 2011 suggested that the response to folic acid supplementation may be more complex. They report that depending on the gene mutation, folic acid supplementation may adversely influence embryonic development and neural tube closure and thus the genetics of an individual may determine whether FA provides a beneficial outcome.

Therefore several reports support the hypothesis that folic acid likely acts through diverse mechanisms to influence neural tube closure (Li et al., 2011; Marean et al., 2011) so in future it will be of interest to determine the mechanistic basis of the specific gene-environment interactions that together influence neural tube closure.

### 3.3 Biomarkers to estimate folate status and intake

Measuring folate intake at the population level would be sufficient to predict NTD occurrence as insufficient folate intake being one of the major cause of NTD. The Food and Agriculture Organization of the United Nations and World Health Organization

(FAO/WHO) Expert Consultation report (FAO/WHO, 1988) suggested that adequate folate status is reflected in a red cell folate level of greater than 150 mg/L. RBC-folate is a effective biomarker that may reflect probable conditions that exist in other cells in the organism and therefore explain the occurrence of NTD (Dary, 2009). Several irrefutable evidences maintain that lower red cell folate, earlier considered as an adequate or normal range, is associated with an increased risk of spina bifida and other NTDs (Kirke et al., 1993). Red cell folate levels higher than 150 µg/L, which are adequate to prevent anaemia are associated with increase risk of NTDs (Daly, 1995; 1997) and colorectal cancer (Mason, 1995; Kim, 2004). Though RBC-folate is a good indicator of the long term folate status, but is influenced by an individual's genetic composition, and the availability of sufficient amounts of iron, zinc, protein, vitamins, and other nutrients which influence the synthesis of RBC and reactions invoving folate (Bailey & Gregory, 1999; Mc Nulty & Scott , 2008).

Apart from red cell folate which is an important index of folate status (Sauberlich, 1995) plasma folate and indicators of haematologic status such as raised mean corpuscular volume, and hypersegmentation of neutrophils remains important indicators of reduced folate status (Lindenbaum et al., 1990). To establish folate intake serum/plasma folate level is a more robust biomarker than RBC-folate, for it reflects the recent folate intake and it is less affected by confounding factors. Though it may vary on a daily basis at individual level, it is satisfactory enough to support population-based folic acid interventions programs. Besides this, the biomarker plasma homo-cysteine is also a very sensitive indicator of folate status and must be added as folate adequacy indicator. But this can be done on an individual basis only after nullifying the chance of a genetic mutation or an inadequate supply of vitamin $B_6$ or vitamin $B_{12}$. In one-carbon metabolism, many pathologies (nutritional and genetic) beyond folate intake can cause abnormalities. Therefore, serum folate should be used along with other biomarkers, such as RBC-folate, blood homocysteine, and others, to identify pathological causes and possible treatments for normalizing abnormal pathways.

## 4. Recommended daily allowance of folate

The US National Academy of Sciences in a series of reports (IOM, 1998) thoroughly evaluated the evidences of folate intake, status in context to health for all age groups and the extra requirements during pregnancy and lactation. Based on the FAO/WHO recommended nutrient intake (RNI), and members of this FAO/WHO expert group the values as recommended dietary allowances (RDAs) were published by the US National Academy of Sciences as the best estimates of folate requirements for healthy individuals and populations. The Recommended Daily Allowance (RDA) for folate recommendations in most countries are therefore set to 400 micrograms (mcg) per day for all adults (Yates et al., 1998). The RDA for folate is expressed in Dietary Folate Equivalents (DFE), which accounts for the difference in absorption between dietary folate and synthetic folic acid, which is more bioavailable (in a form that is easily used by the body).

A woman's folate requirement escalates by 50% during pregnancy with highest in the first trimester of pregnancy. It is important to note that this requirement does not include the additional folate necessary to prevent neural tube defects, as folate intake prior to becoming pregnant largely determines the risk of neural tube defect. Neural tube fully developed between 22 and 28 days after conception (3-4 weeks), during which many women are not even aware about their pregnancy. It is therefore also important for women of childbearing age who are planning a pregnancy or might become pregnant to ensure they consume the recommended quantities of folate for at least one month pre-pregnancy. Researchers have found that 50-70% of NTDs can be prevented if women consume adequate amounts of folate before and in the first trimester of pregnancy. Based on the evidence that multivitamins and foods containing folic acid besides protecting against NTD, also prevent other types of birth defects, including cleft palate and cleft lip and some cardiovascular malformations, the Food and Nutrition Board issued new dietary recommendations for folic acid, recognizing the need for women of childbearing age to get supplemental folic acid, over and above the amounts that are naturally present in foods (Food and Nutrition Board, 1998).

The US Centers for Disease Control (CDC) recommends all women of childbearing age eat a diet high in folic acid or take a multivitamin with 0.4mg of folic acid each day, especially one month prior to conception through the first three months of pregnancy. However, women who have had a previous NTD pregnancy are recommended to take an even higher dosage of folic acid from 0.4mg to 4.0mg, prior to planning a pregnancy. In Canada, the recommendation is to begin three months before pregnancy. The RDA of folate for all pregnant women is 600μg, compared to 400μg for non-pregnant women. As folic acid is also important for lactating women so to fulfill the demands of breastfeeding, the RDA for lactating women in the United States is 500 $\mu$g dietary folate equivalents (DFE) day.

### 4.1 Folic acid supplementation programs

As many pregnancies are unplanned, and neural tube develops in the prelims of pregnancy so NTD prevention is best achieved by adequate daily folic acid intake throughout the reproductive years. Though possible for women to increase their consumption of dietary folates by careful selection of foods, but food folates are about half as bioavailable as synthetic folic acid (Gregory, 1997). The United States Public Health Service recommended that women capable of becoming pregnant should consume 400 ug of folic acid daily (CDC, 1992; Cornel & Erickson, 1997; Penchaszadeh, 2002). The only viable and sustainable preventive strategy for this is fortification of food with folic acid. Fortification of staple food products with synthetic folic acid is an efficient and economical approach to increasing overall folic acid intake and fulfilling RDA.

The intricacy with any fortification programme is that people having low intakes of the fortified food must consume sufficient amount to benefit, whereas those consuming high amounts must be prevented from receiving a potentially harmful dose. An assets of information in folate biochemistry, molecular biology, human and population genetics has been build up that can be used to direct public health decisions on folate interventions. Keeping this in mind, the Food and Drug Administration (1996) mandated the fortification of enriched cereal grain flours with 140 μg synthetic folic acid per 100 grams of grain. Later in 1999 the Ministry of Health of Chile, South America, issued a regulation of folic acid supplementation to the wheat flour premix at a concentration of 2.2 mg/kg of flour (Nazer et al., 2001). This policy was encouraged and implemented by the Pan American Health Organization, the March of Dimes and the CDC with an additional monitoring of its effect on the NTD prevalence (Nazer et al., 2001). As many as 40 countries including United States, Canada, and Israel, have also implemented mass-fortification programs of food supply (usually flour) fortification with folic acid so as to bring folic acid to women of childbearing age so as to prevent folic acid-related birth defects. Such studies showed that fortification programs led to 31% and 16%reduction in prevalence of spina bifida and anencephaly. Some of these programs involve education of mothers-to-be about the importance of taking folic acid supplements prior to conception and during pregnancy (World Health Organization and Food and Agriculture Organization, 2006).

Efficacious amounts of folic acid can also be supplied by both daily (≈100 mg) and weekly (≈400 mg) folic acid supplementation (Adank et al., 2003; Norsworthy et al., 2004; Hao et al., 2008). However, the population dosage should be adjusted based on carefully monitoring of serum folate as biomarker so that the folate and folic acid intakes of most individuals remain within the safety level. Although this is a step ahead to prevent folic acid deficiency but, the actual amount added may not be sufficient to protect against all folic acid-preventable NTDs. Though Vitamin B12 deficiency is rare in women and children, there is apprehension that folic acid dosages exceeding 1000ug (1.0 mg) per day may hamper the Vit B12 diagnosis. Mills et al., (2003) however, indicates that fortification does not lead to a major increase in masking of vitamin B12 deficiency. Hence, the recommended amounts of folic acid obtained from folic acid supplements and food fortification are unlikely to exceed the 1000 ug per day.

## 5. Controversies related to folate versus folic acid fortification

Given the available evidence, the fortification of foods with folic acid is justifiable. It is an effective and inexpensive way to ensure adequate folate levels in all prospective mothers and maximizes the effect of folic acid in preventing NTDs (Kadir & Economides, 2002). Irrespective of folic acid supplementation's benefits for mothers-to-be, there is debate about the necessity of putting folic acid in the food supply. There has been discussion about the long-term effects of food fortification, as well as what effects folic acid may have on the general population, who would also be consuming the fortified foods.

Dietary folate polyglutamates, is enzymatically deconjugated at the mucosal epithelial cell brush border by conjugase to the corresponding monoglutamate forms before absorption (Chandler et al., 1986; Krishnaswamy & Madhavan, 2001). Folic acid and reduced monoglutamyl folates are absorbed mainly in the proximal small intestine (jejunum) by a saturable, carrier-mediated, pH and energy-dependent transport mechanism which, shows a similar affinity for both oxidized (e.g. folic acid) and reduced folate forms (Strum, 1976; Mason, 1990). On passage through the intestinal wall, physiological doses of folic acid undergo biotransformation in the absorptive cells of the upper small intestine to 5-methyltetrahydrofolic acid, the naturally circulating form of folate. Contrary to this, folic acid, the synthetic form which is used in nutritional supplements and fortified foods is very efficiently absorbed by the body (Fig.3.). However, some studies have indicated that oral dosage of folic acid in high doses may overwhelm this conversion pathway, leading to the direct appearance of measurable levels of untransformed folic acid in the systemic circulation of man (Kelly et al., 1997; Wright et al., 2007 ). This indicating a saturation point, is an evidence that intestinal conversion is not a prerequisite for transport, and is arguably indicative of the dividing line between physiological and nonphysiological oral doses of folate.

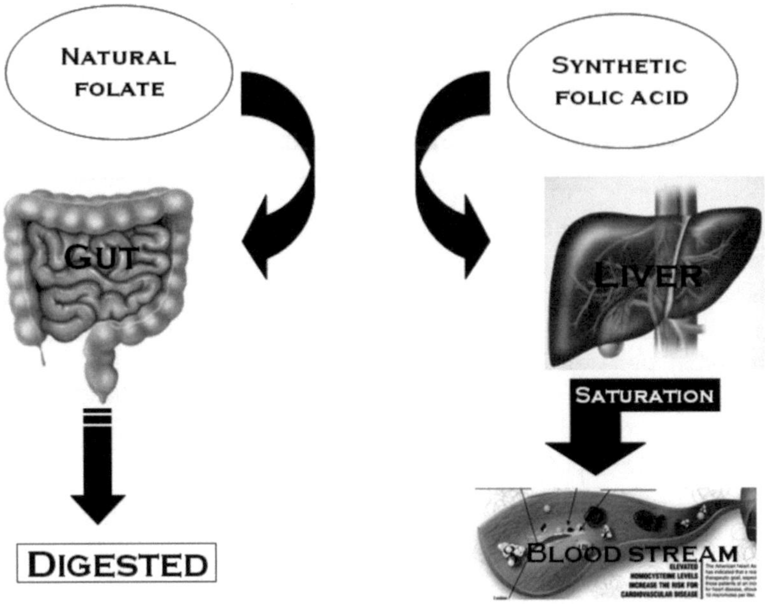


Fig. 3. Fate of natural folate and synthetic folic acid in the gut

Orhvik et al., (2010) determined folate bioavailability after ingestion of breads or a breakfast meal fortified with either folate or folic acid by using a stable-isotope area under the curve and ileostomy model and observed that there is a difference in plasma absorption kinetics for reduced folates and synthetic folic acid administered with the test foods. Also stomal folate contents indicated almost complete bioavailability of labeled folate from the breads or breakfast meal. Therefore, based on a re-appraisal of historical literature it is now hypothesised that folic acid metabolism in man primarily occurs in the liver, on contrary to absorptive cells of the upper small intestine where folate gets metabolized. Therefore due to human liver's low capacity for reduction it eventually gets saturated, resulting in significant and potentially deleterious unmetabolised folic acid entering the systemic circulation. In consequence of limited data available for folate bioavailability of vegetables, fruits, cereal products, and fortified foods, and difficultly in evaluation of bioavailability of food folate Orhvik et al., 2011 recommended to revisie the classical approach of using folic acid as a reference dose for estimating the plasma kinetics and relative bioavailability of food folate. Although a criterion for determining an excessive folate status has not yet been specified, a level above 45 nmol/L has been considered suitable as presence of free-circulating folic acid indicates that the organism's capacity to transform folic acid into folate derivatives has been overwhelmed (Pfeiffer et al., 1997; 2005; Dary , 2009).

A number of studies have shown that this high circulating synthetic folic acid supplements provoke a number of health complaints such as the masking of the early hematological manifestations of vitamin B12 deficiency, leukemia, arthritis, bowel cancer and ectopic pregnancies (Lucock and Yates, 2005; Sweeney et al., 2007; Wright et al., 2007). The other potential risks are interference with folate antagonistic drugs, zinc malabsorption and hypersensitivity reactions (Kadir & Economides, 2002). Though the risk of toxicity and harmful side effects from too much folic acid is low, since it is water soluble and human body excretes any excess that is not absorbed. The tolerable upper intake level for folic acid is 1,000 mcg, reports the Office of Dietary Supplements. Consuming more than this amount may cause adverse effects and mask the absorption of other nutrients.

Therefore before mandatory folic acid fortification is implemented, it is essential that a thorough assessment of all the potential concerns should be addressed precisely to ascertain a true picture of risk/benefit of fortification. To evaluate all the potential benefits and risks and optimal intakes of folic acid for all segments of the population, the physiologic and safety ramifications of lifetime exposure to circulating folic acid need to be elucidated (Kalmbach et al., 2008). Also a minimum efficacious level must be selected that prevent the consequences of folate deficiency yet minimizes the adverse effects associated with excesses.

## 6. Biofortification – A novel natural folate fortification approach

Since the role of the diet and fortified foods is still dubious, determination of the relative efficacy of food folate, folic acid added to foods, and supplemental folic acid alone is one of important question which needs to be answered. As highlighted by FDA, 1996, high intakes of chemically synthesized folic acid, (tolerable upper intake level, 1000 µg $d^{-1}$), can cause several adverse health effects as masking of macrocytic anemia, leukemia, arthritis, bowel cancer. For these reasons, many researchers have been critically evaluating the dietary sources of folates and looking for novel methods to increase concentrations of naturally occurring folate variants in foods instead of supplements and tablets. The enhancement of folate contents in staple food through genetic modification, so-called biofortification, can offer an alternative or at least complement the current methods to enhance intakes of natural food folates (Finglas, 2006). Biofortified crops offer potential advantages over supplementation or fortification strategies as seeds can be re-sown every year from the saved harvest. Recent progress in plant genomics of the model plants (The Arabidopsis Genome Initiative, 2000; Yu et al., 2002), in conjugation with available knowledge of folate biosynthesis biochemistry (Scott et al., 2000), has made feasible the folate enhancement by biofortification.

| Product | Folate (µg $l^{-1}$ ) |
|---|---|
| Milk | 40 ± 10 |
| Buttermilk | 90 ± 20 |
| *Dahi* | 60± 20 |
| Yogurt | 80 ± 20 |
| Acidophilus milk | 50 ± 10 |
| Bifidus milk | 75 ± 15 |

Table 1. Folate concentrations in dairy products and its contribution to the RDI

Besides genetic manipulation, the vegetables (broccoli, cauliflower), legumes (beans, nuts, peas, etc.) leafy greens (such as spinach), citrus fruits, liver (Eitenmiller & Landen, 1999; Forssen et al., 2000; Iyer & Tomar, 2009) milk and fermented dairy products represent an important dietary sources of folates (Lin & Young, 2000; Iyer et al., 2009). However, many dairy products are processed using microbial fermentations in which folate can be synthesized (Table.1), significantly increasing folate concentrations in the final product (Lin & Young, 2000; Iyer & Tomar, 2009). Therefore in some cases, fermented milk products are reported to contain such higher amounts of folate, that with an average serving of the product, the RDA for the vitamin would be met, or exceeded (Sybesma *et al.*, 2003).

This high level is the result of the production of additional folates by bacteria such as as *Lactococcus lactis, S. thermophilus, Leuconostoc species, Bifidobacterium longum* and some strains of *Propionibacteria* (Lin & Young, 2000; Hugenholtz et al., 2002; Crittenden et al., 2003; Papapstoyiannidis et al., 2006; Tomar & Iyer, 2011; Iyer et al., 2011). The ability to produce folate can differ (Table.2) remarkably between different lactic acid bacteria.

| Microbial Species | Total (μg) |
|---|---|
| *Lc. Lactis subsp cremoris* | 92-116 |
| *Lc. Lactis subsp lactis* | 57-291 |
| *L.plantarum* | 45 |
| *L.acidophilus* | 1 |
| *L.casei* subsp *rhamnosus* | -63 |
| *L.delbrueckii* subsp. *bulgaricus* | 54 |
| *P.acidipropionici* | 36 |
| *P.frendenreichii* ssp. *shermanii* | 17-78 |
| *B. adolescents* | 70-110 |
| *S. thermophilus* | 29-202 |
| *Leuconostoc lactis* | 45 |
| *Sacchromyces spp.* | 40 |

Table 2. Folate produced by different microorganisms

Keeping in view the potential risks of fortification with folic acid, fermented milks containing elevated levels of natural form folates seems to be more rationale for fortification purposes (Scott, 1999; Iyer & Tomar, 2011). Fermented milks can be a potential food matrix among dairy products for folate fortification because folate binding proteins of milk improve folate stability and the bioavailability of both 5-methyltetrahydrofolate and folic acid may be enhanced (Jones & Nixon, 2002; Aryana, 2003; Verwei et al., 2003). Hence, is an interesting strategy to increase "natural" folate levels in foods. Hence, an interesting strategy to increase "natural" folate levels in foods is by fermentation fortification by by the judicious selection and exploitation of high folate producing microorganisms. Therefore the application of high folate producing microorganisms could lead to the production of fermented dairy and other food products with increased levels of natural folate and can be a part of strategy for the economic development of novel functional foods with increased nutritional value.

## 7. Conclusion

Over the past half century one of the most exciting scientific developments authenticated by a chain of clinical research studies is the finding that folic acid plays a critical role in protecting against NTD. This article summarizes in brief the more important topics which have been either explored or need to be explored, which have led to the current situation in which all women capable of becoming pregnant are urged to ingest folic acid regularly. Though folate is present in various foods constituting our ordinary diet, yet is insufficient to meet RDA, which makes us vulnerable to folate deficiency. This problem can be addressed either by fortifying foods with folic acids or by use of folate rich foods and fermentation fortification by employing folate synthesizing food grade bacteria to increase the *in situ* folate levels in fermented foods (LeBlanc et al. 2007; Tomar and Iyer, 2011). In consequence to the health benefits associated with increased folate intakes many countries now possess mandatory folate enrichment programs. Although some controversy remains about the adequacy of fortification levels, the adverse effects of synthetic folic acid in contrast to natural food folate and genetic of folate in NTD. Nonetheless, several gaps in knowledge still need to be filled. The most important research need relates to our incomplete understanding of the mechanism and genetics by which the NTD defect occurs and how folate influence it to expand the scientific discussion of best health policy practices. The need for mechanistic knowledge is more so as to identify high-risk subjects and develop more effective interventions with an aim to obtain better results with folic acid supplementation .Besides this there is an urgent need to accurately delineate the dose-response relations of folate and NTD prevention so as to solve the current debate about appropriate levels of food fortification. Development of biofortified staple and vegetable crops with enhanced folate contents and their implementation is urgently required (Finglas, 2006).

Research should also be accompanied by economic feasibility studies that compare biofortification to conventional supplementation and fortification strategies. Simultaneously farmer and consumer acceptance studies should also go hand in hand in order to determine the acceptability of transgenic cereals with enhanced folate levels. Further, more strict regulatory measures for monitoring folic acid content in industrially processed foods and other products should be followed efficiently to complement mass-fortification programs. Apart from all this folic acid education campaigns need to be orchestrated to increase the knowledge about the benefits and sources of folic acid, and especially the correct, periconceptional timing of folic acid intake to reduce the overall incidence of NTDs (Rofai et al., 2011). For successful health campaign research besides identifying and reaching target groups, there is an immense need of awareness programs within high school and university educational system.

## 8. References

Adank.C.; Gree, T.J.; Skeaff, C.M. & Briars, B. (2003).Weekly high-dose folic acid supplementation is effective in lowering serum homocysteine concentrations in women. *Annals of Nutrition and Metabolism,* Vol.47, No.2, (March-April 2003), pp. 55-59, ISSN 1421-9697

Antony, A.C. & Hansen, D.K. (2000). Folate responsive neural tube defects and neurocristopathies. *Teratology,* Vol.62, No. 1, (July 2000),pp. 42-50, ISSN 1096-9926

Aryana, K.J. (2003). Folic acid fortified fat-free plain set yoghurt. *International Journal of Dairy Technology,*Vol. 56, No.4, (November 2003), pp. 219-222, ISSN 1471-0307

Bailey, L.B. & Gregory, J.F. (1999). Folate metabolism and requirements. *Journal of Nutrition,* Vol. 129, No.4, (April 1999), pp. 779-782, ISSN 0022-3166

Barkai, G.; Arbuzova, S.; Berkenstadt ,M.; Heifetz, S. & Cuckle, H. (2003). Frequency of Down's syndrome and neural-tube defects in the same family. *Lancet,* Vol.361, No. 9366,( April 2003), pp. 1331-1335., ISSN 0140-6736.

Barker, D. J. P. & Clark, P. M. (1997). Fetal undernutrition and disease in later life. *Reviews of Reproduction,* Vol. 2, No.2 , (May 1997), pp. 105-112, ISSN 1470-1626

Belkacemi, L.; Nelson, D.M.; Desai, M. & Ross, M.G. (2010). Maternal Undernutrition Influences Placental-Fetal Development. *Biology of Reproduction,* Vol.83, No.3, (September 2010), pp.325-31, ISSN 0006-3363

Benton, D. (2008). Micronutrient status, cognition and behavioral problems in childhood. *European Journal of Nutrition,* Vol. 47, No. 3, (August 2008), pp. 38–50, ISSN 1436-6207.

Botto, L.D.; Moore, C. A.; Khoury, M. J. & Erickson, J. D.(1999) Neural-tube defects. *New England Journal of Medicine,* Vol. 341, No. 20, (November 1999),pp. 1509-1519, ISSN 0028-4793

Brody, T. & Shane, B. (2001) Folic acid. In : *Handbook of vitamins,* R.B. Rucker.; J.W. Suttie.; D.B. McCormick.; L.J. Machlin, (Eds.), 427-462, Marcel Dekker Inc, ISBN 0824783514, New York, United States

Carroll, N.; Pangilinan, F.; Molloy, A.M.; Troendle, J.; Mills, J.L.; Kirke, P.N.; Brody, L.C.; Scott, J.M. & Parle-McDermott, A. (2009). Analysis of the MTHFD1 promoter and risk of neural tube defects. Human Genetics, Vol. 125, No. 3, (April 2009), pp. 247–256, ISSN 0340 6717

CDC (Centers for Disease Control).(1992). Recommendations for the use of folic acid to reduce the number of cases of spina bifida and other neural tube defects. Morbidity and Mortality Weekly Reports, Vol. 41 , (No.RR-14), (September1992).

Chanarin, I. (1979). *The Megaloblastic Anaemia,* Blackwell Scientific Publications , ISBN 0632007605 780632007608,, Oxford.

Chandler, C.J. ; Wang, T.T. & Halsted, C.H. (1986). Pteroylpolyglutamate hydrolase from human jejunal brush borders: Purification and characterization. *Journal of Biological Chemistry,* Vol. 261, No. 2, (January 1986), pp. 928- 933. ISSN 0021-9258

Cornel, M.C. & Erickson, J.D. (1997). Comparison of national policies on periconceptional use of folic acid to prevent spina bifida and anencephaly (SBA). *Teratology,* Vol.55, No. 2, (February 1997), pp.134-137, ISSN 1096-9926

Crittenden, R.G.; Martinez, N.R. & Playne, M.J. (2003). Synthesis and utilization of folate by yogurt starter cultures and probiotic bacteria. *International Journal of Food Microbiology,* Vol. 80, No. 3, (February 2003), pp. 217-222, ISSN 0168-1605

Czeizel, A.E. & Dudás, I. (1992). Prevention of the first occurrence of neural tube defects by periconceptional vitamin supplementation. The New England Journal of Medicine, Vol.327, No.26 ,(December 1992), pp. 1832-1835, ISSN 0028-4793

Czeizel, A.E. (1993). Prevention of congenital abnormalities by periconceptional multivitamin supplementation. *British Medical Journal,* Vol. 306, No.6893 , (June 1993), pp. 1645-1648. ISSN 0959-8138

Daly, L.E.; Kirke, P.N.; Molloy, A.; Weir, D.G. & Scott, J. M. (1995). Folate levels and neural tube defects. Implications for prevention. *The Journal of American Medical Association,* Vol. 274, No. 21, (December 1995), pp.1698–1702, ISSN 0098-7484

Daly, S.; Mills, J.L.; Molloy, A.M; Conley, M.; Lee, Y.J.; Kirke, P.N.; Weir, D.G. & Scott, J.M. (1997). Minimum effective dose of folic acid for food fortification to prevent neural-tube defects. *Lancet,* Vol. 350, No.9092 , (December 1997), pp.1666–1669, ISSN 0140-6736.

Dary, O. (2009). Nutritional interpretation of folic acid interventions. *Nutrition Reviews,* Vol. 67, No.4, (April 2009), pp. 235–244, , ISSN 1753-4887

Datta, V. & Chaturvedi, P. (2000). Congenetial Malformations in Rural Maharasthra. Indian Pediatrics; Vol. 37, No. 9, (September 2000), pp. 998-1001 , ISSN 0019-60061

de Franchis, R.; Sebastio, G.; Mandato, C.; Andria, G. & Mostroiacovo, P. (1995). Spina bifida, 677C-T mutation, and role of folate. *Lancet,* Vol. 346, No. 8991-8992, (December 1995), pp.1703, ISSN 0140-6736

de Marco, P.; Calevo, M.G.; Moroni, A.; Arata, L.; Merello, E.; Finnell, R.H.; Zhu, H.; Andreussi, L.; Cama, A. & Capra, V. (2002). Study of MTHFR and MS polymorphisms as risk factors for NTD in the Italian population. Journal of Human Genetics, Vol. 47, No.6 , (June 2002), pp. 319–324, ISSN 1434-5161

de Wals, P.; Tairou, F.; Van Allen, M.I.; Uh, S.H.; Lowry, R.B.; Sibbald, B.; Evans, J.A.; Hof, M.C.V.; Zimmer, P.; Crowley, M.; Fernandez, B.; Lee, N.S. & Niyonsenga, T. (2007). Reduction in neural-tube defects after folic acid fortification in Canada. New England Journal of Medicine, Vol. 357, No.26, (July 2007), pp.135–142, ISSN 0028-4793

Digra, N. C. (2004). Primary prevention of neural tube defects. *Jammu & Kashmir Sciences,* Vol. 6, No. 1, (January-March 2004), pp. 1-3, ISSN 0972-1177

Doudney, K.; Grinham, J.; Whittaker, J.; Lynch, S.A.; Thompson, D.; Moore, G.E.; Copp, A.J.; Greene, N.D.E. & Stanier, P. (2009). Evaluation of folate metabolism gene polymorphisms as risk factors for open and closed neural tube defects. *American Journal of Medical Genetics,*Vol. 149A, No.7 , (July 2009), pp. 1585–1589, ISSN 1552-4833

Eitenmiller, R.R. & Landen, W.O. (1999). Folate. In: *Vitamin Analysis for the Health and Food Sciences,* R.R. Eitenmiller & W.O. Landen (Eds.), 411-466, CRC Press, , ISBN 0849397715, Boca Raton, United States of America

FAO/WHO.(1988). Requirements of Vitamin A, Iron, Folate and Vitamin $B_{12}$. In: FAO/WHO Expert Consultation. 1988,pp. 51-61. Rome, Italy.

Finglas, P.M.; de Meer, K.; Molloy, A.; Verhoef, P.; Pietrzik, K.; Powers, H.J.; van der Straeten, D.; Ja¨gerstad, M.; Varela-Moreiras, G.; van Vliet, T.; Havenaar, R.; Buttriss, J. & Wright, A.J.A. (2006). Research goals for folate and related B vitamin in Europe. *European Journal of Clinical Nutrition,* Vol. 60, No.2 , (February 2006), pp. 287–294, ISSN: 0954-3007

Finnell, R.H.; Gould, A. & Spiegelstein, O. (2003). Pathobiology and genetics of neural tube defects. *Epilepsia* , Vol. 44, No.3, (June 2003), pp. 14–23, ISSN 1528-1167

Fitzpatrick, A. (2003). (Folic acid): implications for health and disease. *AGRO Food Industry hi-tech,* Vol.14, No. 3,(September 2003), pp. 45–52, ISSN 11206012

Fleming, A. & Copp. A.J. (1998). Embryonic Folate Metabolism and Mouse Neural Tube Defects. *Science,* Vol. 280, No. 5372, (June 1998), pp. 2107-2109, ISSN 0036-8075

Food and Drug Administration, USA. (1996). Folate and neural tube defects. In: *Food standards: food labeling: health claims and label statements, final rule, (21CFR Part 101). Federal Register,* Vol. 61, No. 44, (March 1996), pp. 8752–81.

Forssen, K. M.; Jagerstad, M.I.; Wigertz, K.& Witthoft, C. M. (2000) Folates and Dairy Products: A Critical Update. *Journal of American College of Nutrition,* Vol. 19, No.2 , (April 2000), pp. 100S-110S, ISSN 0731-5724

Frey, L. & Hauser, W.A. (2003). Epidemiology of neural tube defects. *Epilepsia,* Vol. 44, No. 3, ( June 2003) ,pp. 4-13, ISSN 1528-1167

George, L.; Mills, J.L.; Johansson ,A.L.V.; Nordmark, A.; Olander, B.; Granath, F. & Cnattingius, S. (2002). Plasma folate levels and risk of spontaneous abortion. *The Journal of American Medical Association,* Vol. 288, No.15 , (October 2002), pp.1867–73, ISSN 0098-7484.

Goh, Y.I. & Koren, G. (2008). "Folic acid in pregnancy and fetal outcomes". *Journal of Obstet Gynaecol,* Vol.28, No. 1, (January 2008), pp. 3–13, ISSN 0144-3615.

Greene, N.D.; Massa, V. & Copp, A.J. (2009b). Understanding the causes and prevention of neural tube defects: Insights from the splotch mouse model. *Birth Defects Research Part A: Clinical and Molecular Teratology,* Vol. 85, No. 4, (April 2009) pp. 322-330, ISSN 1542-0752.

Gregory, J.F. (1997). Bioavailability of folate. *European Journal of Clinical Nutrition,*Vol. 51, No.1, (January 1997), S54–S59, ISSN 0954-3007.

Hao, L.; Yang, Q-H.; Li, Z.; Bailey, L.B.; Zhu, J.H.; Hu, D.J.; Zhang, B.L.; Erickson, J.D.; Zhang, L.; Gindler, J.; Li, S. & Berry, R. J. (2008). Folate status and homocysteine response to folic acid doses and withdrawal among young Chinese women in a large-scale randomized double-blind trial. *American Journal of Clinical Nutrition,* Vol.88, No.2 , (August 2008), pp. 448–457, ISSN 0002-9165

Harris, M.J. & Juriloff, D.M. (2010). An update to the list of mouse mutants with neural tube closure defects and advances toward a complete genetic perspective of neural tube closure. *Birth Defects Research Part A: Clinical and Molecular Teratology,* Vol. 88, No. 8, (August 2010), pp.653-669, ISSN 1542-0752,

Harris, M.J. (2009) Insights into prevention of human neural tube defects by folic acid arising from consideration of mouse mutants. *Birth Defects Research Part A: Clinical and Molecular Teratology,* Vol. 85, No.4, (April, 2009), pp.331-339, ISSN 1542-0752,

Hendler, S.S., & Rorvik, D. (2001). Resveratrol. In: *PDR for Nutritional Supplements.* Medical Economics™ Thomson Healthcare, 397-401, ISBN 13: 9781563637100, Montvale, New Jersey.

Hibbard, B.M. (1964). The role of folic acid in pregnancy: With particular reference to anaemia, abruption and abortion. *European Journal of Obstetrics & Gynecology and Reproductive Biology,* Vol. 71, No.4 , (August 1964), pp. 529-542, ISSN 0022-3204

Hugenholtz, J., Hunik. J., Santos, H. & Smid, E. (2002). Nutraceuticals production by Propionibacteria. *Lait,* Vol. 82, No.1, (Jan-Feb, 2002), pp.103-111, ISSN 0023-7302

Institute of Medicine.(1998). Dietary Reference Intakes for Thiamin,Riboflavin, Niacin, Vitamin B-6, Folate, Vitamin B-12, Pantothenic Acid, Biotin, and Choline. National Academy Press, Washington, D.C.

Iyer, R. & Tomar, S. K. (2009). Folate: a functional food constituent. *Journal of Food Science,* Vol. 74, No.9, (November/December 2009), pp.114-122, ISSN 1750-3841.

Iyer, R.; Tomar, S.K.; Srivatsa, N. & Singh, R. (2011). Folate Producing *Streptococcus Thermophilus*: *de facto* ideal functional dairy starter, In: *Microbes in the Service of Mankind: Tiny Bugs with Huge Impact,* R. Nagpal, A. Kumar, & R. Singh, (Eds.). In press, I.K. Publishers, New Delhi, India

James, S.J.; Pogribna, M.; Pogribny, I.P.; Melnyk, S.; Hine, R.J.; Gibson, J.B.; Yi, P.; Tafoya, D.L.; Swenson, D.H.; Wilson, V.L. & Gaylor, D.W. (1999). Abnormal folate metabolism and mutation in the methylenetetrahydrofolate reductase gene may be maternal risk factors for Down syndrome. *American Journal of Clinical Nutrition,* Vol. 70, No. 4 ,(October 1999), pp. 495-501, ISSN 0002-9165.

Jaquier, M.; Klein, A. & Boltshauser, E. (2006). Spontaneous pregnancy outcome after prenatal diagnosis of anencephaly, BJOG : *An International Journal of Obstetrics & Gynaecology*. Vol. 113, No. 8, (July 2006), pp. 951-953, ISSN 1471-0528

Jaquier, M.; Klein, A. & Boltshauser, E. (2006). Spontaneous pregnancy outcome after prenatal diagnosis of anencephaly. BJOG: *An International Journal of Obstetrics & Gynaecology*. Vol. 113, No. 8, (July 2006), pp. 951-953, ISSN 1471-0528.

Jones, M.L. & Nixon, P.F. (2002). Tetrahydrofolates are Greatly Stabilized by Binding to Bovine Milk Folate-Binding Protein. *Journal of Nutrition*, Vol. 132, No.9, (September 2002), pp. 2690-2694, ISSN 0022-3166

Kadir, R.A. & Economides, D.L. (2002). Neural tube defects and periconceptional folic acid. *Canadian Medical Association JournalJ*, Vol. 167, No.3 , (August 2002), pp. 255-256, ISSN: 1488-2329

Kalmbach, R.D.; Choumenkovitch, S. F.; Troen, A.M.; D'Agostino, R.; Jacques, P.F. & Selhub, J. (2008). Circulating folic acid in plasma: relation to folic acid fortification. *American Journal of Clinical Nutrition*, Vol. 88, No. 3, (September 2008), pp. 763-768, ISSN 0002-9165

Kelly, P.; McPartlin, J.; Goggins, M.; Weir, D.G. & Scott, J.M. (1997). Unmetabolized folic acid in serum: acute studies in subjects consuming fortified food and supplements. *American Journal of Clinical Nutrition*, Vol. 65, No. 6 ,(June 1997), pp. 1790-1795, ISSN 0002-9165.

Kim, S.Y.; Park, S.Y.; Choi, J.W.; Kim, D.J.; Lee, S.Y.; Lim, J.H.; Han, J.Y.; Ryu, H.M. & Kim, M.H. (2011). Association between MTHFR 1298A>C polymorphism and spontaneous abortion with fetal chromosomal aneuploidy. *American Journal of Reproductive Immunology*, Vol. 66, No.4, (October 2011), pp. 252-258, ISSN 1600-0897

Kim, Y.I. (2004). Will mandatory folic acid fortification prevent or promote cancer? *American Journal of Clinical Nutrition*, Vol. 80, No. 5, (November 2004), pp. 1123-1128, ISSN 0002-9165

Kirke, P.N.; Molloy, A.M.; Daly, L.E.; Burke, H.; Weir, D.G. & Scott, J.M. (1993). Maternal plasma folate and vitamin $B_{12}$ are independent risk factors for neural tube defects. *QJM: An International Journal of Medicine*, Vol 86, No.11 , (November 1993), pp. 86703-86708, ISSN 1460-2725

Koch, M.C.; Stegmann, K.; Ziegler, A.; Schroter, B. & Ermert, A. (1998). Evaluation of the MTHFR C677T allele and the MTHFR gene locus in a German spina bifida population. *European Journal of Pediatrics*, Vol. 157, No.6 , (June 1998), pp. 487-492, ISSN 0340-6199

Konings, E.J.M.; Roomans, H.H.; Dorant, E.; Goldbohm, R.A.; Saris, W.H. & Van Den Brandt, P.A. (2001). Folate intake of the Dutch population according to newly established liquid chromatography data for foods. *American Journal of Clinical Nutrition*, Vol. 73, No.4 , (April 2001), pp. 765-76, ISSN 0002-9165

Krishnaswamy, K. & Madhavan, N.K. (2001). Importance of folate in human nutrition. *British Journal of Nutrition*, Vol. 85, No.2 , (May 2001), pp. S115-S124, ISSN 0007-1145

Kulshteshtra, R.; Nath, L.M. & Upadhyay, P. (1983). Congenital malformations in live born infants in a rural community. *Indian Pediatrics*, Vol. 2, No.1 (January 1983), pp. 45-49, ISSN 0974-7559

LeBlanc, J.G.; Giori, G.S.D.; Smid, E.J.; Hugenholtz, J. & Sesma, F. (2007). Folate production by lactic acid bacteria and other food-grade microorganisms. In: *Communicating Current Research And Educational Topics And Trends In Applied Microbiology*, A. Mendez-Vilas (ed) Vol 1., 329–339, Formatex, ISBN-13: 978-84-611-9422-3, Badajoz, Spain.

Li, C.C.Y.; Cropley, J.E.; Cowley, M.J.; Preiss, T.; Martin, D.I.K. & Suter, C.M. (2011) A Sustained Dietary Change Increases Epigenetic Variation in Isogenic Mice. PLoS Genetics, Vol. 7, No.4, (April 2011), pp. 1-10, ISSN 1553-7404

Lillycrop, K.A.; Phillips, E.S.; Jackson, A.A.; Hanson, M.A. & Burdge, G.C. (2005). Dietary protein restriction of pregnant rats induces and folic acid supplementation prevents epigenetic modification of hepatic gene expression in the offspring. *Journal of Nutrition*, Vol. 135, No. 6 , (June 2005), pp. 1382–1386, ISSN 0022-3166

Lin, M.Y. & Young, C.M. (2000). Folate levels in cultures of lactic acid bacteria. *International Dairy Journal* , Vol.10, No.5, (October 2000) ,pp. 409-414. ISSN 0958-6946

Lindenbaum, J.; Savage, D.G.; Stabler S.P. & Allen, R.H. (1990). Diagnosis of cobalamin deficiency: II. Relative sensitivities of serum cobalamin, methylmalonic acid, and total homo-cysteine concentrations. *American Journal of Haematology*, Vol. 34, No.2 , (June 1990), pp. 99-107, ISSN 1096-8652

Lucock, M. & Yates, Z. (2005). Folic acid-vitamin and panacea or genetic time bomb? *Nature Review Genetics*, Vol. 6, No.4 , (March 2005), pp. 235-240, ISSN 1471-0056)

Marco, P.D.; Merello, E.; Cama, A.; Kibar, Z. & Capra, V. (2011).Human neural tube defects: Genetic causes and prevention, *BioFactors* , Vol. 37, No.4, (July- August 2011),pp. 261–268, ISSN 1872-8081

Marean, A.; Graf, A.; Zhang, Y. & Niswander, L. (2011). Folic acid supplementation can adversely affect murine neural tube closure and embryonic survival. *Human Molecular Genetics* (June 2011), doi: 10.1093/hmg/ddr289, ISSN 1460-2083.

Mason, J. B. (1990). Intestinal transport of monoglutamyl folates in mammalian systems. In :*Contemporary issues in clinical nutrition*, 13. Folic acid metabolism in health and disease, M.F. Picciano.; E.L.R. Stokstad. & J.F. Gregory. (Eds.), 47-63, Wiley-Liss Inc., ISBN 0471567442, New York, United States

Mason, J. B. (1995). Folate status. Effects on carcinogenesis. In: *Folate in health and disease* , L.B. Baily (Ed.), 316-378, Marcel Dekker, ISBN 1420071246, New York, United States

Mathers, J. C.; Strathdee, G. & Relton, C. L. (2010). Induction of epigenetic alterations by dietary and other environmental factors. *Advances in Genetics*, Vol. 71, No. , (August 2011), pp. 3-39, ISBN: 978-0-12-380864-6

McNulty, H. & Scott, J. M. (2008). Intake and status of folate and related B-vitamins: considerations and challenges in achieving optimal status. *British Journal of Nutrition*. Vol. 99, No.3, (February 2008), pp S48–S54, ISSN 0007-1145

Merchant, S. M. (1989). Indian Council of Medical Research Center, *Annual Report*, pp. 27,Mumbai, India

Mills, J.L.; von Kohorn, I.; Conley, M.R.; Zeller, J.A.; Cox, C.; Williamson, R.E. & Dufour, D.R. (2003). Low vitamin B12 concentrations in patients without anaemia: the effect of folic acid fortification of grain. *American Journal of Clinical Nutrition*, Vol. 77, No. 6, (June 2003), pp 1474–1477, ISSN 0002-9165

Nazer, J.H.; Lopez-Camelo, J. & Castilla, E.E. (2001). ECLAMC: Results of thirty years of epidemiological surveillance of neural tube defects. *Revista Médica de Chile,* Vol. 129, No.5 , (May 2001), pp.531-539, ISSN 0034-9887

Nicholas, D.E.G.; Stanier, P. & Copp, A.J. (2009). Genetics of human neural tube defects. *Human Molecular Genetics* , Vol. 18, No. R2, (October 2009), pp R113-R129., ISSN 0964-6906

Norsworthy, B.; Skeaff, C.M.; Adank, C. & Green, T.J. (2004). Effects of once-a- week or daily folic acid supplementation on red blood cell folate concentrations in women. *European Journal of Clinical Nutrition,* Vol. 58, No. 3, (March 2004), pp. 548–554, ISSN 0954-3007

O'Brien, M.M.; Kiely, M.; Harrington, K.E.; Robson, P.J.; Strain, J.J. & Flynn, A. (2001). The North/South Ireland Food Consumption Survey: vitamin intakes in 18-64-year-old adults. *Public Health Nutrition,* Vol.4, No. 5A, (October 2001), pp. 1069–79, ISSN 1368-9800

Ohrvik, V.E. & Witthoft, C.M. (2011). Human Folate Bioavailability. *Nutrients,* Vol. 3, No.4 , (April, 2011), pp. 475-490, ISSN 2072-6643

Ohrvik, V.E.; Buttner, B.E.; Rychlik, M.; Lundin, E. & Witthoft, C.M. (2010). Folate Bioavailability from Breads and a Meal Assessed with a Human stable-isotope area under the curve and ileostomy model. *American Journal of Clinical Nutrition,* Vol. 92, No. 3, (September 2010), pp. 532–538, ISSN 0002-9165

Papapstoyiannidis, G.; Polychroniadou, A.; Michaelidou, A.M. & Alichandis, E. (2006). Fermented Milks Fortified with B-group Vitamins: Vitamin Stability and Effect on Resulting Products. *Food Science and Technology International,* Vol. 12, No. 6 , (December, 2006), pp. 521-529, ISSN 1082-0132

Patterson, D. (2008). Folate metabolism and the risk of Down syndrome. *Down Syndrome Research and Practice* , Vol. 12, No.2, (October 2008),pp. 93-97, ISSN 0968-7912

Penchaszadeh, V.B. (2002). Preventing Congenital Anomalies in Developing Countries. *Community Genet ics,* Vol. 5, No. 1, (September 2002), pp. 61-69, ISSN 978-3-8055-7479-2

Pfeiffer, C.M.; Caudill, S.P.; Gunter, E.W.; Osterloh, J. & Sampson, E.J. (2005). Biochemical indicators of B vitamin status in the US population after folic acid fortification: results from the National Health and Nutrition Examination Survey 1999–2000. *American Journal of Clinical Nutrition,* Vol. 82, No.2 , (August 2005),pp.442–450, ISSN 0002-9165

Pfeiffer, C.M.; Rogers, L.M.; Bailey, L.B.; Gregory, J.F. (1997). Absorption of Folate from Fortified Cereal-Grain Products and of Supplemental Folate Consumed with or Without Food Determined Using a Dual-Label Stable-Isotope Protocol. *American Journal of Clinical Nutrition,* Vol. 66, No. 6, (December, 1997), pp. 1388–1397, ISSN 0002-9165

Pitkin, R.M. (2007). Folate and neural tube defects. *American Journal of Clinical Nutrition,* Vol. 85, No.1 ,(January 2007), pp.285S–288S, ISSN: 1938-3207

Pulikkunnel, S.T. & Thomas, S.V.(2005). Neural Tube Defects: Pathogenesis and Folate Metabolism. *Journal of the Association of Physicians of India,* Vol. 53,(February 2005), pp.127-135, ISSN 0004-5772

Redmer, D.A.; Wallace, J.M.& Reynolds. L.P. (2004). Effect of nutrient intake during pregnancy on fetal and placental growth and vascular development. *Domestic Animal Endocrinology,* Vol. 27, No. 3, (October 2004), pp. 199-217, ISSN 0739-7240

Rofail, D.; Colligs, A.; Abetz, L.; Lindemann, M. & Maguire. L. (2011). Factors contributing to the success of folic acid public health campaigns. *Journal of Public Health.* doi:10.1093/pubmed/fdr048, (July 2011), pp. 1-10, ISSN 1741-3842

Saborio, M. (1992). Experience in providing genetic services in Costa Rica. *Birth Defects Orig Art Ser,* Vol. 28, No. 3, pp. 96-102, .

Sadler, T.W. (2005). Embryology of Neural Tube Development. American Journal of Medical Genetics Part C , Vol. 135C, No. 1 ,( May 2005), pp. 2-8 , ISSN: 1552-4825

Sauberlich, H. (1995). Folate status in the US Population groups. In: *Folate in Health and Disease.* L.Bailey,(Ed.), 171-194, Marcel Dekker, ISBN : 1420071246, New York, United States.

Sauberlich, H.E.; Kretsch, M.J.; Skala, J.H.; Johnson, H. & Taylor, P.C. (1987). Folate requirement and metabolism in nonpregnant women. *American Journal of Clinical Nutrition,* Vol. 46, No. 6 , (December 1987), pp. 1016-1028, ISSN: 1938-3207

Scott , J. M. (1999). Folate and vitamin B12. *Proceedings of the Nutrition Society, Vol.* 58, No. 2, (May 1999), pp. 441-448, ISSN 0029-6651

Scott, J. & Weir, D. (1994). Folate/vitamin B12 inter-relationships.*Essays in Biochemistry,* Vol. 28, No.1, pp. 63–72, ISSN 00711365

Scott, J.; Rebeille, F. & Fletcher, J. (2000). Folic acid and folates: the feasibility for nutritional enhancement in plant foods. *Journal* of the *Science* of *Food* and *Agriculture.* Vol. 80, No.7, (May 2000), pp. 795–824, ISSN 1097-0010

Shils, L.; Maurice, E.; James, A.; Olson, S. & Shike, M. (1994). *Modern Nutrition in Health and Disease* , Lea & Febiger, ISBN 0812117522, Philadelphia, Pennsylvania

Smithells, R.W.; Sheppard, S. & Schorah, C.J. (1976). Vitamin deficiencies and neural tube defects. *Archives of Disease in Childhood,* Vol. 51, No.12 , (December 1976), pp. 944-950, ISSN 14682044

Strum, W.B. (1979). Enzymatic reduction and methylation of folate following pH-dependant, carrier-mediated transport in rat jejunum. *Biochimica et Biophysica Acta,* Vol. 554, No. 1 , (June 1979), pp. 249–257, ISSN 0005-2736.

Sugden, M. C. & Holness, M. J. (2002). Gender-specific programming of insulin secretion and action. *Journal of Endocrinology,* Vol. 175, No.3 , (December 2002), pp. 757-767, ISSN 0022-0795

Swain, S.; Agarwal, A., Bhatia, B.D. (1994). Congential malformations at birth. Indian Pediatrics, Vol. 31, No. 10, (October 1994), pp. 1187-1191, ISSN 0974-7559

Sweeney, M.R.; McPartlin , J. & Scott, J. (2007). Folic acid fortification and public health: Report on threshold doses above which unmetabolised folic acid appear in serum. *BMC Public Health,* Vol. 7, No. 41, (March 2007) doi:10.1186/1471-2458-7-41, ISSN 1471-2458

Sybesma, W.; Starrenburg, M.; Kleerebezem, M.; Mierau, I.; de Vos, W.M. & Hugenholtz, J. (2003). Increased production of folate by metabolic engineering of *Lactococcus lactis. Applied Environmental Microbiology,* Vol. 69, No. 6 , (June 2003), pp.3069–3076, ISSN 0099-2240

The Arabidopsis Genome Initiative. (2000). Analysis of the genome sequence of the flowering plant *Arabidopsis thaliana. Nature,* Vol. 408, No. 6814 , (December 2000), pp. 796–815, ISSN 0028-0836

Tomar, S.K. & Iyer, R. (2011). Folate production by lactic acid bacteria. In: *Functional Dairy Foods: Concepts and Applications,* S.K.Tomar .; R. Singh.; A. K. Singh .; S. Arora. & R.R.B.Singh, (Eds.), 9-21, Satish Serial Publishing House, ISBN 8189304909, Delhi, India

Van der Put, N.M.J.; Steegers-Theunissen, R.P.M.; Frosst ,P.; Trijbels, F.J.M.; Eskes, T.K.A.B.; Van den Heuvel, L.P.; Mariman, E.C.M.; Den Heyer, M.; Rozen, R. & Blom, H.J. (1995). Mutated methylenetetrahydrofolate reductase as a risk factor for spina bifida. Lancet, Vol. 346, No. 8982 , (October 1995), pp.1070–1071, ISSN 0140-6736

Van der Put, N.M.J.; Van Straaten, H.W.; Trijbels, F.J. & Blom, H.J. (2001). Folate, homocysteine and neural tube defects: an overview. *Experimental Biology* and *Medicine,* Vol. 226, No. 4 , (April 2001), pp. 243–270, ISSN 1573-822

Verhaar, M.C.; Stroes, E. & Rabelink, T.J. (2002).Folates and cardiovascular disease. Arteriosclerosis, *Thrombosis,* and *Vascular Biology,* Vol. 22, No.1 , (January 2002), pp. 6-13, ISSN 1524-4636

Verhoef, P.; Stampfer, M.J. & Rimm, E.B. (1998). Folate and coronary heart disease. Curr Opin Lipidol, Vol. 9, No 1. ,(February 1998), pp. 17-22, ISSN 0957-9672.

Verwei, M.; Arkbage, K.; Havenaar, R.; van den Berg, H.; Witthoft, C. & Schaafsma, G. (2003). Folic acid and 5-methyltetrahydrofolate in fortified milk are bioaccessible as determined in a dynamic in vitro gastrointestinal model. *Journal of Nutrition,* Vol. 133, No. 7, (July 2003),pp. 2377-2383, ISSN 0022-3166

Wald, N.; Sneddon, J.; Densem, J.; Frost, C.; Stone, R. & MRC Vitamin Study Research Group. (1991). Prevention of neural tube defects: Results of the Medical Research Council Vitamin Study. *Lancet,* Vol. 338, No. 8760, (July 1991), pp.131-137, ISSN 0140-6736

Waterland, R. A. & Jirtle, R. L. (2004). Early nutrition, epigenetic changes at transposons and imprinted genes, and enhanced susceptibility to adult chronic diseases. *Nutrition,* Vol. 20, No.1 , (January 2004), pp. 63-68, ISSN 1475-2891

Werler, M.M.; Shapiro, S. & Mitchell, A.A.(1993). Periconceptional Folic Acid Exposure and Risk of Occurrent Neural Tube Defects. *The Journal of American Medical Association,* Vol. 269, No.10, (March 1993), pp. 1257-1261, ISSN 0098-7484.

World Health Organization and Food and Agriculture Organization. (2006). Guidelines on Food Fortifi cation with Micronutrients. Geneva: World Health Organization and Food and Agriculture Organization of the United Nations; ISBN 92 4 159401 2, Geneva, United States

Wright, J.; Dainty, J. & Finglas, P.(2007). Folic acid metabolism in human subjects revisited: potential implications for proposed mandatory folic acid fortification in the UK. *British Journal of Nutrition,* Vol. 98, No. 4, (July 2007), pp.665-666, ISSN 0007-1145

Wu, F.; Bazer, W.; Wallace, J. M.; & Spencer, T. E. (2006). Intrauterine growth retardation: Implications for the animal sciences. *Journal of Animal Science,* Vol. 84, No. 9 , pp. 2316-2337, ISSN 0021-8812

Wu, G.; Bazer, F.W.; Cudd, T.A.; Meininger, C.J. & Spencer, T.E.(2004). Maternal nutrition and fetal development. *Journal of Nutrition,* Vol. 134, No. 9, (September 2004), pp. 2169–2172, ISSN 0022-3166

Xiao, K.Z.; Zhang, Z.Y.; Su, Y.M.; Liu, F.Q.; Yan, Z.Z.; Jiang, Z.Q.; Zhou, S.F.; He, W.G.; Wang, B.Y. & Jiang, H.P. (1990). Central nervous system congenital malformations, especially neural tube defects in 29 provinces, metropolitan cities and autonomous regions of China: Chinese Birth Defects Monitoring Program. *International Journal of Epidemiology*, Vol. 19, No.4, (December 1990),pp. 978-982, ISSN 0300-5771

Yang, Q.; Cogswell, M.E.; Hamner, H.C.; Carriquiry, A.; Bailey, L.B.; Pfeiffer, C.M. & Berry, R.J. (2010). Folic acid source, usual intake, and folate and vitamin B-12 status in US adults: National Health and Nutrition Examination Survey (NHANES) 2003–2006. *The American Journal of Clinical Nutrition*, Vol. 91, No. 1, (January 2010), pp. 64–72, ISSN 0002-9165

Yates, A.; Schlicker, S. & Suitor, C.(1998). Dietary reference intakes: the new basis for recommendations for calcium and related nutrients, B vitamins, and choline. *Journal of the American Dietetic Association,* Vol. 98, No. 6, (June 1998), pp. 699-706, ISSN 0002-8223

Yu, J.; Hu, S.N.; Wang, J.; Wong, G.K.S.; Li, S.G.; Liu, B. et al. (2002). A draft sequence of the rice genome (Oryza *saliva* L. ssp *indica*). *Science, Vol.* 296, No. 5565, (April 2002), pp. 79–92, ISSN 0036-8075

# Part 2

# Genetics of Neural Tube Defects

8

# Advances in Genetics of Non Syndromic Neural Tube Defects

Patrizia De Marco
*Neurosurgery Department*
*G. Gaslini Institute, Genoa,*
*Italy*

## 1. Introduction

This chapter revisits established and emerging information on the causes of the human Neural Tube Defects (NTD). These congenital malformations, affecting 1 per 1000 births, have adverse consequences that afflict society as well as the affected individuals. The mechanisms by which they arise are still unknown.

Investigators have focused their efforts in many research fields (developmental and metabolic pathways and animal models) to understand the mechanisms underlying the etiology of these devasting defects. Nevertheless, few candidate genes have proved to have significant impact on the development of NTDs. Moreover, the existing body of literature is still fragmented and constrained by limited size, lack of power, and lack of replicated and independent studies.

The review attempts to describe the results obtained by the analysis of candidate genes from three types of evidences: developmental pathway and biochemical pathways (folate metabolism). The update of the literature includes the most recent findings.

This chapter aims to improve the knowledge of the readers on a such complex multifactorial disease outlining that, even though the remarkable recent progresses, further studies are needed to clarify the molecular basis of NTDs.

The knowledge of the etiology con help us in developing strategies for prevention of the NTDs, by the identification of parents who have a higher chance of having an affected child. In these families it may be possible to clarify the mode of inheritance and estimate the recurrence risk of the disorder. Actually, we are far to have immediate clinical benefits for NTDs, but providing clinicians with a better knowledge of the development of the disease, we could speed up the search for a focused prevention and a more complete familial counselling.

Neural tube defects (NTDs) are congenital malformations that involve failure of the neural tube closure during the early phases of development at any level of the rostro-caudal axis. The incidence of NTDs in European countries excluding UK and Ireland was 0.1-0.6 per 1000 births in the period 1989-2002. [1] Each year, more than 4500 pregnancies in the European Union are affected by NTDs. [2]

In order to gain insights into the embryonic basis of NTDs, it is important to understand the morphogenetic processes and the underlying molecular mechanisms involving the neural tube closure. Neurulation begins with formation of the neural plate, a thickening of the ectoderm on the dorsal surface of the post-gastrulation embryo. Neurulation occurs in a two-part process: i) primary neurulation (weeks 3-4) resulting in formation of the neural tube that will develop into brain and most of spinal cord; ii) secondary neurulation (weeks 5-6) that creates the neural tube caudal to the mid-sacral region. [3] During the primary neurulation, the neural plate is subject to shaping and folding, with fusion along the midline to form the tube. The secondary neural tube is derived from a population of mesenchymal cells, the tail bud, which undergo proliferation and condensation followed by cavitation and fusion with the primary neural tube. [4] Neurulation is driven by redundant mechanisms both at the tissue and cellular level. [5]. Active processes required for neural tube closure include convergent extension cell movements, expansion of the cranial mesenchyme, contraction of actin filaments, bending of the neural plate, and adhesion of the neural folds. Insight into these mechanisms are being provided by the many mouse models in which NTDs occur as a result of genetic mutations. [6] Neural tube closure is a discontinuous process and proceed bi-directionally in a zipper-like fashion. Five closure sites exist in human embryos and on the basis of the study of clinical cases, van Allen et al. [7] proposed a multisite model in which the initial site of closure starts at the rhomboencephalic segment and the caudal end is the last to close.

There are several different types of NTDs. The distribution of different types may vary in different populations and can also vary by the birth prevalence of the defects. [8] The most common classification includes anencephaly, myelomeningocele (also called spina bifida) and encephalocele. Craniorachischisis and iniencephaly are considered to be rarer in most populations. NTDs group includes other conditions, broadly described as occult spinal dysraphisms (lipoma, tight filum terminale) and some complex dysraphic states as diastematomelia, spinal segmental dysgenesis, and caudal regression syndrome. [9] Failure of the closure at any level of the body axis leads to open NTDs where the affected nervous tissues are exposed to the surface. Failure of the secondary neurulation leads to closed forms of NTDs, where the defect is covered by the skin and it is not exposed to the surface of the body.

The majority of NTD cases are non syndromic or isolated NTDs, meaning that the NTD is the only defect. A number of anomalies including clubfoot, deformation of the lower limbs, hydrocephalus and Arnold Chiari II malformation have been widely accepted as secondary abnormalities that may accompany NTDs. Aetiology of non syndromic NTDs is multifactorial with both environmental and genetic factors implicated. Non syndromic NTDs have an important genetic component and it is important that research is focused at determining the basis of this genetic aetiology. The aim of this chapter is provide evidences for genetic contribution to non syndromc NTDs along with the discussion of different approaches for identifying such genes. The identification of genetic factors for NTDs is a relatively a new area of research. In fact, thare are many different mutations in mice resulting in NTDs, but only few well characterized genetic factors in humans. Here we provide an overview of the major causative genes and the more recent genetic advances emerging thanks to the powerful tool of mouse models.

## 2. Evidence for genetic contribution of non syndromic NTDs

There are strong evidence supporting a genetic component to NTDs. NTDs can be associated with various chromosome rearrangements, the most common include trisomy 13, trisomy 18, tetraploidy, and deletions involving chromosomes 2, 3, 11, 13, 22. Genetic syndromes with NTDs include Meckel-Gruber syndrome and Currarino syndrome. [10] Overall hereditabilty in NTDs is estimated to be 60% with multiple genes involved. Recurrence risk for sibling is 2-5%, which represents up to 50-fold increased risk respect to that observed in the general population [11]. Positive family history families with many affected children have implied an autosomal recessive model of inheritance. [12] Inspection of multiplex families demonstrated that affected relative pairs are related at either the second- or third-degree, suggesting oligogenic inheritance. [13]. The recurrence risk and the inheritance pattern in families have been demonstrated to follow a multifactorial threshold model in which the liability to these malformations follows a normal distribution pattern: additive effects of several genetic and environmental factors cumulate to increase the liability until a threshold value beyond which the phenotype become expressed. Twin studies demonstrated that concordance rate is relatively low among cotwins of affected cases. [11]. Recurrences in families in which the case is affected with spina bifida tend to be spina bifida and families; recurrence in families in which the case is anencephaly tend to be anencephaly. [14-15] However, one third of recurrent cases involve a NTDs phenotype that is different from the cases phenotype. This intra-familial heterogeneity may be the consequence of the pleiotropic effect of a underlying causative gene. NTD occurrence vary among different ethnic groups and it is unknown if this population-specific incidence is due to differences in the frequency of risk-associated alleles or to specific dietary habits or exposures. The highest incidence is in Northern China (7/1000) and the lowest in Japan (0.1/1000). In Europe, the highest rate is reported in Ireland (3/1000). Furthemore, an Irish study demonstrated that predisposing genetic factors may be transmitted from the mother's side of the family. [16] Another important line of evidence for a genetic basis for NTDs comes from the numerous mouse models, both spontaneous and induced via a gene-driven process. [17].

## 3. Identification of susceptibility genes involved in NTDs

The number and identity of genes predisposing to NTDs remain unknown. Once genes implicated in the development of NTDs are identified, it will be essential to understand potential additive or multiplicative effects of genetic and environmental factors. Candidate genes for NTDs can be classified into two categories according to how they have been identified: biological and positional. Candidate genes based on biological plausibility have resulted from research done in animal models and from biological pathways important for NTDs. Candidate genes can also be identified through positional techniques via chromosomal rearrangements in NTD patients or genomic screen in linkage analysis.

A number of genes have been identified from research done in experimental animals, most notably from mouse models. The mouse model remains one of the most well studied animal models for NTDs. More than 190 genes in mouse produce varying NTDs phenotypes. [17]. There are both naturally occurring and induced strains of mice. The two most common mouse phenotypes are exencephaly, that is comparable to human anencephaly, and craniorachoischisis, in which the neural tube remains open along the entire body axis. The mouse system is useful for the study of NTDs because the genetic map of mouse is noted and many of the human homologues are known. Moreover, mouse has a short gestational period and does not require the same ethical considerations as the studies in humans. Another advantage is that both genetic and environmental factors may be studied. For example three mouse mutants have been demonstrated to have a reduced risk for NTDs after maternal folate supplementation: *crooked* (*Cd*), *splotch* (*Sp*) and *cartilage homeoprotein1* (*Cart1*). [17] Nevertheless, there are obvious differences between mouse and human, so that it is possible that genes contributing to NTDs in mouse not always do the same in humans. The majority of human NTDs are isolated a show a multifactorial inheritance. In contrast, NTDs in mouse are a lethal condition in the homozygous knock-out state and NTDs is a part of a larger syndrome. Mice have a four-sites model of neural tube closure. In humans controversies have been arisen about the number of closure sites , although there is a general agreement on the presence of rostral and caudal sites. The majority of candidate genes from mouse are involved in a wide range of functions, in crucial steps of neurulation and only few are implicated in cellular functions such as genome stability and DNA repair. Despite a such long list of candidate genes, studies failed to show positive association in humans. Another system that can be used is the zebrafish (*Brachydanio rerio*), that is a cost-effective model system for studying NTDs since fertilized eggs can develop rapidly into transparent embryos, allowing all stages of vertebrate development to be visualized easily. [18] Zebrafish has proven to be very useful for studying embryological processes, including morphogenesis, lineage specification, and mechanisms of acquired cell fate. Furthemore, assays have been developed to perform both gain and loss of function experiments. Partial loss of function phenotypes can be generated by microinjection of antisense morphplino. [19] A forward genetic approach (random mutagenesis) will led to identification of potential NTDs genes. Such a screen would be useful in expanding the collection of potential NTDs risk genes.

The approach for identifying positional candidate genes is through a genomic screen in which genetic markers at known locations are tested in families with two or more affected individuals. Thanks to advances in the density and polymorphisms of genetic markers, highthroughput genotyping methods, and powered statistical genetic linkage analysis, it is possible to perform large-scale investigation of human complex traits such as NTDs. Regions with excess sharing of alleles among affected individuals are considered region of interest and may harbour genes that predispose to NTDs. Few studies have performed genome-wide linkage studies in families with multi le affected individuals, given the scarcity of these large families. In fact, high morbidity and mortality rates associate with the disorder, and pregnancy termination after case identification are factors that limit the ascertainment of multiplex families. [20] A recent genomic screen was performed on 44 multiplex American NTDs families identifying linkage to chromosome 7 and 10. Two candidate genes (Meox2 and Twist1 ) were identified on chromosome 7 and three candidates (FGFR2, GFRA1, Pax2) were found on critical region of the chromosome 10. [21]

Statistical test are employed to assess evidence of allelic association for NTDs. Infact allelic association is population-specific. There are two methods of testing allelic association in NTDs candidate genes: case-control and family-based studies. Traditionally, NTDs studies have employed case-control studies, where the allelic frequency in an unrelated group of patients are comparated to a group of controls individuals. This study can be flawed, if the controls are not properly matched with patients for age, gender, and geographic origin. This population admixture may result in biased results and spurious associations. In family based studies, the frequencies of alleles transmitted by a parent to the affected child are compared with that of the allele not transmitted. The family studies can also detect a paternal or maternal effect. The most used family-based test is the Transmission disequilibrium test (TDT). [22] When one parent is not available for the analysis unaffected sibling can be used as controls. Association studies in patients with NTDs were often underpowered by a small sample size, leading to inconsistent results. Larger cohorts of patients and controls are needed to reach definitive conclusion regarding the role of the most of studied genes. Meta-analysis for variants of genes are also warrented.

## 4. Genetic variations in folate metabolism

A large number of experimental and observational clinical research studies over the past half century demonstrated that folic acid supplementation decreases both the occurrence and recurrence risk of NTDs by approximately 70%. [23-24] The recommended intakes are 4 mg/day for high risk women and 0.4 mg/day for all others. Maternal periconceptional folate supplementation may act to overcome insufficient maternal folate levels. However, in most cases, mothers of affected foetuses have either normal folate status or are, at most, mildly folate-deficient, arguing against maternal folate deficiency as a major causative factor. [25-26] Alternatively, it is postulated that supplemental folic acid may act to overcome an underlying defect in folate metabolism that results from a genetic mutation in the mother or in the foetus. Although a protective effect of folate is recognized, the mechanism by which some women develop low folate levels and predispose their offspring to NTDs and other congenital malformation is still debated.

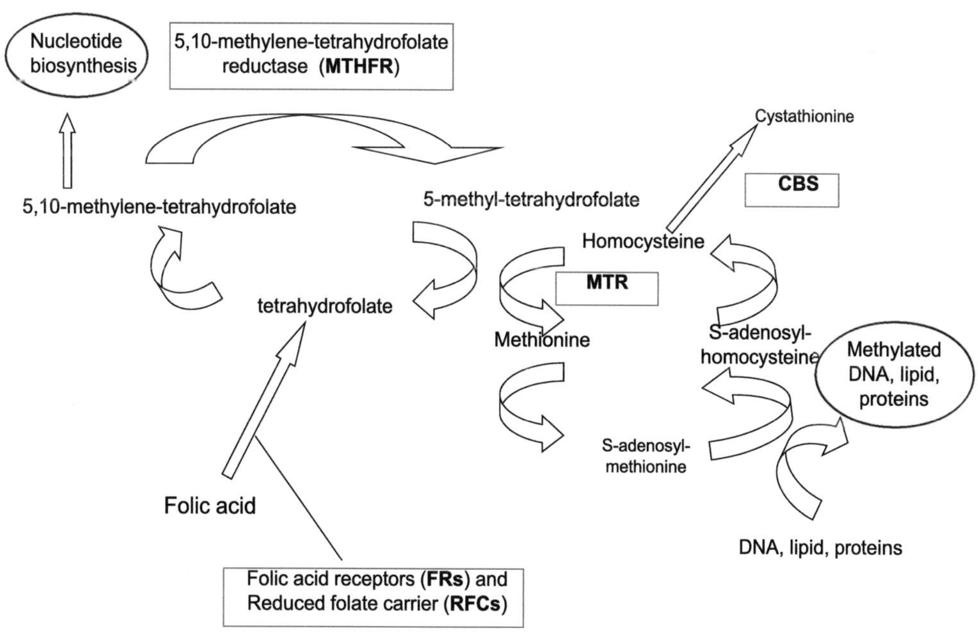


Fig. 1. Folate and homocysteine metabolism

Folic acid is a water soluble B vitamin that partecipates in transfer of single-carbon units in several critical pathways (Figure 1). These pathways include synthesis or catabolism of amino acids (serine, glycine, histidine, and methionine) and synthesis of nucleotides. Through their role in methionine synthesis, folates are also critical for the methylation cycle, since methionine is the methyl donor for many important methylation reactions, including DNA methylation. Folate-dependent conversion of homocysteine to methionine begins early in development in all tissues and provides a link between folate and homocysteine metabolism. An elevation of plasma homocysteine, mild hyperhomocysteinemia, has become recognized as a risk factor for NTDs [25, 27].

Proteins that mediate, or are functionally associated with, folate metabolism have provided candidates for genetic analysis in human NTDs. There are over 25 proteins involved in the folate and closed-related homocysteine pathways. Several of the corresponding genes have been examined as risk factors for NTDs, but few have showed a positive association (Table 1).

| Variant | Association with NTDs risk |
|---|---|
| MTHFR C677T | + |
| MTHFR A298C | +/- |
| MTHFR C116T | + (only in one study) |
| MTHFR G1793A | + (only in one study) |
| MTHFD1 G19658A | + |
| MTHHD1L 781-6823ATT(7-9) | + |
| MTR A2756G | - |
| MTRR A66G | + (in mothers with low levels of vitamin B12) |
| CBS 844ins68 | + |
| BHMT G742A | + |
| RFC-1 A80G | + |
| FR alpha/Betas | + |
| TCII A67G; G280A; A701G; C776G; C1043T; G1196A | + |
| GCPII C1561T | - |

Table 1. Variants of genes involved in folate and homocysteine metabolism studied for association with NTDs risk

Methylenetetrahydrofolate reductase (MTHFR) converts 5,10methyleneTHF to 5-mthylTHF, the methyl donor for homocysteine conversion to methionine. The 677C→T variant converts an alanine residue to a valine residue. Biochemical studied confirmed that this variant is characterized by residual activity after heating. [28] The variant is extremely common, with homozygosity frequencies ranging between 5% and 15% in many populations. [29] The association of the mutant 677T/T genotype with hyperhomocysteinemia occurs only in individuals with low folate status. Folate has been shown to stabilize the mutant human enzyme and should prevent hyperhomocysteinemia in mutant individuals [30]. The MTHFR 677T/T Homozygous mutant genotype first emerged as a possible risk factor for NTDs in some populations [31-33], even if other studies failed to demonstrate an association. [34-35] Two meta-analysis were performed in 1997 [36] and 2000 [29]. The latter study found a pooled odds ratio for cases 677T/T homozygous cases of 1.7 (95%CI 1.4-2.2), with a pooled attributable fraction of NTDs cases of 6%. A second mutation in the *MTHFR* gene

(1298A→C) has also been positively associated with NTDs [37-39]. The 1298 variant is in strong linkage disequilibrium with the 677 variant, such that 1298C and 677T changes are rarely seen on the same allele. Therefore, the two mutations can occur on separate alleles in the same individual who may be predisposed to hyperhomocysteinemia, if folate status is low. Compound heterozygosity for the 677T and 1298C alleles (677C/T/1298A/C) has been suggested to increase the risk, although the results have been conflicting. [37, 40-41] Moreover, a very recent report identified other two polymorphisms of *MTHFR* gene a 116C→T (P39P) and 1793G→A (R594Q). A possible association between NTDs cases and these two new polymorphisms was found; further analysis demonstrated that this association is driven by the linkage disequilibrium with the 677C→T NTD risk factor [42]. The MTHFR 677 variant has been suggested to account for approximately 10% of the NTDs risk. [29]. Since up to 70% of NTD cases may be prevented by the folate, other variants in folate-related genes have to be involved.

Given its important role in folate metabolism, the trifunctional enzyme methylenetetrahydrofolate dehydrogenase/methenyltetrahydrofolate cyclohydrolase/ formyltetrahydrofolate synthetase (*MTHFD1*) may play a role in NTD pathogenesis. Brody et al. demonstrated that the polymorphism 1958G→A (R653Q) within the *MTHFD1* gene resulting in the substitution of a conserved arginine by glutamine is a maternal risk factor for NTDs. [43] Mothers who possess two copies of the Q allele have an increased risk of an NTD-affected pregnancy. There was also a suggestion that the Q allele decreases fetal viability. Very recently, the impact of the *MTHFD1* 1958G>A polymorphism on NTD risk was elevaluated in the Italian population both by case-control and family-based studies. An increased risk was found for the heterozygous 1958G/A (OR=1.69; P=0.04) and homozygous 1958A/A (OR=1.91; P=0.02) genotypes in the children. The risk of an NTD-affected pregnancy of the mothers was increased 1.67-fold (P=0.04) only when a dominant effect (1958G/A or 1958A/A vs 1958G/G) of the 1958A allele was analysed. Family-based tests also confirmed a significant excess of transmission of the 1958A allele to affected individuals, demonstrating that this variant is a genetic risk factor for Italian NTD cases. [44] A potential role of the mitochondrial paralogue MTHFD1L as candidate gene for NTDs association has been also investigated. In particular, a common triallelic deletion/insertion variant 781-6823ATT(7-9) which influences splicing efficiency was tested and a significant incresead risk for allele 1 [ATT(7)] was identified. [45]

The methionine synthase (MTR), a vitamin $B_{12}$-dependent enzyme, utilizes 5-methyltetrahydrofolate, generated by MTHFR, for homocysteine remethylation to methionine. A polymorphism of the MTR gene, the 2756A→G (D919G) that lead to the substitution of an aspartic acid with a glycine residue, has been studied in several studies, but the majority have not reported a significant association [36, 40, 46-48].

A common variant in the gene methionine synthase reductases (MTRR), the 66A→G (I22M), that converts a isoleucine into a methionine residue, has been shown to confer a four-fold increased risk for NTDs in mothers having low vitamin $B_{12}$ levels [49]. Other studies have also suggested an effect on NTDs risk, both for mothers and children with 66GG mutant genotype, but interactions with nutrients has not been examined. [50-51]. The MTRR mutant genotype combined with MTHFR mutant genotype conferred a significant four-fold increased risk in children [49]. An interaction of MTR and MTRR genotypes has also recently reported. [50]

Cystathionine beta synthase (CBS) catalyzes the first step in the transsulfuration pathway of homocysteine. The 68-bp insertion in the exon 8 of the gene appeared to be associated with an increased risk in several studies. [46, 52-53]. Multiplicative interaction of the CBS 68-bp insertion with the homozygosity for the MTHFR 677C→T variant was showed to confer a five-fold increased risk for NTDs children, The MTHFR mutation alone had a two-fold increased risk, whereas there was no risk for CBS mutant genotype alone. [54].

Betaine homocysteine methyltransferase (BHMT) catalyzes homocysteine remethylation to methione, using betaine as the methyl donor. Homozygosity for the BHMT R239Q variant is associated with a decreased risk in mother and children [55]. The 80GG genotype for the 80A→G variant of the reduced folate carrier (RFC1), which transports 5-methyltetrahydrofolate across the plasma membrane, confers an increased risk for mothers with low red blood cell folate [55] and for children whose mothers do not use vitamins [56]. A recent study by Rothenberg et al. showed that some mothers with a NTDs-pregnancy produce autoantibodies that bind to folate receptors (FRs) on the placental membrane [57] The authors suggest that folate supplementation would bypass autoantibody formation that mediates the placental FRs blockage.

Several variants have been identified in trancobalamin II (*TCII*) gene (67A→G, 280G→A, 701A→G, 776C→G, 1043C→T, 1196G→A), but none of the SNPs were associated with a significant increased risk for NTD. Among them, three *TCII* SNPs (67A→G, 776C→G, 1196G→A) affected the transcobalamin concentration, even if these variants only partially accounted for the reduced proportion of vitamin $B_{12}$. [58].

The glutamate carboxypeptidase II (GCPII) is localized in the jejunum and catalyzes the conversion of folate polyglutamates to monoglutamates prior to absorption. The GCPII C1561T (H475Y) variant was identified and studied as risk factor for NTDs, but no study demonstrated an association. [59-60]

In general, there are many different polymorphism in genes invoved in folate transport or metabolism that have been identified and studied for association with NTDs risk, but data are not yet convincing for most of them. The only one well characterized genetic risk factor is the MTHFR C677T. Many studies are biased by small sample size and insufficient statistical power. The interaction between genes and non genetic factors is an intriguing area of investigation, but it requires larger cohort of patients and controls (Table 2).

| | |
|---|---|
| MS A2756G/MTHFR C677T | (Morrison et al., 1998) |
| MS A2756G/MTRR A66G | (Zhu et al., 2003) |
| MTRR A66G/MTHFR C677T | (Relton et al., 2004) |
| MTRR A66G/FGCP C1561T | (Relton et al., 2004) |
| MTRR A66G/MTHFD1 G1958A | (van der Put et al., 1997; Hol et al., 1998) |
| MTHFR A1298C/RFC-1 A80G | (DeMarco et al., 2003) |
| RFC-1 A80G/CBS 844ins68 | (Relton et al., 2004) |
| MTFR C677T/CBS 31 bp VNTR | (Afman et al., 2003) |
| MTHFR C677T/CBS 844ins68 | (Botto and Mastroiacovo 1998; de Franchis et al. 2002;Relton et al., 2004) |

Table 2. Gene-gene interactions between variants of genes involved in folate/homocysteine metabolism

## 5. From animal models to humans

Mouse mutant strains that exhibit NTDs have arisen by spontaneous mutations, or are the result of mutagen- and gene-trapped induced mutations. Other mutants have arisen through manipulation of an already identified and characterized gene that is manipulated to alter its function. The majority of the known mouse models are those generated by gene knock-out technology, that mainly develop cranial defects. [17, 61-62] The penetrance of NTDs in mouse models is frequently affected by both genetic background and environmental influences. Mouse mutant genes produce NTDs, for the most part, when they are homozygous. Mouse with double heterozygosity for two mutant genes also develop NTDs, demonstrating that gene-gene interaction may promote the development of NTDs. [63] A variety of exogenous agents when administrated to embryos exert teratogenic effects with production of abnormalities that include NTDs. Drugs, chemicals, or other substances extraneous to pregnancy cause NTDs. In addition, molecules derived from maternal metabolism, such those produced in maternal diseases condition, may induce NTDs. For example, elevated glucose and ketone body concentrations, as found in diabetes mellitus, increased the NTD risk. [64] Teratogens interact directly with genetic mutant effects in the causation of NTDs. The frequency of exencephaly in the *curly tail* strain is elevated by administration of all-trans retinoic acid. [65] This demonstrates that exogenous agents can exacerbating the severity of the phenotype interacting with a genetic mutation. An exogenous agent that ameliorates the genetic predisposition to NTDs in mouse models is a candidate therapeutic agent. Several NTDs mouse mutant, *Sp, Cart1, Cd, Splotch,* have shown to interact with folic acid, exhibiting a reduction of NTDs incidence. [66-68] But not all mouse models are folate responsive, demonstrating that there is a proportion of NTDs defects that require another preventive therapy. Inositol was shown preventive in folate-resistante mouse models, such as *curly tail* strain, an action that operates via stimulation of protein kinase C activity. [69]

Many of the genes that are mutated or disrupted in NTD mouse models are now being identified. Few genes have been identified as contributing to human NTD aetiology. Recently, animal models demonstrated an essential role of for the planar cell polarity (PCP) signaling pathway in the process of the convergent extension. Sistematic analysis of human homologues PCP genes is giving promising results for our understanding of molecular basis of human NTDs.

## 6. Genes of PCP pathway and NTDs

Several studies showed that early, during embryogenesis of CNS, the major driving force essential to the shaping of the neural plate is a process which is referred to as convergent extension (CE). This is a morphogenetic process by which cells elongate medio-laterally and intercalate with other neighboring cells forming a longer and narrower array. This changes lead to the conversion of an initially wide and short neural plate into a narrow and elongated one. [70] A crucial role in CE has been assigned to the Planar Cell Polarity (PCP) pathway, a highly conserved, non-canonical Wnt-frizzled-dishevelled signaling cascade (Figure 2). PCP signaling plays a key role in establishing and maintaining polarity in the plane of epithelia in Drosophila and in epithelial and non-epithelial tissues in vertebrates.

[71-72] Genetic studies of mutants affecting complex structures in the fly have identified a group of proteins referred to as "core PCP" components, that include transmembrane proteins such as Frizzled (Fz), Strabismus/Van Gogh (Stbm/Vang) and Flamingo (Fmi), as well as cytoplasmic proteins, including Dishevelled (Dsh/Dvl), Prickle (Pk), and Diego (Dgo). [73-74] Downstream of the core PCP members, additional factors mediate the PCP signaling in different tissues, the so-called "PCP effectors", that include the proteins Inturned, Fuzzy and Fritz. [75-77] Evidence for the involvement of the PCP pathway in CE process in vertebrate has emerged from studies of a wide range of mutants of orthologs of Drosophila PCP genes in several animal models such as zebrafish, Xenopus and mouse. [78-83] In mouse, *Loop-tail* (*Lp*) was the first mutant to implicate a role of PCP pathway and CE process in NTD pathogenesis. [84-85] *Lp* heterozygotes are characterized by a "looped" tail appearance, while homozygotes develop a severe NTD resembling human craniorachischisis. [86] NTD in *Lp* is caused by independent missense mutations S464N (*Lp*) and D255E (*Lpm1Jus*), localized in the proposed C-terminal cytoplasmic domain of a gene, now referred to as Van Gogh-like 2 (Vangl2). [84-85; 87] A novel experimentally induced allele, *Lp* (*m2Jus*), having a missense mutation, R259L, in Vangl2 has been recently reported. This mutation segregates in a recessive manner, with all heterozygotes appearing normal, and 47% of homozygotes showing a looped-tail. Homozygous *Lp* (*m2Jus*) embryos showed spina bifida in 12%. [88] Seven other mutant mice carrying mutations in some of PCP genes and fail to complete neural tube closure leading to craniorachischisis have been described; they include: *circle-tail* (*Crc*), *crash* (*Crsh*), *Ptk7*, and *dishevelled1*$^{-/-}$/*dishevelled2*$^{-/-}$ (*Dvl1*$^{-/-}$/*Dvl2*$^{-/-}$), *Frizzled3*$^{-/-}$/*Frizzled6*$^{-/-}$ (*Fzd3*$^{-/-}$/*Fzd6*$^{-/-}$), *dishevelled3/Lp* (Dvl3$^{+/-}$/*Lp*/+) double-knockout mice, and *Fuzzy*. [89-94] The *Crsh* mouse harbors a mutation in Celsr1 that encodes a protein orthologous to Drosophila Flamingo. [93] Like Vangl2, this gene functions in the PCP pathway. In the *Crc* mouse, a point mutation was identified introducing a stop codon into the apical cell polarity gene scribble (Scrb1), a PDZ domain-containing gene that is the ortholog of Drosophila scribble. [95] Scribble was not known, at a first time, to be a PCP component in Drosophila. However, a polarity defect is observed in the inner ear of the Crc mice, suggesting a role for Scrb1 in establishment of polarity in vertebrates. [96] A mutation in the protein tyrosine kinase 7 (Ptk7) gene, wich encodes a conserved transmembrane protein with tyrosine kinase homology, disrupts neural tube closure and stereociliary bundle orientation and shows genetic interaction with *Lp*. [93] Double null homozygous embryos for both dishevelled1 and dishevelled2 genes (*Dvl1*$^{-/-}$/*Dvl2*$^{-/-}$) as well as Frizzled3 and Frizzled6 genes (*Fzd3*$^{-/-}$/*Fzd6*$^{-/-}$), two members of highly homologous seven-pass receptor family, also exhibit NTDs that closely resemble the craniorachischisis observed in single knock-out mice. [91, 97] Although neurulation appeared normal in both Dvl3$^{-/-}$ and *LtapLp*/+ mutants, combined mutants Dvl3$^{+/-}$/*LtapLp*/+ displayed incomplete neural tube closure. [94] *Fuzzy* knockout mice exhibit both NTDs and defective primary cilia. [98] The exact mechanism by which the PCP pathway regulates CE cellular movements remains poorly understood. A recent study reported that PCP signalling was requested for re-establishing cell polarity that is transiently lost in dividing cells during neurulation. In fact, during mitosis, dividing cells loose their polarized features threatening the overall organization of the developing tissue; PCP signaling acts through quickly repolarization of the daughter cells and directs their integration into the neuroepithelium. [99] Evidence for an intrinsic role of ciliogenesis in PCP is derived from study of Bardet-Biedl syndrome

(BBS), a genetically heterogeneous human disorder with pleiotropic manifestations including obesity, polydactily, endocrine dysfunction, cystic renal disease, progressive photoreceptor degeneration and hearing loss. [100-101] BBS genes share the common features that the encoded proteins localized to the cilium or its cellular anchor, the basal body. [102] Targeted disruption of Bbs1, Bbs4 or Bbs6 in mouse lead to phenotype shared with PCP mutants, including NTDs (14% of Bbs4$^{-/-}$ mice display exencephaly) [103]. A second link between PCP and cilia has come from the identification of the mouse Inversin (Invs) gene, which encodes a large adaptor-like protein with homology to Drosophila PCP protein Diego. Recent studies in zebrafish and Xenopus embryos revealed that knock-down of Invs disrupts CE process. [104] The subcellular localization of inversin is complex and dynamic, and includes the basal bodies, primary cilia and, during metaphase and anaphase, the spindle poles. [105-107] A recent study in Xenopus demonstrated a link between ciliogenesis, Hedgehog signalling (HH) and PCP [108]. Disruption of orthologs of two Drosophila PCP effectors, Inturned (In) and Fuzzy (Fy), leads to failure of ciliogenesis, resulting from incorrect orientation of ciliary microtubules. In Xenopus, the absence of In and Fy elicited prominent rostral NTDs in addition to more caudal NTDs, predicted to result from disruption of PCP signalling. These caudal defects were shown to arise from failure of CE in the neural plate, whereas the rostral defects were shown to stem from a failure of Hedgehog signalling. [108]. Finally, it is tempting to speculate that both PCP and Hedgehog phenotypes may be linked in humans to NTDs. Mutations in two genes, MKS1 and MKS3, that were predicted to be involved in cilia formation have been recently found in patients with Meckel syndrome (MKS), characterized by bilateral renal cystic dysplasia, central nervous system malformations, bilateral upper and lower limb polydactyly and fibrocystic changes of the liver. [109-112]. The gene mutated in type 1 MKS encodes a protein associated with the base of the cilium in vertebrates and nematodes. Loss of function of mouse Mks1 results in an accurate model of human MKS, with structural abnormalities in the neural tube, biliary duct, limb patterning, bone development and the kidney that mirror the human syndrome. Analysis of patterning in the neural tube and the limb demonstrates altered Hedgehog pathway signaling underlies some MKS defects.[113]

## 7. PCP pathway and human NTDs

In humans mutations in VANGL1 and VANGL2 genes cause NTDs and abrogate the physical interaction between VANGL proteins and other members of PCP pathway. In a first study three Italian patients who were heterozygotes for missense mutations of VANGL1 (V239I, R274Q, and M328T) were identified. The V239I mutation was identified in a girl with a severe form of caudal regression The girl's mother also carried the mutation, but showed no clinical signs of NTDs. Her brother having a milder form of the disorder, a dermal sinus, also carried the V239I mutation. The V239I mutation was absent in the father, in the maternal aunt and in the maternal grandparents, indicating that it had arisen *de novo* in the germline of one of the maternal grandparents or somatically in the mother, with subsequent transmission through the mother's germline. Valine at position 239 is located in the fourth predicted transmembrane domain of the VANGL1 protein. It is invariant and part of a 'VLLE' motif, which is conserved across all known VANGL proteins. In vitro studies demonstrated that V239I mutation abrogated interaction between VANGL1 and their binding partners, Dvl1, Dvl2, and Dvl3. The R274Q mutation was found in a girl with myelomeningocele. Her mother, who carried the R274Q mutation, and maternal aunt had vertebral schisis, a minimal sign of NTD. Arg274 is in the cytoplasmic domain of VANGL1 and is invariant in all known orthologs except in C. elegans, in which it is replaced by glutamate. The M328T mutation was carried by a child with myelomeningocele, hydrocephalus, and Chiari II malformation. M328T mutation occurs in the predicted cytoplasmic domain of VANGL1. We did not detect these variants in 150 ancestrally matched controls. Thus, these are the first genetic mutations clearly linked to NTDs such as spina bifida in humans. [114].

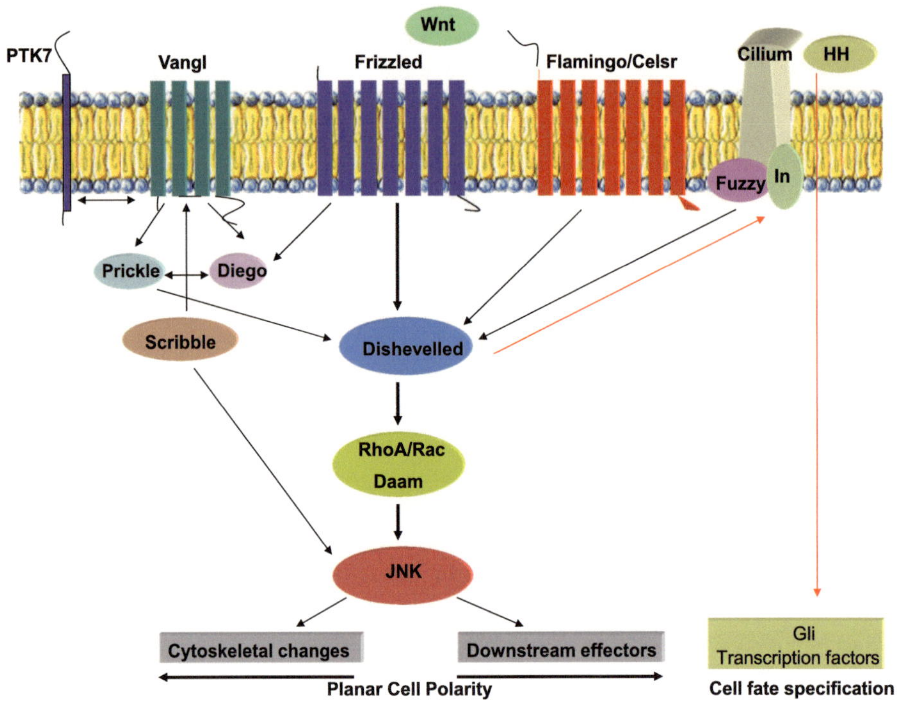


Fig. 2. Planar Cell Polarity (PCP) pathway.

Wnt proteins bind to its receptors, Frizzled (Fz), leading to recruitment and activation of Dishevelled, that is a multimodule protein PCP activation requires formation of a multimodule protein-complex including two transmembrane proteins, Vangl (1/2) and Flamingo/Celsr, and three cytoplasmic proteins, Dishevelled, Diego and Prickle. These proteins acquire an asymmetric localization at the plasma membrane that is crucial for proper PCP signaling. Scribble is a cytoplasmic protein binds to and genetically interacts with Vangl, suggesting a role in PCP signaling. Ptk7 receptor is a regulator and shows genetic interaction with Vangl. Downstream effectors include small GTPases Rho or Rac, which are active when bound to GTP. The Formin homology protein, Daam1, as an important link between Dishevelled and the Rho GTPase for cytoskeletal modulation. Alternatively, Dvl can initiate Rac signaling and its downstream effector c-Jun N-terminal kinase (JNK) that promote sites of actin polymerization modulating lamellipodia extension. Inturned (In) and Fuzzy that are down-stream regulator of PCP pathway do influence convergent extension and they also are broadly required for Hedgehog (HH) signaling

Validation of the potential pathogenic effect of VANGL1 V239I, M328T, and R274Q mutations *in vivo* was performed by investigating their effect on CE in zebrafish. Knocking down the expression of tri, the ortholog of Vangl2, using an antisense morpholino (MO), led to a defective CE manifested by a shortened body axis and widened somites. Co-injection of the human VANGL1 with the tri-MO was able to partially rescue the tri-MO induced phenotype in zebrafish. In contrast, co-injection of V239I and M328T, failed to rescue this phenotype. Overexpression studies evaluating the ability of the human VANGL1 alleles to induce a CE phenotype when injected at high doses in zebrafish embryos have been carried out. While overexpressing the wild-type allele led to a severely defective CE, overexpression of either V239I and M328T variants failed to do so. Thus, results from both tri-MO knockdown/rescue results and overexpression assays suggest that these two variants most likely represent "loss-of-function" alleles that affect protein function during embryonic development. [115].

Overall, human VANGL1 gene has been sequenced in a cohort of 810 NTD patients with various ethnic origin. Eight missense mutations both in familial (V239I, R274Q, S83L, and R181E) and sporadic (M238T, F153S, L202F, and A404S) cases have been identified. These mutations affect evolutionary conserved amino residues that are distributed along the entire length of the VANGL1 protein. Since these many of these variants do not represent obvious null mutations (like stop codon, deletions), functional experiments are needed to investigate their effect on the protein function. All mutations detected so far in VANGL1 in NTDs are heterozygous, leading to the speculation that these variants may act as partial loss of function alleles and interact with other environmental and genetic factors to cause the NTD phenotype. The finding of VANGL1 mutations in both open and closed NTDs support this hypothesis of common underlying molecular mechanisms. [116]

Sequencing of *VANGL2* in the same cohort of patients led to the identification of six novel heterozygous missense mutations in seven patients, that could be pathogenic based on genetic and initial validation data [117]. Four of these mutations, R135W, R177H, L242V, R270H, were predicted to be damaging to protein function using bioinformatics' tools, and two others, T247M and R482H, affect highly conserved residues across evolution. Five mutations were identified in patients affected with closed spinal NTDs, suggesting that VANGL2 mutations may predispose to NTDs is approximately 2.5% of closed spinal NTDs. A Chinese study recently reported the identification of three other missense mutations in VANGL2 in fetuses with a cranial NTDs: S84F, R353C , and F437S. [118]

Recently, three non-synonymous Fuzzy amino acid substitutions in some patients with NTDs have been identified, resulting in alteration of the length of primary cilia and cell movement. Since Fuzzy knockout mice exhibit both NTDs and defective primary cilia and Fuzzy is expressed in the emerging neural tube, mutations in Fuzzy may account for a subset of NTDs in humans. [98]

Thus, the evidence is accumulating for an important contribution of PCP genes to the pathogenesis of human NTDs, necessitating a detailed analysis of other not yet explored PCP genes in large cohorts of patients.

## 8. Conclusions

NTDs are a group of severe congenital malformations having a profound physical, emotional, and financial effects on families and communities. Despite their importance in terms both of human suffering and cost to the health care system, the causes of most cases of NTDs are not known. There is growing evidence that many NTDs have a genetic background. Elucidation of genetic causes predisposing to NTDs are important challenge in light of preconception care program that aim to reduce reproductive risks before conception and to improve the chance for a healthy birth outcome. Further, the genetic screening done for research setting may become available for diagnostic purposes, allowing to identify the predisposition before conception and to provide reproductive options to minimize the chance of having affected children in the future.

## 9. References

[1] EUROCAT Working Group: Surveillance of Congenital anomalies in Europe 1980-1999. 2002. EUROCAT, University of Ulster, Report No.: 8.

[2] Busby A, Abramsky L, Dolk H, Armstrong B, Addor MC, Anneren G, Armstrong N, Baguette A, Barisic I, Berghold A, Bianca S, Braz P, Calzolari E, Christiansen M, Cocchi G, Daltveit AK, De Walle H, Edwards G, Gatt M, Gener B, Gillerot Y, Gjergja R, Goujard J, Haeusler M, Latos-Bielenska A, McDonnell R, Neville A, Olars B, Portillo I, Ritvanen A, Robert-Gnansia E, Rösch C, Scarano G, Steinbicker V. 2005. Preventing neural tube defects in Europe: a missed opportunity. Repro Toxic 20 (3): 393-402.

[3] Schoenwolf GC, Smith JL. 2000. Mechanisms of neurulation. Methods Mol Biol 136 125-134.

[4] Catala M. Genetic control of caudal development. 2002. Clin Genet 61: 89-96.

[5] Colas J.F. and Schoenwolf. 2001. Towards a cellular and molecular understanding of neurulation. Dev Dyn 221, 117-145.

[6] Copp AJ, Greene ND, Murdoch JN: 2003. The genetic basis of mammalian neurulation. Nat Rev genet 4: 784-793.

[7] van Allen MI, Kalousek DK, Chernoff GF, Juroff D, Harris M, McGillivray BC, Young S-L, Langlois S, MacLeod PM, Chitayat D, et al.. 1993. Evidence for multi-site closure of the neural tube in humans. Am J Med Genet 47, 723-743.

[8] Botto LD, Moore CA, Khoury MJ, Erickson JD. 1999. Neural-tube defects. New England Journal of Medicine 341: 1509-1519.

[9] Rossi A, Cama A, Piatelli G, Ravegnani M, Biancheri R, Tortori-Donati P. 2004. Spinal dysraphism: MR imaging rationale. J Neuroradiol 31: 3-24.

[10] O'Reilly GC, Shields LE. Karyotyping for isolated neural tube defects.2000. A report of two cases. J Reprod Med 45:950-952.

[11] Elwood JM, Little J, Elwood JH. 1992. Epidemiology and control of neural tube defects. Oxford:Oxford University Press.

[12] Fuhrmann W, Seeger W, Böhm R. 1971. Apparently monogenic inheritance of anencephaly and spina bifida in a kindred. Hum Genet 13(3) :241-243.

[13] Partington MD, McLone DG. 1995. Hereditary factors in the etiology of neural tube defects. Results of a survey. Pediatr Neurosurg. 23(6): 311-316.

[14] Toriello HV, Higgins JV. 1985. Possible causal heterogeneity in spina bifida cystica. Am J Med Genet. 21(1): 13-20.

[15] Garabedian BH, Fraser FC. 1993. Upper and lower neural tube defects: an alternate hypothesis. J Med Genet 30(10): 849-51.
[16] Byrne J, Carolan S. 2006. Adverse reproductive outcomes among pregnancies of aunts and (spouses of) uncles in Irish families with neural tube defects. Am J Med Genet A 140(1):52-61.
[17] Juriloff DM, Harris MJ. 2000. Mouse models for neural tube closure defects. Hum Mol Genet. 19(6): 993-1000.
[18] Udvadia AJ, Linney E. 2003. Windows into development: historic, current, and future perspectives on transgenic zebrafish. Dev Biol 256(1):1-17.
[19] Wienholds E, Schulte-Merker S, Walderich B, Plasterk RH. 2002. Target-selected inactivation of the zebrafish rag1 gene. Science 297:99-102.
[20] Sebold CD, Melvin EC, Siegel D, Mehltretter L, Enterline DS, Nye JS, Kessler J, Bassuk A, Speer MC, George TM; NTD Collaborative Group. 2005. Recurrence risks for neural tube defects in siblings of patients with lipomyelomeningocele.Genet Med 7(1):64-67.
[21] Rampersaud E, Bassuk AG, Enterline DS, George TM, Siegel DG, Melvin EC, Aben J, Allen J, Aylsworth A, Brei T, Bodurtha J, Buran C, Floyd LE, Hammock P, Iskandar B, Ito J, Kessler JA, Lasarsky N, Mack P, Mackey J, McLone D, Meeropol E, Mehltretter L, Mitchell LE, Oakes WJ, Nye JS, Powell C, Sawin K, Stevenson R, Walker M, West SG, Worley G, Gilbert JR, Speer MC. 2005. Whole genomewide linkage screen for neural tube defects reveals regions of interest on chromosomes 7 and 10. J Med Genet 42(12):940-946.
[22] Spielman RS, McGinnis RE, Ewens WJ. 1993. Transmission test for linkage disequilibrium: the insulin gene region and insulin-dependent diabetes mellitus (IDDM). Am J Hum Genet 52(3):506-16.
[23] MRC Vitamin Study Group. 1991. Prevention of neural tube defects: results of the Medical Research Council Vitamin Study. MRC Vitamin Study research Group. Lancet 338, 131-137.
[24] Czeizel AE, Dudas I .1992. Prevention of the first occurence of neural-tube defects by periconceptional vitamin supllementation. N Engl J Med 327, 1832-1835.
[25] Mills JL, Scott JM, Kirke PN, McPartlin JM, Conley MR, Weir DG, Molloy AM, Lee YJ. 1996. Homocysteine and neural tube defects. J Nutr 126(3):756S-760S.
[26] Scott JM. 1999. Folate and vitamin B12 Proc Nutr Soc58(2):441-448.
[27] Steegers-Theunissen RP, Boers GH, Trijbels FJ, Finkelstein JD, Blom HJ, Thomas CM, Borm GF, Wouters MG, Eskes TK. 1994. Maternal hyperhomocysteinemia: a risk factor for neural-tube defects? Metabolism ;43(12):1475-80.
[28] Frost P, Blom HJ, Milos R et al. 1995. A candidate genetic risk factor for vascular disease: a common mutation in methylenetetrahydrofolate reductase. Nature Genet 10: 111–113.
[29] Botto LD, Yang Q. 2000. 5,10-Methylenetetrahydrofolate reductase gene variants and congenital anomalies: a HuGE review. Am J Epidemiol. 151: 862-877.
[30] Malinow MR, Nieto FJ, Kruger WD, Duell PB, Hess DL, Gluckman RA, Block PC, Holzgang CR, Anderson PH, Seltzer D, Upson B, Lin QR. 1997. The effects of folic acid supplementation on plasma total homocysteine are modulated by

multivitamin use and methylenetetrahydrofolate reductase genotypes. Arterioscler Thromb Vasc Biol 17(6):1157-1162.

[31] Van der Put NM, Steegers-Theunissen RP, Frosst P, Trijbels FJ, Eskes TK, van den Heuvel LP, Mariman EC, den Heyer M, Rozen R, Blom HJ. 1995. Mutated methylenetetrahydrofolate reductase as risk factor for spina bifida. Lancet 346:1070-1071.

[32] Ou CY, Stevenson RE, Brown VK, Schwart CE, Allen WP, Khoury MJ, Rozen R, Oakley GP, Adams MJ. 1996. Methylenetetrahydrofolate reductase genetic polymorphism as a risk factor for neural tube defects. Am J Med Genet 63: 610-614.

[33] Christensen B, Arbour L, Tran P, Leclerc D, Sabbaghian N, Platt R, Gilfix BM, Rosenblatt DS, Gravel RA, Forbes P, Rozen R. 1999. Genetic polymorphisms in methylenetetrahydrofolate reductase and methionine synthase, folate levels in red blood cells, and risk of neural tube defects. Am J Med Genet 84: 151-157.

[34] Koch MC, Stegmann K, Ziegler A, Schroter B, Ermert A. 1998. Evaluation of the MTHFR C677T allele and the MTHFR gene locus in a German spina bifida population. Eur J Pediatr 157: 487-492.

[35] Gonzales-Herrera L, Garcia-Escalante G, Castillo-Zapata I, Canto-Herrera J, Caballos-Quintal J, Pinto-Escalante D, Diaz-Rubio F, Del Angel RM, Orozco-Orozco L. 2002. Frequency of the thermolabile vatiant C677T in the MTHFR gene and lack of association with neural tube defects in the State of Yucatan, Mexico. Clin Genet 62: 394-398.

[36] van der Put NM, Eskes TK, Blom HJ. 1997. Is the common 677C-->T mutation in the methylenetetrahydrofolate reductase gene a risk factor for neural tube defects? A meta-analysis. QJM. 90(2):111-115.

[37] van der Put NM., Gabreels F, Stevens EM., Smeitink JA, Trijbels FJ, Eskes TK, van den Heuvel LP, Blom H.J. 1998. A second common mutation in the methylenetetrahydrofolate reductase gene: an additional risk factor for neural-tube defects? Am J Hum Genet 62: 1044-1051.

[38] Weisberg I, Tran P, Christensen B, Sibani S, Rozen R. 1998. A second genetic polymorphism in methylenetetrahydrofolate reductase (MTHFR) associated with decreased enzyme activity. Mol Genet Metab 64: 169-172.

[39] De Marco P, Calevo MG, Moroni A, Arata L, Merello E, Finnell RH, Zhu H., Andreussi L, Cama A, Capra V. 2002. Study of MTHFR and MS polymorphisms as risk factors for NTD in the Italian population. J Hum Genet 47: 319-324.

[40] Trembath D, Sherbondy AL, Vandyke DC, Shaw GM, Todoroff K, Lammer EJ, Finnell RH, Marker S, Lerner G, Murray JC. 1999. Analysis of select folate pathway genes, PAX3, and human T in a Midwestern neural tube defect population. Teratology 59(5):331-341.

[41] Richter B, Stegmann K, Röper B, Böddeker I, Ngo ET, Koch MC. 2001. Interaction of folate and homocysteine pathway genotypes evaluated in susceptibility to neural tube defects (NTD) in a German population. J Hum Genet 46(3):105-109.

[42] O'Leary VB, Mills JL, Parle-McDermott A, Pangilinan F, Molly AM, Cox C, Weiler A, Conley M, Kirke PN, Scott JM, Brody LC. 2005. Screening for new MTHFR polymorphisms and NTD risk. Am J Med Genet 138: 99-106.

[43] Brody LC, Conley M, Cox C, Kirke PN, McKeever MP, Mills JL, Molloy AM, O'Leary VB, Parle-McDermott A, Scott JM, Swanson DA. 2002. A polymorphism, R653Q, in the trifunctional enzyme methylenetetrahydrofolate dehydrogenase/ methenyltetrahydrofolate cyclohydrolase/formyltetrahydrofolate synthetase is a maternal genetic risk factor for neural tube defects: report of the Birth Defects Research Group. Am J Hum Genet 71:1207-1215.
[44] De Marco P, Merello E, Calevo MG, Mascelli S, Raso A, Cama A, Capra V. 2006. Evaluation of methylenetetrhydrofolate-dehydrogenase 1958G>A polymorphism for neural tube defect risk. J Hum Genet 51: 98-103.
[45] Pearle-McDermott A, Pangilinan F, O'Brien KK, Mills JL, Magee AM, Troendle J, Sutton M, Scott JM, Kirke PN, Molloy AM, Brody LC. 2009. A common variant in MTHFD1L is associated with neural tube defects and mRNA splicing efficiency. Hum Mutat 30(12): 1650-1656.
[46] Morrison K, Papapetrou C, Hol FA, Mariman EC, Lynch SA, Burn J, Edwards YH. 1998. Susceptibility to spina bifida; an association study of five candidate genes. Ann Hum Genet 62: 379-396.
[47] Brody LC, Baker PJ, Chines PS, Musick A, Molloy AM, Swanson DA, Kirke PN, Ghosh S, Scott JM, Mills JL. 1999. Methionine synthase: high-resolution mapping of the human gene and evaluation as a candidate locus for neural tube defects. Mol Genet Metab 1999 67(4):324-333.
[48] Johanning GL, Tamura T, Johnston KE, Wenstrom KD. Comorbidity of 5,10-methylenetetrahydrofolate reductase and methionine synthase gene polymorphisms and risk for neural tube defects. 2000. J Med Genet 37(12):949-951.
[49] Wilson A, Platt R, Wu Q, Leclerc D, Christensen B, Yang H, Gravel RA, Rozen R. A common variant in methionine synthase reductase combined with low cobalamin (vitamin B12) increases risk for spina bifida. 1999. Mol Genet Metab 67(4):317-323.
[50] Zhu H, Wicker NJ, Shaw GM, Lammer EJ, Hendricks K, Suarez L, Canfield M, Finnell RH. 2003. Homocysteine remethylation enzyme polymorphisms and increased risks for neural tube defects. Mol Genet Metab 78(3):216-221.
[51] Guéant-Rodriguez RM, Rendeli C, Namour B, Venuti L, Romano A, Anello G, Bosco P, Debard R, Gérard P, Viola M, Salvaggio E, Guéant JL. 2003. Transcobalamin and methionine synthase reductase mutated polymorphisms aggravate the risk of neural tube defects in humans. Neurosci Lett 344(3):189-192.
[52] Ramsbottom D, Scott JM, Molloy A, Weir DG, Kirke PN, Mills JL, Gallagher PM, Whitehead AS. 1997. Are common mutations of cystathionine beta-synthase involved in the aetiology of neural tube defects? Clin Genet 51(1):39-42.
[53] Speer MC, Nye J, McLone D, Worley G, Melvin EC, Viles KD, Franklin A, Drake C, Mackey J, George TM. 1999. Possible interaction of genotypes at cystathionine beta-synthase and methylenetetrahydrofolate reductase (MTHFR) in neural tube defects. NTD Collaborative Group.Clin Genet 56(2):142-144.
[54] Botto LD, Mastroiacovo P. 1998. Exploring gene-gene interactions in the etiology of neural tube defects. Clin Genet 53(6):456-459.

[55] Morin I, Platt R, Weisberg I, Sabbaghian N, Wu Q, Garrow TA, Rozen R. 2003. Common variant in betaine-homocysteine methyltransferase (BHMT) and risk for spina bifida. Am J Med Genet A119A(2):172-176.
[56] Shaw GM, Lammer EJ, Zhu H, Baker MW, Neri E, Finnell RH. 2002. Maternal periconceptional vitamin use, genetic variation of infant reduced folate carrier (A80G), and risk of spina bifida. Am J Med Genet 108(1):1-6.
[57] Rothenberg SP, da Costa MP, Sequeira JM, Cracco J, Roberts JL, Weedon J, Quadros EV. 2004. Autoantibodies against folate receptors in women with a pregnancy complicated by a neural-tube defect. N Engl J Med. 350(2):134-142.
[58] Afman LA, Van Der Put NM, Thomas CM, Trijbels JM, Blom HJ. 2001. Reduced vitamin B12 binding by transcobalamin II increases the risk of neural tube defects. QJM 94(3):159-166.
[59] Vieira AR, Trembath D, Vandyke DC, Murray JC, Marker S, Lerner G, Bonner E, Speer M. 2002. Studies with His475Tyr glutamate carboxipeptidase II polymorphism and neural tube defects. Am J Med Genet 111(2):218-219.
[60] Afman LA, Trijbels FJ, Blom HJ. 2003. The H475Y polymorphism in the glutamate carboxypeptidase II gene increases plasma folate without affecting the risk for neural tube defects in humans. J Nutr 133(1):75-77.
[61] Juriloff DM, Harris MJ. 2000.Mouse models for neural tube closure defects. Hum Mol Genet 9(6):993-1000.
[62] Harris MJ, Juriloff DM. 2007. Mouse mutants with neural tube closure defects and their role in understanding human neural tube defects. Birth Defects Res A Clin Mol Teratol 79(3):187-210.
[63] Estibeiro JP, Brook FA, Copp AJ. 1993. Interaction between splotch (Sp) and curly tail (ct) mouse mutants in the embryonic development of neural tube defects. Development 119(1):113-121.
[64] Sadler TW, Hunter ES 3rd, Wynn RE, Phillips LS. 1989. Evidence for multifactorial origin of diabetes-induced embryopathies. Diabetes 38(1):70-74.
[65] Tom C, Juriloff DM, Harris MJ. 1991. Studies of the effect of retinoic acid on anterior neural tube closure in mice genetically liable to exencephaly. Teratology 43(1):27-40.
[66] Zhao Q, Behringer RR, de Crombrugghe B. 1996. Prenatal folic acid treatment suppresses acrania and meroanencephaly in mice mutant for the Cart1 homeobox gene. Nat Genet13(3):275-283.
[67] Fleming A, Copp AJ. 1998. Embryonic folate metabolism and mouse neural tube defects. Science 280(5372):2107-2109.
[68] Gefrides LA, Bennett GD, Finnell RH. 2002. Effects of folate supplementation on the risk of spontaneous and induced neural tube defects in Splotch mice. Teratology 65(2):63-69.
[69] Greene ND, Copp AJ. 1997. Inositol prevents folate-resistant neural tube defects in the mouse. Nat Med 3(1):60-66.
[70] Wallingford JB, Harland RM. 2002. Neural tube closure requires Dishevelled-dependent convergent extension of the midline. Development 129, 5815-5825.

[71] Strutt D. 2003. Frizzled signalling and cell polarisation in Drosophila and vertebrates. Development 130:4501-4513.
[72] Klein TJ, Mlodzik M. 2005. Planar cell polarization: an emerging model points in the right direction. Annu Cell Dev Biol 21: 155-176.
[73] Jenny A, Mlodzik M. 2006. Planar cell polarity signaling: a common mechanism for cellular polarization. Mt Sinai J Med 73:738-750.
[74] Jones C, Chen P. 2007. Planar cell polarity signaling in vertebrates. Bioessays 29 (2):120-32.
[75] Adler PN. 2002. Planar signaling and morphogenesis in Drosophila. Dev Cell 2:525-535.
[76] Adler PN, Zhu CM, Stone D. 2004. Inturned localizes to the proximal side of wing cells under the instruction of upstream planar polarity proteins. Current Biology 14: 2046-2051.
[77] Collier S, Lee H, Burgess R, Adler P. 2005. 40 repeat protein fritz links cytoskeletal planar polarity to frizzled subcellular localization in the drosophila epidermis. Genetics 169: 2035-2045.
[78] Wallingford JB. 2005. Neural tube closure and neural tube defects: studies in animal models reveal known knowns and known unknowns. Am J Med Genet C Semin Med Genet 135:59-68.
[79] Barrow JR. 2006. Wnt/PCP signaling: a veritable polar star in establishing patterns of polarity in embryonic tissues. Semin cell Dev Biol 17 (2): 185-93.
[80] Montcouquiol M, Crenshaw EB III, Kelley MW. 2006. Noncanonical Wnt signaling and neural polarity. Annu Rev Neurosci 29:363-386.
[81] Wallingford JB, Rowning BA, Vogeli KM. 2000. Dishevelled controls cell polarity during Xenopus gastrulation. Nature 405:81-85.
[82] Tada M, Smith JC. 2000. Xwnt11 is a target of Xenopus Brachyury: regulation of gastrulation movements via Dishevelled, but not through the canonical Wnt pathway. Development 127: 2227-2238
[83] Heisenberg CP, Tada M, Rauch GJ, Saude L, Concha ML, Geisler R, Stemple DL, Smith JC, and Wilson SW. 2000. Silberblick/Wnt11 mediates convergent extension movements during zebrafish gastrulation. Nature 405: 76-81
[84] Kibar Z, Vogan KJ, Groulx N, Groulx N, Justice MJ, Underhill DA, Gros P. 2001. Ltap, a mammalian homolog of Drosophila Strabismus/Van Gogh, is altered in the mouse neural tube mutant Loop-tail. Nat Genet 28:251-255.
[85] Murdoch JN, Doudney K, Paternotte C, Copp AJ, Stenier P. 2001. Severe neural tube defects in the loop-tail mouse result from mutation of Lpp1, a novel gene involved in floor plate specification. Hum Mol Genet 10: 2593-2601.
[86] Stein K, Rudin IA. 1953. Development of mice homozygous for the gene for looped-tail. J hered 44: 59-69.
[87] Kibar Z, Underhill DA, Canonne-Hergaux F, Gauthier S, Justice MJ, Gros P. 2001. Identification of a new chemically induced allele (Lp(m1Jus)) at the loop-tail locus: morphology, histology, and genetic mapping. Genomics 72:331-337.

[88] Guyot MC, Bosoi CM, Kharfallah F, Reynolds A, Drapeau P, Justice M, Gros P, Kibar Z. 2011. A novel hypomorphic Looptail allele at the planar cell polarity Vangl2 gene. Dev Dyn. 2011 240(4):839-849
[89] Smith LJ and Stein JK. 1962. Axial elongation in the mouse and its retardation in homozygous loop tail mice. J mbryol Exp Morphol 10: 73-87.
[90] Murdoch JN, Rachel RA, Shah S, Beermann F, Stanier P, Mason Ca, Copp AJ. 2001. Circletail, a new mouse mutant with severe neural tube defects: chromosomal localization and interaction with the loop-tail mutation. Genomics 78:55-63.
[91] Hamblet NS, Lijam N, Ruiz-Lozano P. 2002. Dishevelled 2 is essential for cardiac outflow tract development, somite segmentation and neural tube closure. Development 129:5827-5838
[92] Curtin JA, Quint E, Tsipouri V, Arkell RM, Cattanach B, Copp AJ, Henderson DJ, Spurr N, Stanier P, Fisher EM, Nolan PM, Steel KP, Brown SD, Gray IC, Murdoch JN. 2003. Mutation of Celsr1 disrupts planar polarity of inner ear hair cells and causes severe neural tube defects in the mouse. Curr Biol 13:1129-1133.
[93] Lu X, Borchers AG, Jolicoeur C, Rayburn H, Baker JC, Tessier-Lavigne M. 2004. PTK7/CCK-4 is a novel regulator of planar cell polarity in vertebrates. Nature 430: 93-98.
[94] Etheridge SL, Ray S, Li S, Hamblet NS, Lijam N, Tsang M, Greer J, Kardos N, Wang J, Sussman DJ, Chen P, Wynshaw-Boris A. 2008. Murine dishevelled 3 functions in redundant pathways with dishevelled 1 and 2 in normal cardiac outflow tract, cochlea, and neural tube development. PLoS Genet 4(11):e1000259.
[95] Murdoch JN, Henderson DJ, Doudney K, Gaston-Massuet C, Philipps HM, Paternotte C, Arkell R, Stanier P, Copp AJ. 2003. Disruption of scribble (Scrb1) causes severe neural tube defects in the circletail mouse. Hum Mol Genet 12:87-98.
[96] Montcouquiol M, Rachel RA, Lanford PJ, Copeland NG, jenkins NA, Kelley MW. 2003. Identification of Vangl2 and Scrb1 as planar polarity genes in mammals. Nature 423:173-177.
[97] Wang Y, Guo N, Nathans J. 2006. The role of Frizzled3 and Frizzled6 in neural tube closure and in the planar polarity of inner-ear sensory hair cells. J Neurosci 26:2147-2156.
[98] Seo JH, Zilber Y, Babayeva S, Liu J, Kyriakopoulos P, De Marco P, Merello E, Capra V, Gros P, Torban E. 2011. Mutations in the planar cell polarity gene, Fuzzy, are associated with neural tube defects in humans. Hum Mol Genet. 2011 Aug 25.
[99] Ciruna B, Jenny A, Lee D, Mlodzik M, Schier AF. 2006. Planar cell polarity signalling couples cell division and morphogenesis during neurulation. Nature 439:220-224.
[100] Bisgrove BW, Yost HJ. 2006. The roles of cilia in developmental disorders and disease. Development 133: 4131-4143.
[101] Davis EE, Brueckner M, Katsanis N. 2006. The emerging complexity of the vertebrate cilium: New functional roles for an ancient organelle. Developmental Cell 11: 9-19.
[102] Ansley SJ, Badano JL, Blacque OE, Hill J, Hoskins BE, Leitch CC, Kim JC, Ross AJ, Eichers ER, Teslovich TM, Mah AK, Johnsen RC, Cavender JC, Lewis RA, Leroux MR, Beales PL, and Katsanis N. 2003. Basal body dysfunction is a likely cause of pleiotropic Bardet-Biedl syndrome. Nature 425: 628-633.

[103] Ross AJ, May-Simera H, Eichers ER, Kai M, Hill J, Jagger D J, Leitch CC, Chapple JP, Munro PM, Fisher S, Tan PL, Phillips HM, Leroux MR, Henderson DJ, Murdoch JN, Copp AJ, Eliot MM, Lupski JR, Kemp DT, Dollfus H, Tada M, Katsanis N, forge A, Bales PL. 2005. Disruption of Bardet-Biedl syndrome ciliary proteins perturbs planar cell polarity in vertebrates. Nature Genet 37: 1135-1140.

[104] Simons M, Gloy J, Ganner A, Bullerkotte A, Bashkurov M, Kronig C, Schermer B, Benzing T, Cabello OA, Jenny A, Mlodzik M, Polok B, Driever W, Obara T, Walz G. 2005. Inversin, the gene product mutated in nephronophthisis type II, functions as a molecular switch between Wnt signaling pathways. Nat Genet 37:537-543

[105] Morgan D, Goodship J, Essner JJ, Vogan KJ, Turnpenny L, Yost HJ, Tabin CJ, Strachan T. 2002. The left-right determinant inversin has highly conserved ankyrin repeat and IQ domains and interacts with calmodulin. Human Genetics 110: 377-384.

[106] Watanabe D, Saijoh Y, Nonaka S, Sasaki G, Ikawa Y, Yokoyama T, Hamada H. 2003. The left-right determinant Inversin is a component of node monocilia and other 9+0 cilia. Development 130: 1725-1734.

[107] Eley L, Turnpenny L, Yates LM, Craighead AS, Morgan D, Whistler C, Goodship JA, Strachan T. 2004. A perspective on inversin. Cell Biology International 28: 119-124

[108] Park TJ, Haigo SL, Wallingford JB. 2006. Ciliogenesis defects in embryos lacking inturned or fuzzy function are associated with failure of planar cell polarity and Hedgehog signaling. Nat Genet 38 (3): 303-11.

[109] Ahdab-Barmada, M.; Claassen, D. 1990. A distinctive triad of malformations of the central nervous system in the Meckel-Gruber syndrome. J Neuropath Exp Neurol 49: 610-620.

[110] Salonen R, Paavola P. 1998. Meckel syndrome. Journal of Medical Genetics 35: 497-501.

[111] Smith U, Pasha S, Cox P, Attie-Bitach T, Maher ER, Johnson CA. 2005. Fine-mapping the MKS3 locus for Meckel-Gruber syndrome. Journal of Medical Genetics 42: S107

[112] Kyttälä M, Tallila J, Salonen R, Kopra O, Kohlschmidt N, Pavola-Sakki P, Peltonen L, Kestila M. 2006. MKS1, encoding a component of the flagellar apparatus basal body proteome, is mutated in Meckel syndrome. Nat Genet 38:155-157.

[113] Weatherbee SD, Niswander LA, Anderson KV. 2009. A mouse model for Meckel syndrome reveals Mks1 is required for ciliogenesis and Hedgehog signaling. Hum Mol Genet 18(23):4565-4575.

[114] Kibar Z, Torban E, Mc Dearmid JR, Reynolds A, Mathieu M, kirillova I, De Marco P, Merello E, Hayes JM, Wallingford JB, Drapeau P, Capra V, Gros P. 2007. Mutations in VANGL1 associated in neural-tube defects. N Engl J Med 361(14): 1432-1437.

[115] Reynolds A, McDearmid JR, Lachance S, De Marco P, Merello E, Capra V, Gros P, Drapeau P, Kibar Z. 2010. VANGL1 rare variants associated with neural tube defects affect convergent extension in zebrafish. Mech Dev 127:385-392.

[116] Kibar Z, Bosoi CM, Kooistra M, Salem S, Finnell RH, De Marco P, Merello E, Bassuk AG, Capra V, Gros P. 2009. Novel Mutations in VANGL1 in Neural Tube Defects. Hum Mutat 30:E706-E715.

[117] Kibar Z, Salem S, Bosoi CM, Pauwels E, De Marco P, Merello E, Bassuk AG, Capra V, Gros P. 2010. Contribution of VANGL2 mutations to isolated neural tube defects. Clin Genet 2011 80(1):76-82.
[118] Lei YP, Zhang T, Li H, Wu BL, Jin L, Wang HY. 2010. VANGL2 mutations in human cranial neural-tube defects N Engl J Med 362:2232-2235.

# 9

# Neural Tube Defects in Algeria

Bakhouche Houcher[1], Samia Begag[1], Yonca Egin[2] and Nejat Akar[2]
[1]*Faculty of Sciences, Department of Biology University of Sétif, Sétif*
[2]*Department of Pediatric Molecular Genetics,*
*University Medical School, Ankara,*
[1]*Algeria*
[2]*Turkey*

## 1. Introduction

Neural tube defects (NTD) are severe congenital malformations and can be fatal. These malformations constitute one of the principal causes of mortality and morbidity in childhood. Classically, NTD have been divided into two main groups: (a) defects affecting cranial structures, such as anencephaly and encephalocele, and (b) defects involving spinal structures (spina bifida) (Verrotti et al., 2006). In newer classification schemes for the NTD, encephalocele shows more similarities to spina bifida or anencephaly than it shows differences with respect to characteristics, temporal trend and the impact of fortification (Rowland et al., 2006).

In recent years, various clinical and experimental studies have demonstrated that folic acid supplementation during the periconceptional period can prevent the occurrence and recurrence of NTD (Czeizel and Dudas, 1992). Thus, a low folate status is associated with an increased NTD risk. Up to 70% of human NTD can be prevented by folate supplementation during the periconceptional period (Czeizel and Dudas, 1992; MRC Vitamin Study Research Group, 1991).

Both genetic and environmental factors such as the maternal vitamin status have been proposed to affect the risk for NTD (Copp et al., 1990). The incidence is nearly 1 in 1,000 births, but various numbers have been reported from different countries (Botto, 2000). At present, the exact mechanism through which folic acid works remains unknown (Morrison et al., 1998). It is known that folic acid plays an important role in the homocysteine metabolism, in which 5-methylene-tetrahydrofolate (THF), formed upon reduction of 5,10-methyl-THF by the enzyme methylene-THF reductase (MTHFR), donates its methyl group via the vitamin- $B_{12}$-dependent enzyme methionine synthase to homocysteine to form methionine. Another major pathway of homocysteine metabolism is the transsulfuration pathway, in which homocysteine is irreversibly condensed with serine to cystathionine by the vitamin $B_6$-dependent enzyme cystathionine β-synthase (Afman et al., 2003).

The genetic risk factors for NTDs have been intensively studied in recent years. As a result, numerous candidate genes associated with folate metabolism have been studied in detail and their association with NTD, including MTHFR (Selhub et al., 1993). The prevalence of

MTHFR C677T genotypes varies among different ethnic groups. It is low in Africa, whereas in Europe and North America it ranges between 5% and 15%, thereby suggesting regional differences in the MTHFR C677T distribution (Almawi et al., 2004). For example, a high prevalence of the TT genotype was reported for Mexico (34.8%) (Mutchinick et al., 1999), Italy (21.4%) (D'Angelo et al., 2000) and France (16.8%), while lower prevalences were reported for Thailand (1.4%) and India (2.0%).

There are several studies that have found a positive association between NTD and the common mutation C677T of MTHFR, and other studies that have not found such an association. Van der Put et al. (1995) discovered that a common genetic defect in the *MTHFR* gene, the C677T mutation, resulting in a reduced but not an abolished enzyme activity, is a genetic risk factor for spina bifida. The C677T mutation is associated with a 2- to 4-fold increased risk if an NTD mother is homozygous for this mutation.

Data from several association studies on different ethnic groups have resulted in conflicting conclusions about the role of the C677T mutation of the MTHFR gene, as a risk factor for NTD (Rampersaud et al., 2003).

In the present study, we aimed to determine the prevalence of the MTHFR C677T polymorphism in the Algerian population and evaluated their impact on NTD individuals and their relatives.

## 2. Patients and methods

### 2.1 Study population

The study was a retrospective review of the medical case notes over a 3-year period. Infants born with a NTD were identified from the University Maternity Hospital of Sétif (Algeria) database. The following items are routinely collected for each case: birth date, sex, single or multiple birth, presence of additional congenital malformations, mother's county of residence and birth date. The proportion of all congenital anomalies on the register accounted for by NTD was calculated. Prevalence (birth) rates per 1,000 births were examined each year for 3 year study period. The following factors were compared by type of NTD: prevalence, sex ratio, mother's age and season of birth. It was not possible to identify stillbirths with NTD born at home and we have no data on prenatal diagnosis of NTD by ultrasound among our patients.

### 2.2 Sample collection and DNA extraction

The total study group consisted of 71 mothers and 27 fathers. A group of 147 apparently healthy adult (82 women and 65 men) were used as control group. Peripheral blood samples were collected by venipuncture, collected in test tubes which contained EDTA as an anticoagulant and maintained frozen at -20°C until extraction of DNA and genotyping. The research protocol was approved by the Sétif Medical Faculty Ethics Committee.

DNA extraction was performed using the conventional phenol-chloroform method. After haemolysis of the blood in hypotonic solution, the DNA was isolated by using a simple proteinase K treatment at 65°C in the presence of SDS, followed by ammonium actetate precipitation of debris and ethanol precipitation of the DNA. Then, DNA amount and DNA purity were quantified for each DNA sample by spectrophotometry (Nanodrop ND-1000). DNA samples were stored at -4°C until use.

### 2.3 Polymorphism analysis by LightCycler PCR® and melting curve analysis

The genetic analysis of the MTHFR C677T polymorphism was performed by real-time polymerase chain reaction (PCR) via a melting curve analysis performed on a Light Cycler (Roche Molecular Biochemicals, Mannheim, Germany) in borosilicate capillaries with an MTHFR C677T polymorphism detection kit (Roche Molecular Biochemicals). Primers and fluorescence-labelled hybridization probes designed were used. The primer sequences were: 5′-TGGCAGGTTACCCCAAAGG-3' (forward) and 5'-TGATGCCCATGTCGGTGC-3' (reverse) and hybridization probe sequences were:
5′-TGAGGCTGACCTGAAGCACTTGAAGCACTTGAAGGAGAAGGTGTCT-3′-Flu and 5′-LC-640-CGG GAG CCG ATT TCA TCA T-3′-PHO (TIB Molbiol, Berlin Germany).

The 20.0 µl amplification reaction was prepared, containing 5.0 µl genomic DNA, 1.6 µl Mg, 4.0 µl Reagent Mix (Specific primers and probe, Tib molbion), 2 µl Fast Start DNA master HybProbe (Roche Diagnostics Mannheim, Germany), 7.4 µl H2O (PCR-grade).

Cycling conditions for MTHFR were initial denaturation at 95°C for 10 min, followed by 45 cycles with denaturation at 95°C for 5 s, annealing at 60°C for 10 s and extension at 72°C for 15 s. After amplification, melting curves have been generated following denaturation of the reaction at 95°C for 20s, holding the sample at 40°C for 20s and then slowly heating the sample to 85°C with a ramp rate of 0.2°C/s and simultaneous monitoring of fluorescence decline.

The identification of the *MTHFR* genotype has been performed by an analysis of the melting peaks of the run of the real-time PCR. The presence of just 1 melting peak at 63.0°C indicates a wild-type genotype, 2 melting peaks at 54.5°C and 63.0°C indicate a heterozygous mutant, and 1 melting peak at 54.5°C indicates a homozygous mutant (fig. 1).

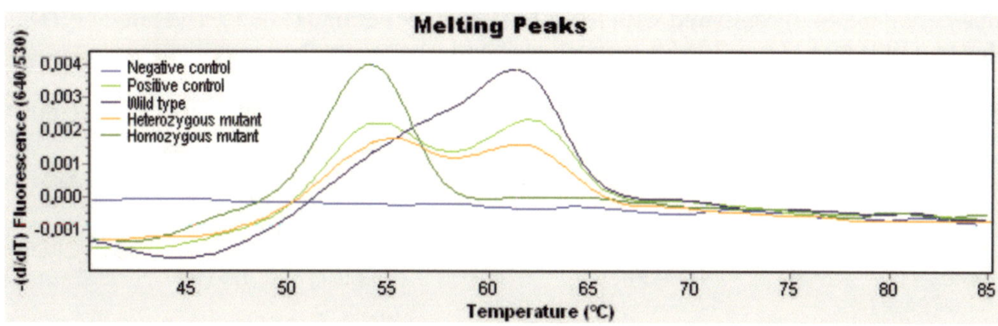


Fig. 1. Melting-curve analysis was performed analyze the MTHFR C677T polymorphism

### 2.4 Statistical analysis

Comparisons of NTD between sex and/or between mother's age and of genotype and allele frequencies between cases and control subjects were done by a $\chi^2$ test. Allele frequencies were deduced from genotype distribution Statistical significance was accepted at $p < 0.05$. The odds ratios (OR) as well as their 95% CI were computed to assess strength of association, if any, between different genotypes and NTD. We calculated the OR and associated 95% CI for individuals who were homozygous for the thermolabile variant at MTHFR (TT).

## 3. Results

The annual prevalence of all types of NTDs during the 3 years treated in the Service of Pediatrics and Genocology-Obstetrics at Sétif Hospital (Algeria), was 7.3, 8.2 and 7.1 NTD cases per 1000 live births and fetal deaths. The total NTDs numbered 215 and the total live births and fetal deaths were around 28,500. Therefore, the incidence of NTD at Sétif Hospital is 7.5 per 1,000 births.

Of the total NTD cases, there where 122 (56.7%) with spina bifida, 69 (32.1%) with anencephaly, 1 (0.5%) with encephalocele and 23 (10.7%) with spina bifida and anencephaly; the corresponding birth prevalence per 1000 births was 4.35 for spina bifida, 2.42 for anencephaly, 0.70 for spina bifida and anencephaly and 0.03 for encephalocoele.

Table 1. shows the characteristics of cohorts of the different types of NTD. The sex distribution among NTD cases was significantly different, 126 (58.6%) females, 88 (40.9%) males ($p < 0.05$) and one (0.5%) unknown or indeterminate. There were also significant differences between the type of NTD with regard to the female to male sex ratio. The female sex ratio was significantly higher for anencephalics (1.76) and spina bifida and anecephalics (4.0) compared with spina bifida (1.1) ($p < 0.05$). Of all NTD cases studied, hundred and seventeen (54.4%) cases died in utero and 4 cases (1.9%) unknown. The trend had not significantly changed for spina bifida and anencephaly during the 3 year period. The spina bifida/anencephaly ratio for the 3 year period was 1.77 (122/69).

Of the 215 NTD cases in the study, there were 64 (29.8%) with associated hydrocephalus anomalies. This study shows 13% (28/215) of the parents with affected newborns had consanguineous marriages. The rate of affected newborns was highest in mothers aged between 31-35 years (21.9%) (Tab. 1). Seasonal variation in the birth prevalence of NTD during the 3 year period was observed. Birth prevalence of NTD was higher in the January-June period (58.14%) compared with the July-December period (41.86%). The rate of NTD in May and June was 13.5 and 15.8% respectively, and was higher than for other months.

| Variable | Type of defect | | | | Total | $\chi^2$ | *P*-value |
|---|---|---|---|---|---|---|---|
| | Spina bifida | Anencephaly | Spina bifida +Anencephaly | Encephalocele | | | |
| | No. (%) | No. (%) | No. (%) | No. (%) | No. (%) | | |
| Sex | | | | | | | |
| Male | 59 (67.0) | 25 (28.4) | 4 (4.5) | 0 (0.0) | 88 (100) | 5.02 | 0.05 |
| Female | 65 (51.6) | 44 (34.9) | 16 (12.7) | 1 (0.8) | 126 (100) | | |
| Mother's age (y) | | | | | | | |
| 20 | 4 (57.1) | 1 (14.3) | 2 (28.6) | 0 (0.0) | 7 (100) | 14.28 | 0.01 |
| 21-25 | 24 (60.0) | 11 (27.5) | 5 (125) | 0 (0.0) | 40 (100) | | |
| 26-30 | 23 (67.6) | 9 (22.5) | 2 (59) | 0 (0.0) | 34 (100) | | |
| 31-35 | 20 (42.5) | 22 (46.8) | 5 (10.6) | 0 (0.0) | 47 (100) | | |
| 36 | 21 (56.7) | 13 (35.1) | 2 (5.4) | 1 (2.7) | 37 (100) | | |
| Consanguinity | 16 (57.1) | 9 (32.1) | 3 (10.7) | 0 (0.0) | 28 (100) | | |
| Death | 30 (25.6) | 64 (54.7) | 23 (19.6) | 0 (0.0) | 117 (100) | | |

Table 1. Characteristics of cohorts of the different types of NTD.

The observed frequencies of the various genotypes and alleles of C677T polymorphisms in the *MTHFR* gene are shown in Table 2. Forty-two (46%) out of 92 mothers analysed for the C677T polymorphism carried the T allele and 15 (16%) were homozygotes (table 2). Finally, 5 (10%) out of 48 fathers had the TT genotype and 22 (46%) were heterozygotes (Tab. 2). In the control mothers group (n = 82), 35 (43%) were heterozygotes (table 3). In the control mothers group (n = 82), 35 (43%) were heterozygotes and 14 (17%) were homozygotes (table 2). These frequencies were not significantly different from those observed in a sample of the general population (n = 147) (table 3).

There was no statistically significant difference between the genotype and allele frequencies of C677T polymorphisms in mothers with a previous child with NTD compared with mother controls. The allele frequencies for the MTHFR C677T polymorphism were similar in case mothers and control mothers, with approximate allele frequencies of 0.6 and 0.3 for C and T alleles, respectively (table 2). Comparisons of genotype frequencies between case mothers and controls did not reveal any statistically significant differences (tables 2, 3).

The frequency of C677T homozygotes in the couple was higher in mothers with a previous child with NTD than in corresponding controls (19 vs. 14%), but the difference was not statistically significant. The OR was 2.05 (95% CI: 0.78-5.41) (table 2). The frequency of T alleles too was higher in case mothers compared to controls (45 vs. 34%; OR = 1.55; 95% CI: 0.97-2.48), but the differences in frequencies were statistically insignificant (table 3).

| | Control mothers (n = 82) | Case mothers (n = 92) | OR |
|---|---|---|---|
| CC | 33 (0.40) | 35 (0.38) | 1 |
| CT | 35 (0.43) | 42 (0.46) | 1.13 (0.59-2.17) |
| TT | 14 (0.17) | 15 (0.16) | 1.01 (0.42-2.41) |
| C | 101 ( 0.62) | 112 (0.61) | 1 |
| T | 63 (0.38) | 72 (0.39) | 1.03 (0.67-1.59) |

Table 2. Genotype and allele frequency of the MTHFR C677T polymorphism among control mothers and mothers with a previous child with NTD. Values in parentheses denote allele frequencies (columns 2 and 3) or 95% CI (column 4)

| Variable | Controls (n = 147) | NTD mothers (n = 48) | NTD fathers (n = 48) | $OR_{NTD}$ mothers[1] | $OR_{NTD}$ fathers[1] |
|---|---|---|---|---|---|
| Genotype | | | | | |
| CC | 67 (0.46) | 14 (0.29) | 21 (0.44) | 1 | 1 |
| CT | 59 (0.40) | 25 (0.52) | 22 (0.46) | 2.03 (0.97-4.26) | 1.19 (0.6-2.38) |
| TT | 21 (0.14) | 9 (0.19) | 5 (0.10) | 2.05 (0.78-5.41) | 0.76(0.26-2.26) |
| Allele C | 193 (0.66) | 53 (0.55) | 64 (0.67) | 1 | 1 |
| Allele T | 101 (0.34) | 43 (0.45) | 32 (0.33) | 1.55 (0.97-2.48) | 0.96 (0.59-1.56) |

Values in parentheses denote allelic frequencies unless otherwise specified.
[1]OR (95% CI) versus controls.

Table 3. Genotype distribution and allelic frequency of the MTHFR C677T polymorphism among mothers and fathers of cases with a previous child with NTD and controls.

## 4. Discussion

Neural tube defects are a worldwide problem, affecting an estimated 300,000 or more fetus or infants each year (The Centers for Disease Control and prevention (CDC), 1998). The reported annual percentage fall in the rates of NTD was 3.1-7.7% for the United States and 10.6% for the United Kingdom (Windham & Edmands, 1982). Unfortunately we do not have previous data from our area or in all Algeria for comparison. This is the first report regarding NTD in Sétif (Algeria). Our study showed the incidence was 7.5 cases per 1,000. The trend over the 3 years remained fairly constant. Our rate is higher than studies in other countries such as Canada where it was 1.41/1,000 (DeWalls et al., 1992; Murphy, 1992; Van Allen et al., 1992; Wilson & Van Allen , 1993), in the United States of America 0.93 to 1.46/1,000 (Hendricks et al., 1999; Stevenson et al., 2000), in Germany 1.50/1,000 (Koch & Fuhrmann, 1984), in Holland 0.58/1,000 (Eurocat Working Group, 1991), in the North of England 1.79/1,000 (Rankin et al., 2000), in France 1,000 (Alembik et al., 1995; Candito & Van Obberghen, 2001), in Italy 0.36/1,000 (Eurocat Working Group, 1991), in South Africa 1.74/1,000 (Buccimazza et al., 1994), in Turkey 3.01/1,000 (Tuncbilek et al., 1999), in Jordan 1.63/1000 (Daoud et al., 1996), Palestine 5.49/1000 (Dudin, 1997), in United Arab Emirates 1.23/1000 (Samson, 2003), in Tunisia 2.2/1000 (Khrouf et al., 1986) and in Iran 2.87/1,000 (Golalipour et al., 2007). A higher prevalence in comparison with our results was observed in China 10.23-13.87/1000 (Dai et al., 2002; Li et al., 2006; Xiao et al., 1990) and Egypt 13.8/1000 (Samaha et al., 1995).

Spina bifida was the most common NTD in our study, which agrees with other studies (Golalipour et al., 2007; Harris & James, 1997; Soumaya et al., 2001; Wasant & Sathienkijkanchai, 2005), followed by anencephaly and encephalocele. The spina bifida to anencephalic ratio is similar to that reported by other workers (McDonnell et al., 1999). Our research was shown that more than half of mortality is a consequence of anencephaly (Eurocat Working Group, 1991).

In our study, there were 64 spina bifida (29.8%) with associated hydrocephalus anomalies. The etiology of congenital hydrocephalus is extremely heterogeneous and for instance it may be secondary to an open neural tube defect (Williamson et al., 1984). In general, patients with spina bifida, not including anencephaly and encephalocele, will have 80 to 85% chance of developing hydrocephallus (Rintoul et al., 2002). Also, it has been suggested that there is an increased risk for hydrocephalus in families with a propositus affected with NTD (Cohen et al., 1979).

As reported in many other studies (Lary & Paulozzi, 2001; Rittler et al., 2004), we also observed a significant females predominance. Regarding sex differences, our results indicate that the rate of NTD was higher in females than males (male to female ratio = 0.70). Others had reported 0.73 (Daoud et al., 1996), 0.78 (Golalipour et al., 2007; Stevenson et al., 2000) and 0.85 (Samson, 2003), or even a male predominance 1.07 (Wasant & Sathienkijkanchai, 2005). The predominance of female anencephalic births over males in our study is similar to that seen in other countries and likewise the slight female predominance in spina bifida births (McDonnell et al., 1999).

Our research showed that the highest rate of affected newborns was in mothers aged 31-35 years (21.9%), with 3.2% in mothers aged 16-20 years and 9.76% aged 36-40 years. Our observation is different from other studies which show a linear relation between the rate of NTD and increasing maternal age (Golalipour et al., 2007) or which show, a U-shaped curve with a higher risk among younger mothers and higher rates in mothers aged over 35 years (Hendricks et al., 1999; Li et al., 2006). It may be due to factors such as lower rate of marriage under 20 years (sometimes even more than 25 years of age) and can be attributed to the use of contraceptive drugs using over 35 years.

In this study a seasonal variation in the birth prevalence of NTD was observed, it was higher in the January-June period compared with July-December period, then is similar to that reported by Mc Donnell et al. (1999). Some research has shown a predominance of NTD births in winter months particularly in October to December and January to March (Golalipour et al., 2007; Office for Population Censuses and Surveys, 1998). Our research has shown that rate of NTD was higher in May with a peak in June. In Ireland the peak prevalence was in April (McDonnell et al., 1999) and in Northern Iran it was in December (Golalipour et al., 2007). The seasonal variations in the birth prevalence and the peak of NTD observed in our population were difficult to compare with those of previous studies, which were performed in countries where income, seasonal changes in diet is completely different. The high prevalence of NTD it may be attributed to the low dietary intake of folate in our women population (Houcher et al., 2003) and related with the seasonal variation of folate consumption. For example, the folate dietary intake of Havanan men was lowest in June and July, which contrasts with improvement in folate intake in June and July observed in Gambian women ( Bates et al., 1994), and with the increase in serum folate concentration during the summer observed in British men (Clarke et al., 1998).

It has shown that the rate of consanguineous marriage is high in NTD births (Murshid, 2000). In different Middle Eastern countries the rate of consanguineous marriages varies from 23.3% to 57.9% (Khoury & Massad, 1992; Teebi, 1994) The incidence of consanguineous marriage in Algeria was 23-34% (Benallegue & Kedji 1984; Zaoui & Biemont, 2002) and the frequency of consanguineous marriage rates were 40.5 and 30.6% in rural and urban settings, respectively (Zaoui & Biemont, 2002). First-cousin marriages constitute almost one-third of all marriages in many Arab countries (Hamamy et al., 2005). First-cousin marriage in Algeria was 10-16% (Zaoui & Biemont, 2002). In our study 13% of parents with affected newborns had consanguineous marriage (first-cousin). In families with children born with neural tube defects, the consanguinity rate was much higher than observed in the general population (Jaber et al., 2004; Khrouf et al., 1986; Zlotogora, 1997). The relatively high proportion of first cousin marriages among parents of individuals with neural tube defects suggests that some of these cases are due to monogenic disorders (Zlotogora, 1997). We were not able to confirm the suggestion that there is an increase risk for NTD in children born of consanguineous parents. The possibility that consanguinity could be a risk factor for NTD in a population requires further research (Murshid, 2000; Rajab et al., 1998).

Numerous articles have been published regarding the effect of folic acid intake on the reduction or prevention of NTD (Frey & Hauser, 2003; Li et al., 2006; Morin et al., 2001; Smithells et al., 1980; Stevenson et al., 2000). Intake of 0.4 mg per day of folic acid in the periconceptional period reduces the risk of NTD by 30-100% (Berry et al., 1999; Czeizel and Dudas, 1992; MRC Vitamin Study Research Group, 1991; Ray et al., 2002). Several studies have suggested that low vitamin B12 levels may be associated with an increased risk for

NTD (Candito et al., 2004; Kirke et al., 2004; Williams et al., 2005). Our NTD group showed a higher risk of NTD among our women population, which may in part be attributable to a lower daily folate intake of women in our previous report; it revealed a large proportion of women (69%) presenting with less than the Reference Nutrient Intake (RNI) for folate (Houcher et al., 2003). Possibly, the most important finding from this study was the very low periconceptional use of folic acid-containing vitamins among our women population. Only 2.4% women in our population consumed multivitamins daily (Houcher et al., 2003).

NTD is recognized to have a complex etiology, involving both environmental and genetic factors. The *MTHFR* gene is chosen for study because of its direct catalytic interaction with homocysteine, cobalamin and folate, which predicted risk factors in NTD (Kirke et al., 1993; van der Put et al., 1997). It has been shown that homozygosity for the common C677T mutation in the *MTHFR* gene is a genetic risk factor for NTD in man (van der Put et al., 1995; Ou et al., 1995).

The association between the C677T variant in the *MTHFR* gene and NTD is controversial in several populations worldwide. Our research is the first in Algeria, which studied NTD patients in order to determine the association of the T allele with NTD in the region of Sétif, where NTD are highly prevalent (Houcher et al., 2008). The MTHFR C677T gene polymorphism was neutral in our population. We found the same prevalence of the 677T *MTHFR* allele in mothers as in controls and in the general population. Our results on Algerian NTD mothers did not show a significant association for any group, suggesting that the thermolabile variant C677T in the MTHFR gene is not a risk factor for NTD for a mother to have NTD offspring. These data are not in agreement with those of others (Grandone et al., 2006), who reported a higher prevalence in mothers than in controls and in the general population. However, no association was found for mothers of offspring with NTD in Italy or in Ireland, two countries with a higher 677 T allele frequency (De Marco et al., 2002; Kirke et 2004).

Thus, homozygosity for *MTHFR 677T* may only be a risk factor for NTD in some ethnic groups and not in others (Papapetrou et al., 1996). The divergence between populations raises the question whether dietary factors could play a significant interactive role in C677T mutations. There is evidence that the risk for NTD in association with the *MTHFR* genotypes might vary depending on the nutritional status (Gonzalez-Herrera et al., 2002) and, especially, due to low levels of red cell folate (Martinez de Villarreal et al., 2001). It is also relevant to note that the incidence of the C677T variant differs markedly amongst populations. These differences do not correlate with the incidence of NTD; for example, the frequency of homozygosity for the 677T allele is 8.3% in Ireland where the prevalence of NTD is high, and 16% in Italy where the NTD prevalence is low (Morrison et al., 1998).

Davalos et al (2000), who included among their cases the mothers and fathers of children affected by NTD, also found no differences between the cases and the control groups concerning the maternal genotype or allelic frequencies. We found that mothers who are homozygous for the C677T mutation, have a 4-fold higher risk of having a child with an NTD. Thus, the *MTHFR* genotype of the father also contributes to the risk of NTD (Blom, 1998)

The thermolabile MTHFR C677T variant is a risk factor for NTD in some but not all populations (Botto and Yang, 2000) and is associated with low folate and elevated homocysteine levels. The high prevalence of the *MTHFR 677T* allele (17%) (Bourouba et al., 2009), the higher risk of NTD (7.5 per 1,000 births) (Houcher et al., 2008) and lower daily folate intake (69%) of less than the reference nutrient intake for folate (Houcher et al., 2003), i.e. a combination of genetic and nutritional factors, may therefore play a role in the NTD rate in this region of Algeria, although the mechanism, by which the genotype or folate status increases the risk of NTD is not clear.

Our results support the hypothesis by Shields et al. (1999), which upholds that the 677T allele may only be a risk factor in populations with a poor folate diet, which could explain the lack of consistency among studies. Molloy et al. (1997) observed a decreased red cell folate in individuals that were homozygous for the C677T mutation. Consequently, the MTHFR A1298C variant was found to increase the risk of spina bifida when combined with MTHFR C677T alteration (Akar et al., 2000). However, it cannot be excluded that mutations of folate receptor genes correlate with NTD (De Marco et al., 2000) and can be involved in NTD etiology (Heil et al, 1999).

Currently, the molecular analysis in case of NTD is based on the examination of mutation (polymorphism) in genes, which is why it is difficult to determine their genetic basis. It seems that NTD diagnosis will be based on single nucleotide polymorphism analysis (Gos and Szpecht-Potocka, 2002). It has been established that the dihydrofolate reductase (DHFR) 19-bp intron deletion allele has a significant protective association by reducing the risk of woman having NTD of offspring in the Irish population (Parle-McDermott et al., 2007). Very recently, it has been reported that NTD mothers homozygous for the 19-bp del allele have a 2.04-fold greater risk compared to the controls in the Turkish population (Akar et al., 2008). In addition, Au et al. (2008) also found that several genes for glucose transport and metabolism are potential risk factors for meningomyolocele.

Several studies even pointed out that a folate intake high enough to prevent NTD cannot be achieved by a diet of folate-rich nutrition. Only intake of folate supplements or fortified foods such as flour and cereals can achieve these recommended daily values (van der Put et al., 1998). In terms of public health, we think that the most important finding from this study is the very low periconceptional use of folic-acid-containing vitamins among our population of women.

## 5. Conclusion

According to our findings genetic factors, interfamilial marriage and nutritional factors as folate deficiency may play a role in the NTD rate in this region of Algeria, although the mechanism, by which the genotype or folate status increases the risk of NTD, is not clear. So further investigations are needed, and we recommend that a central registry be set up to record NTD occurring in the Sétif region.

Several studies even pointed out that a folate intake high enough to prevent NTD cannot be achieved by a diet of folate-rich nutrition. Only intake of folate supplements or fortified foods such as flour and cereals can achieve these recommended daily values. In terms of public health, we think that the most important finding from this study is the very low periconceptional use of folic-acid-containing vitamins among our population of women.

## 6. Acknowledgment

This study was supported in part by Ankara University, Turkey. We extend our special thanks to the personnel of the newborns and delivery sections at the Setif University Maternity Hospital, Algeria, and the families who participated in this study.

## 7. References

Afman, LA. ; Lievers, KJA. ; Kluijtmans, LAJ. ; Trijbels, FJM. & Blom, HJ. (2003). Gene-gene interaction between the cystathionine β-synthase 31 base pair variable number of tandem repeats and the methylenetetrahydrofolate reductase 677C>T polymorphism on homocysteine levels and risk for neural tube defects. *Mol Gent Metab*, Vol.78, pp. 211-215, ISSN 1096-7192

Akar, N.; Akar, E.; Deda, G. & Arsan, S. (2000). Spina bifida and common mutations at the homocysteine metabolism pathway. *Clin Genet*, Vol.57, pp. 230-231, ISSN 0009-9163

Akar, N.; Akar, E.; Eğin, Y.; Deda, G.; Arsan, S. & Ekim, M. (2008). Neural tube defects and 19 bp deletion within intron-1 of dihydrofolate reductase gene. *Turk J Med Sci*, Vol.38, pp. 383-386, ISSN 1300-0144

Alembik, Y.; Dott, B.; Roth, MP. & Stoll, C. (1995). Prevalence of neural tube defects in northeastern France, 1979-1992 impact of prenatal diagnosis. *Ann Genet*, Vol.38, pp. 49-53, ISNN 0003-3995

Almawi, WY.; Finan, RR.; Tamim, H.; Daccache, JL. & Irani-Hakime, N. (2004). Differences in the frequency of the C677T mutation in the methylenetetrahydrofolate reductase (MTHFR) gene among the Lebanese population. *Am J Hematol*, Vol.76, pp. 85-87, ISSN 0361-8609

Au, KS.; Tran, PX.; Tsai, CC.; O'Byrne, MR.; Lin, J-I.; Morrison, AC.; Hampson, AW.; Cirino, P.; Fletcher, JM.; Ostermaier, KK.; Tyerman, GH.; Doebel, S. & Northrup, H. (2008). Characteristics of a spina bifida population including north American Caucasian and Hispanic individuals. *Birth Defects Research A* , Vol.82, pp. 692-700, ISNN 1542-0752

Bates, CJ.; Prentice, AM.; & Paul, AA. (1994). Seasonal variations in vitamins A, C, riboflavin and folate intake and status of pregnant and lactating women in a rural Gambian community: some possible implications. *Eur J Clin Nutr*, Vol.48, pp. 660-668, ISSN 0954-3007

Benallegue, A. & Kedji, F. (1984). Consanguinité et santé publique: Une étude algérienne. *Arch Fr Pédiatr*, Vol.41, pp. 435-40, ISSN 0003-9764

Berry, RJ.; Li, Z.; Erickson, JD.; Li, S.; Moore, CA.; Wang, H.; Mulinare, J.; Zhao, P.; Wong, LY.; Gindler, J.; Hong, SX. & Correa, A. (1999). Prevention of neural tube defects with folic acid in China. China-U.S. Collaborative Project for Neural Tube Defect Prevention. *N Engl J Med*, Vol.341, pp. 1485-1490, ISNN 0028-4793

Blom, HJ. (1998). Mutated 5,10-methylenetetrahydrofolatereductase and moderate hyperhomocysteinemia. *Eur J Pediatr*, Vol.157, pp. S131-S134, ISSN 0340-6199

Botto, LD. & Yang, Q. (2000). 5,10-Methylenetetrahydrofolate reductase gene variants and congenital anomalies: a HuGe review. *Am J Epidemiol*, Vol.151, pp. 862-877, ISSN 0002-9262

Bourouba, R., Houcher, B., Djabi, F., Egin, Y. & Akar, N. (2009). The prevalence of methylenetetrahydrofolate reductase 677 C-T, factor V 1691 G-A, and prothrombin

20210 G-A mutations in healthy populations in Sétif, Algeria. *Clin Appl Thromb Hemost*, Vol.15, pp. 529-534, ISNN 1076-0296

Buccimazza, S. ; Molteno, C. ; Dunne, T. & Viljoen, DL. (1994). Prevalence of neural tube defects in Cape Town, South Africa. *Teratology*, Vol.50, pp. 194-199, ISNN 0040-3709

Candito, M.; Houcher, B.; Boisson, C.; Abbellard, A.; Demarcq, MJ.; Gueant, JL.; Benhacine, K.; Gérard, P. & Van Obberghen, E. (2004). Neural tube defects and vitamin B12 : a report of three cases. *Ann Biol Clin (Paris)*, Vol.62, pp. 235-238, ISSN 0003-3898

Candito, M. & , Van Obberghen E. (2001). Folates, vitamine B12, homocystéine et anomalies du tube neural. *Ann Biol Clin (Paris)*, Vol.59, pp. 111-112, ISNN 0003-3898

Clarke, R.; Woodhouse, P.; Ulvik, A.; Frost, C.; Sherliker, P.; Refsum, H.; Ueland, PM. & Khaw, KT. (1998). Variability and determinants of total homocysteine concentrations in plasma in an elderly population. *Clin Chem*, Vol.44, pp. 102-107, ISSN 1530-8561

Cohen, T.; Stern, E. & Rosenman, A. (1979). Sub risk of neural tube defect. Is prenatal diagnosis indicated in pregnancies following the birth of a hydrocephalic child? *J Med Genet*, Vol.16, pp. 14-16, ISNN0022-2593

Copp, AJ.; Brook, FA.; Estibeiro, JP.; Shum, AS. & Cockroft DL. (1990). The embryonic development of mammalian neural tube defects. *Progr Neurobiol*, Vol.35, pp. 363-403, ISNN 0301-0082

Czeizel, AE. & Dudas, I. (1992). Prevention of the first occurrence of neural tube defects by periconceptional vitamin supplementation. *N Engl J Med*, Vol.327, pp. 1832-1835, ISSN 0028-4793

Dai, L.; Zhu, J.; Zhou, G.; Wang, Y.; Wu, J.; Miao, L. & Liang, J. (2002). Dynamic monitoring of neural tube defects in China during 1996 to 2000. *Chinese J Prevent Med*, Vol.36, pp. 402-405, ISNN 0253-9624

D'Angelo, A. ; Coppola, A. ; Madonna, P. ; Fermo, L., Pagano, A. ; Mazzola, G. ; Galli, L. & Cerbone, AM. (2000). The role of vitamin B12 in fasting hyperhomocysteinemia and its interaction with the homozygous C677T mutation of the methylenetetrahydrofolate reductase (MTHFR) gene. A case-control study of patients with early-onset thrombotic events. *Thromb Haemost*, Vol.83, pp. 563-70, ISSN 0340-6245

Daoud, AS.; Al-Kaysi, F.; El-Shanti, H.; Batieha, A.; Obeidat, A. & Al-Sheyyab, M. (1996). Neural tube defects in Northern Jordan. *Saud Med J*, Vol.17, pp. 78-81, ISSN 0379-5284

Davalos, IP.; Olivares, N.; Castillo, MT.; Cantu, JM.; Ibarra, B.; Sandoval, L.; Moran, MC.; Gallegos, MP., Chakraborty, R. & Rivas F. (2000). The C677T polymorphism of the methylenetetrahydrofolate reductase gene in Mexican mestizo neural tube defect parents, control mestizo and native populations. *Ann Genet*, Vol.43, pp. 89-92, ISSN 0003-3995

De Marco, P.; Calevo, MG.; Moroni, A.; Arata, L.; Merello, E.; Finnell, RH.; Zhu, H.; Andreussi, L.; Cama, A. & Capra, V. (2002). Study of MTHFR and MS polymorphisms as risk factors for NTD in the Italian population. *J Hum Genet*,Vol.47, pp. 319-324, ISSN 0002-9297

DeWalls, P.; Trochet, C. & Pinsonneaut, L. (1992). Prevalence of neural tube defect in the province of Quebec. *Can J Pub Health*, Vol.90, pp. 237-239, ISSN 0008-4263

Dudin, A. (1997). Neural tube defects in Palestinians: a hospital based study. *Ann Trop Pediatr*, Vol.17, pp. 217-22, ISSN 0272-4936

Eurocat Working Group. (1991). Prevalence of neural tube defects in 20 regions of Europe and the impact of prenatal diagnosis 1980- 86. *J Epidemiol Community Health*, Vol.45, pp. 52-8, ISNN 0143-005X

Frey, L. & Hauser, WA. (2003). Epidemiology of neural tube defects. *Epilepsia*, Vol.44, pp. 4-13, ISNN 0013-9580.

Golalipour, MJ.; Mobasheri, E.; Vakili, MA. ; & Keshtkar, AA. (2007). Epidemiology of neural tube defects in Northern Iran, 1998-2003. *Eastern Mediterr Health J*, Vol.3, pp. 560-566, ISSN 1020-3397

Gonzalez-Herrera, L.; Garcia-Escalante, G. & Castillo-Zapata, I. (2002). Frequency of the thermolable variant C677T in the MTHFR gene and lack of association with neural tube defects in the State of the Yucatan, Mexico. *Clin Genet*, Vol.62, pp. 394-398, ISSN 0009-9163

Gos, M. & Szpecht-Potocka, A. (2002). Genetic basis of neural tube defects. II. Genes correlated with folate and methionine metabolism. *J Appl Genet*, Vol.43, pp.511-524, ISSN 1234-1983

Grandone, E.; Corrao, AM.; Colaizzo, D.; Vecchione, G.; Girgenti, CD.; Paladini, D.; Sardella, L.; Pellegrino, M.; Zelante, L.; Martinelli, P. & Margaglione, M. (2006). Homocysteine metabolism in families from southern Italy with neural tube defects: role of genetic and nutritional determinants. *Prenat Diagn*, Vol.26, pp.1-5, ISSN 0197-3851

Hamamy, H.; Jamhawi, L.; Al-Darawsheh, J.; & Ajlouni, K. (2005). Consanguineous marriages in Jordan: Why is the rate changing with time? *Clin Genet*, Vol.67, pp. 511-516, ISSN 0009-9163

Harris, JA. & James, L. (1997). State-by-state cost of birth defects-1992. *Teratology*, Vol.56, pp. 11-16, ISSN 0040-3709

Heil, SG.; van der Put, NMJ.; Trijbels, FJ.; Gabreels, FJ. & Blom, HJ. (1999). Molecular genetic analysis of human folate receptors in neural tube defects. *Eur J Hum Genet*, Vol.7, pp. 393-396, ISSN 1018-4813

Hendricks, KA.; Nuno, OM.; Suarez, L.; & Larsen R. (2001). Effects of hyperinsulinemia and obesity on risk of neural tube defects among Mexican Americans. *Epidemiology*, Vol.12, pp. 630-635, ISSN 1044-3983

Hendricks, KA.; Simpson, JS. & Larsen, RD. (1999) Neural tube defect along the texas-Mexico border, 1993-1995. *Am J Epidemiol*, Vol.149, pp. 1119-27, ISSN 0002-9262

Houcher, B.; Bourouba, R.; Djabi, F. & Houcher, Z. (2008). The prevalence of neural tube defects in Setif university maternity hospital, Algeria-3 years review (2004-2006). *Pteridines*, Vol.19, pp. 12-18, ISSN 0933-4807

Houcher, B.; Potier de Courcy, G.; Candito, M.; van Obberghen, E. & Naimi, D. (2003). Nutritional assessment of folate status in a population of Setif, Algeria. *Pteridines*, Vol.14, pp. 138-142, ISSN 0933-4807

Jaber, L.; Karim, IA.; Jawdat, AM.; Fausi, M. & Merlob, P. (2004). Awareness of folic acid for prevention of neural tube defects in a community with high prevalence of consanguineous marriages. *Ann Genet*, Vol.47, pp. 69-75, ISSN 0003-3995

Khoury, SA. & Massad, D. (1992). Consanguineous marriage in Jordan. *Am J Med Genet*, Vol.43, pp. 769-775, ISSN 1552-4825

Khrouf, N. ; Spang, R. ; Podgorna, T. ; Miled, SB.; Moussaoui, M.; & Chibani, M. (1986). Malformations in 10,000 consecutive births in Tunis. *Acta Paediatr Scand*, Vol.75, pp. 534-539, ISNN 0001-656X

Kirke, PN.; Mills, J.; Molloy, AM.; Brody, LC.; O'Leary, VB.; Daly, L.; Murray, S.; Conley, M.; Mayne, PD.; Smith, O. & Scott, JM. (2004). Impact of the MTHFR C677T polymorphism on the risk of neural tube defect case-control study. *BMJ*, Vol.328, pp. 1535-1536, ISSN 0959-8146

Kirke, PN.; Molloy, AM.; Daly, LE.; Burke, H.; Weir, DG. & Scott, JM. (1993). Maternal plasma folate and vitamin B12 are independent risk factors for neural tube defects. *Q J Med*, Vol.86, pp. 703-708, ISSN 1460-2725

Koch, M. & Fuhrmann, W. (1984). Epidemiology of neural tube defects in Germany. *Hum Genet*, Vol.68, pp. 97-103, ISSN 0340-6717

Lary, JM. & Paulozzi, LJ. (2001). Sex differences in the prevalence of human birth defects: a population-based study. *Teratology*, Vol.64, pp. 237-51, ISSN 0040-3709

Li, Z. ; Ren, A. ; Zhang, L. ; Ye, R.; Li, S.; Zheng, J.; Hong, S.; Wang, T. & Li, Z. (2006). Extremely high prevalence of neural tube defects in a 4-county area in Shanxi province, China. *Birth Defects Res A Clin Mol Teratol*, Vol.76, pp. 237-240, ISSN 1542-0752

Martinez de Villarreal, L.; Delgado-Enciso, I. ; Valdez-Leal, R. ; Ortiz-Lopez, R. ; Rojas-Martinez, A. ; Limon-Benavides, C. ; Sanchez-Pena, MA. ; Ancer-Rodriguez, J. ; Barrera-Saldana, HA. & Villarreal-Perez, JZl. (2001). Folate levels and $N^5$,$N^{10}$-Methylenetetrahydrofolate reductase genotype (MTHFR) in mothers of offspring with neural tube defects: a case-control study. *Arch medical Res*, Vol.32, pp. 277-282, ISSN 0188-4409

McDonnell, RJ.; Johnson, Z.; Delaney, V.; & Dack P. (1999). East Ireland 1980-1994: epidemiology of neural tube defects. *J Epidemiol Community Health*, Vol.53, pp. 782-8, ISSN 0143-005X

Molloy, A.; Daly, S.; Mills, J.; Kirke, PN.; Whitehead, AS.; Ramsbottom, D.; Conley, MR.; Weir, DG. & Scott, JM. (1997). Thermolabile variant of 5,10-methylenetetrahydrofolate reductase associated with low red-cell folates: implications for folate intake recommendations. *Lancet*, Vol.349, pp. 1591-1593, ISSN 0140-6736

Morin, VI.; Mondor, M. & Willson, RD. (2001). Knowledge on periconceptional use of folic acid in women of Brithsh Columbia. *Fetal Diagn. Ther*, Vol.16, pp. 111-115, ISNN 1015-3837

Morrison, K.; Papapetrou, C.; Hol, FA.; Mariman, ECM.; Lynch, SA.; Burn, J. & Edwards, YH. (1998). Susceptibility to spina bifida; an association study of five candidate genes. *Ann Hum Genet*, Vol.62, pp. 379-396, ISSN 0003-4800

MRC Vitamin Study Research Group. (1991). Prevention of neural tube defects: results of the Medical Research Council Vitamin Study. *Lancet*, Vol.338, pp. 131-137, ISSN 0140-6736

Murphy, PA. (1992). Periconceptional supplementation with folic acid: does it prevent neural defects? *J Nurse-Midwifery*, Vol.37, pp. 25-32, ISSN 0091-2182

Murshid, WR. (2000). Spina bifida in Saudi Arabia : is consanguinity among the parents a risk factor ? *Pediatric neurosurgery*, Vol.32, pp.10-12, ISSN1016-2291

Mutchinick, OM. ; Lopez, MA. ; Luna, L. ; Maxman, J. & Babinsky, VE. (1999). High prevalence of the thermolabile methylenetetrahydrofolate reductase variant in Mexico: a country with a very high prevalence of neural tube defects. *Mol Genet Metab*, Vol.68, pp. 461-467, ISSN 1096-7192

Office for Population Censuses and Surveys. (1988). Congenital malformation statistics: notifications 1981-85. London: HMSO, ISBN 0116912251

Ou, CY.; Stevenson, RE.; Brown, VK.; Schwartz, CE.; Allen, WP.; Khoury; MJ., Rozen, R. & Oakley, GP. Jr. (1995). C677T homozygosity associated with thermolabile 5,10-methylenetetrahydrofolate reductase as a risk factor for neural tube defects. *Am J Hum Genet*, Vol.57, pp. 223, ISSN 0002-9297

Papapetrou, C.; Lynch, SA.; Burn, J. & Edwards, YH. (1996). Methylenetetrahydrofolate reductase and neural tube defects. Lancet, Vol.348, pp. 58, ISSN 0140-6736

Parle-McDermott, A.; Pangilinan, F.; Mills, JL.; Kirke PN.; Gibney, ER.; Troendle, J.; O'Leary, VB.; Molloy, AM.; Conley, M.; Scott, JM. & Brody, LC. (2007). The 19-bp deletion polymorphism in intron-1 of dihydrofolate reductase (DHFR) may decrease rather than increase risk for spina bifida in the Irish population. *Am J Med Genet A*, Vol.143, pp. 1174-1180, ISSN 1552-4825

Rajab, A. ; Vaishnav, A. ; Freeman, NV. & Patton, MA. (1998). Neural tube defects and congenital hydrocephalus in the Sultanate of Oman. *J Trop Pediatr*, Vol.44, pp. 300-303, ISSN 0142-6338

Rampersaud, E.; Melvin, EC.; Siegel, D.; Mehltretter, I.; Dickerson, ME.; George, TM.; Enterline, D.; Nye, JS.& Speer, MC. (2003). Updated investigations of the role of methylenetetrahydrofolate reductase in human neural tube defects. NTD Collaborative group. *Clin Genet*, Vol.63, pp. 210-214, ISNN 0009-9163

Rankin, J.; Glinianaia, S. & Brown, R. (2000). The changing prevalence of neural tube defects: a population-based study in the north of England, 1984-96. Northern Congenital Abnormality Survey Steering Group. *Peadiatr Perinat Epidemiol*, Vol.14, pp. 104-110, ISSN 0269-5022

Ray, JG. ; Meier, C. ; Vermeulen, MJ. ; Boss, S.; Wyatt, PR.; & Cole, DE. (2002). Association of neural tube defects and folic acid food fortification in Canada. *Lancet*, Vol.360, pp. 2047-8, ISSN 0140-6736

Rintoul, NE. ; Sutton, LN. ; Hubbard, AM. ; Cohen, B.; Melchionni, J.; Pasquariello, PS. & Adzick, NS. (2002). A new look at myelomeningoceles: functional level, vertebral level, shunting, and the implications for fetal intervention. *Pediatrics*, Vol.109, pp. 409-413, ISSN 0031-4005

Rittler, M.; Lopez, CJ. & Castilla, EE. (2004). Sex ratio and associated risk factors for 50 congenital anomaly types: clues for causal heterogeneity. *Birth Defects Res A Clin Mol Teratol*, Vol.70, pp. 13-19, ISNN 15420752

Rowland, CA.; Correa, A.; Cragan, JD. & Alverson, CJ. (2006). Are encepaloceles neural tube defects? *Pediatrics*, Vol. 118, pp. 916-923, ISSN 0031-4005

Samaha, I. ; Rady, M. ; Nabhan, A. & Gadallah, M. (1995). The prevalence of congenital malformations at birth in Ain Shams University Maternity Hospital Cairo, Egypt, 1994. *J Egypt Public Health Assoc*, Vol.70, pp. 595-608, ISSN 0013-2446

Samson, GR. (2003). The incidence and demography of neural tube defects in Abu Dhabi, United Arab Emirates (1992-1999). *J Torp Pediatr*, Vol.49, pp. 256-257, ISSN 0142-6338

Selhub, J.; Jacques, PF.; Wilson, PWF.; Rush, D. & Rosenberg, IH. (1993). Vitamin status and intake as primary determinants of homocysteinemia in an elderly population. *JAMA*, Vol.270, pp. 2693-2698. ISSN 0098-7484

Shields, DC.; Kirke, PN.; Mills, JL.; Ramsbottom, D.; Molloy, AM.; Burke, H.; Weir DG.; Scott, JM. & Whitehead, AS. (1999). The 'thermolabile' variant of methylenetetrahydrofolate reductase and neural tube defects: an evaluation of genetic risk and the relative importance of the genotypes of the embryo and the mother. *Am J Hum Genet*, Vol.64, pp. 1045-1055, ISSN 0002-9297

Smithells, RW.; Sheppard, S.; Schorah, CJ.; Seller, MJ.; Nevin, NC.; Harris, R.; Read, AP. & Fielding, DW. (1980). Possible prevention of neural tube defects by periconceptional vitamin supplementation. *Lancet*, Vol.1, pp. 339-40, ISSN 0140-6736

Soumaya, SG. ; Aida, M. ; Sami, M. ; Khaled, N.; Med Badis, C.; Sami, J.; Ezedine, S.; Zohra, M.; Issam, L.; Faouzia, Z.; Hedi, R.; Hela, C. & Naima, K. (2001). Encephalocele: 26 retrospective cases at the maternal and neonatal center of La Rabta, Tunis. *Tunis Med*, Vol.79, pp. 51-53, ISSN 0041-4131

Stevenson, RE. ; Allen, WP. ; Pai, GS.; Best, R.; Seaver, LH.; Dean, J. & Thompson, S. (2000). Decline in prevalence of neural tube defects in a high-risk region of the United States. *Pediatrics*, Vol.106, pp. 677-683, ISSN 0031-4005

The Centers for Disease Control and prevention (CDC). (1998). Preventing Neural Tube Birth Defects: A Prevention Model and Resource Guide. Atlanta, GA 30333.

Tuncbilek, E.; Boduroglo, K. & Alikasifoglu, M. (1999). Neural tube defects in Turkey: prevalence distribution and risk factors. *Turk J Pediatr*, Vol.41, pp. 299-305, ISNN 0041-4301

Van Allen, MI.; Fraser, FC. ; Dallaire, L.; Allason, J.; McLeod, DR.; Andermann, E. & Friedman, JM. (1993). Recommendations on the use of folic acid supplementation to prevent the recurrence of neural tube defects. Clinical Teratology Committee, Canadian College of MedicalGeneticists. *Can Med Assoc J*, Vol.149, pp. 1239-1243, ISSN 0820-3946

van der Put, NMJ.; Gabreëls, F.; Stevens, EMB.; Smeitink, JAM.; Trijbels, FJM.; Eskes, T.; van den Heuvel, LP. & Blom, HJ. (1998). A second common mutation in the methylenetetrahydrofolate reductase gene: an additional risk factor for neural tube defects? *Am J Hum Genet*, 1998; Vol.62, pp. 1044-1051, ISSN 0002-9297

van der Put, NMJ.; Steegers-Theunissen, RPM.; Frosst, P.; Trijbels, FJM.; Eskes, TKAB.; van den Heuvel, LP.; Mariman, ECM.; den Heyer, M.; Rozen, R. & Blom, HJ. (1995). Mutated methylenetetrahydrofolate reductase as a risk factor for spina bifida. *Lancet*, Vol.346, pp. 1071-1072. ISSN 0140-6736

van der Put, NMJ.; Thomas, CMG.; Eskes, TKA.; Trijbels, FJM.; Steegers-Teunissen, RPM.; Mariman, ECM.; de Graaf-Hess, A.; Smeitink, JAM. & Blom, HJ. (1997). Altered folate and vitamin B12 metabolism in families with spina bifida offspring. *Q J Med*, Vol.90, pp. 505-510, ISSN 1460-2725

Verrotti, A.; Tana, M.; Pelliccia, P.; Chiarelli, F. & Latini, G. (2006). Recent advances on neural tube defects with special reference to valproic acid. *Endocer Metab Immune Disord Drug Targets*, Vol.6, pp. 25-31, ISSN 1871-5303

Wasant, P. &, Sathienkijkanchai, A. (2005). Neural tube defects at Siriraj hospital, Bangkok, Thailand-10 years review (1990-1999). *J Med Assoc Tha*, Vol.88, pp. 92-99, ISSN 0125-2208

Williams, LJ. ; Rasmussen, SA. ; Flores, A.; Kirby, RS. & Edmonds, LD. (2005). Decline in the prevalence of spina bifida and anencephaly by race/ethnicity: 1995-2002. *Pediatrics*, Vol.116, pp. 580-6, ISSN 0031-4005

Williamson, RA.; Schauberger, CW.; Varner, MW.; & Aschenbrener, CA. (1984). Heterogeneity of prenatal onset hydrocephalus: Management and counseling implications. *Am J Med Genet*, Vol. 17, pp. 497-504, ISSN 0148-7299

Wilson, RD. & Van Allen, MI. (1993). Recommendations on the use of folic acid for the prevention of neural tube defects. *J Soc Obstet Gynecol*, Vol.15, pp. 41-44, ISSN 1488-2329

Windham, GC. & Edmands, LD. (1982). Current trends in the incidence of neural tube defects. *Pediatrics*, Vol.70, pp. 333-337, ISNN 0031-4005.

Xiao, KZ. ; Zhang, ZY. ; Su, YM. ; Liu, FQ. ; Yan, ZZ.; Jiang, ZQ.; Zhou, SF.; He, WG.; Wang, BY. & Jiang, HP. (1990). Central nervous system congenital malformations, especially neural tube defects in 29 provinces, metropolitan cities and autonomous regions of China: Chinese Birth Defects Monotoring Program. *Int J Epidemiol*, Vol.19, pp. 978-982, ISSN 0300-5771

Zaoui, S. & Biemont, C. (2002). Frequency of consanguineous unions in the Tlemcen area (West Algeria). *Santé*, Vol.12, pp. 289-295, ISSN 1157-5999

Zlotogora, J. (1997). Genetic disorders among Palestinian Arabs: 1. Effects of consanguinity. *Am J Med Genet*, Vol.68, pp. 472-475, ISSN 1532-4825

10

# Association of *A80G* Polymorphism in the *RFC1* Gene with the Risk for Having Spina Bifida-Affected Offspring in Southeast Mexico and Interaction with *C677T-MTHFR*

Lizbeth González-Herrera et al.*
*Laboratorio de Genética. Centro de Investigaciones Regionales.*
*Universidad Autónoma de Yucatán. Mérida, Yucatán,*
*Departamento de Toxicología del Centro de Investigaciones y Estudios Avanzados,*
*Distrito Federal*
*Mexico*

## 1. Introduction

Spina bifida (SB) is one of the most prevalent congenital anomalies known as neural tube defects (NTD) in Yucatan, at Southeast Mexico. NTD results from failures of normal neural tube closure between the third and fourth week of embryonic development (Chen, 2008; Ramirez-Espitia et al., 2003). The majority of NTD cases can be categorized as either anencephaly with a lack of closure in the region of the head; or spina bifida with a lack of closure below the head (Au et al., 2010). SB refers to defects in the vertebral arches that obligatorily accompany open lesions. When the neural folds remain open, the sclerotome is unable to cover the neuroepithelium and skeletogenesis occurs abnormally, leaving the midline exposed (Greene & Copp, 2009). SB encompasses several subgroups of defects including the protrusion of the nervous tissue and its covering through a defect in the vertebrae named myelomeningocele, meningocele, and lipomeningocele. Myelomeningocele is by far the most common, accounting for greater than 90% of SB cases (Au et al., 2010). Wide variations in SB prevalence based on geography, race/ethnicity, and socioeconomic level suggest that genetic and environmental factors contribute to its etiology (Chen, 2008). Maternal folate status is critical for proper neural tube closure during embryogenesis. However epidemiological studies suggest that factors other than maternal deficiency of folic acid are involved in the etiology of SB. Numerous environmental and genetic influences

* Orlando Vargas-Sierra, Silvina Contreras-Capetillo, Gerardo Pérez-Mendoza, Ileana Castillo-Zapata, Doris Pinto-Escalante, Thelma Canto de Cetina and Betzabet Quintanilla-Vega
*Laboratorio de Genética. Centro de Investigaciones Regionales.*
*Universidad Autónoma de Yucatán. Mérida, Yucatán,*
*Departamento de Toxicología del Centro de Investigaciones y Estudios Avanzados,*
*Distrito Federal*
*Mexico*

contribute to NTD etiology; accumulating evidence from population-based studies which has demonstrated that folate status is a significant determinant of NTD risk.

Since the observation that periconceptional folic acid supplementation reduces the risk of having a NTD-affected pregnancy by 50–70% (Czeizel & Dudas, 1992; MRC, 1991); and the identification of the C677T SNP in the *MTHFR* gene as the first genetic risk factor of NTD (Whitehead et al, 1995); research has focused on genetic variation in genes encoding for the enzymes involved in the folate cycles and the closely-related homocysteine (Hcy) metabolism. Folate metabolism cross-regulates a complex network of basic biological pathways vital to growth, differentiation, and proliferation of cells. These processes include folate recycling, methionine metabolism, trans-sulfuration, synthesis of purines and pyrimidines, synthesis of serine/glycine, biomolecule methylation, membrane lipid synthesis, and drug metabolism. Neural tube formation involves intricately synchronized cell-cycle activities of the cells composing the neural plate and neighboring tissues. Abnormal activity of genes affecting the balance of the aforementioned biological activities can lead to failure of the neural tube to close appropriately resulting in NTDs. Completion of neural tube closure requires the precise coordination of cell proliferation, survival, differentiation, and migration events; any one of these events could feasibly be disrupted by impairments in folate metabolism (Beudin & Stover, 2007).

Polymorphisms in genes controlling folate–homocysteine metabolism have been suggested as predisposing factors and susceptibility candidates for SB. However, in Yucatan, Mexico, no association between NTD and two common polymorphisms, C677T and A198C of the methylentetrahydrofolate reductase (*MTHFR)* gene was found (Gonzalez-Herrera et al., 2002, 2007). Mutations in the *MTHFR* gene can only partially explain the protective effect of folate against NTD. Therefore, other defects in folate metabolism, such as defective folate receptors and carriers, could also be causes of NTD. Dietary folates mainly exist as polyglutamates. As the uptake and transport of folates in the body occurs as monoglutamates, the dietary polyglutamated folates have to be deconjugated to monoglutamates before absorption. The enzyme responsible for this deconjugation is folylpoly-γ-glutamate carboxypeptidase, which is associated with the intestinal apical brush border and is encoded by the glutamate carboxypeptidase II (*GCPII*) gene. After the deconjugation process the folate monoglutamates are absorbed in the proximal small intestine via a mechanism that involves reduced folate carrier (van der Linden et al., 2006). Ingested folate is hydrolyzed into monoglutamate forms in the intestine by means of a specialized carrier-mediated process, with a protein named the reduced-folate carrier (RFC-1), which only transports the reduced form of folate, including the physiological substrate 5-methyltetrahydrofolate. RFC-1 is a bidirectional anion exchanger that mediates folate delivery into a variety of cells of different origin. A polymorphism, A80G substitution, in exon 2 of the *RFC-1* gene has been identified; that leads to the replacement of a histidine, CAG by an arginine, CGG, (Whetstine et al., 2001; Chango et al., 2000). Mutation of *RFC-1 80* AA to RFC-1 GG could impair folate transport from maternal blood to the fetus. So, the homozygous genotype (GG) could be a biologically plausible risk of NTDs. The A80G polymorphism has been demonstrated as a genetic risk factor for NTDs in both patients and their mothers (De Marco et al., 2003, Shang et al., 2008). Additional studies demonstrated that this variant may interact with low folate status and *MTHFR* mutations to increase NTDs risk. A study in a Chinese population has reported an increased NTD risk in patients with the GG genotype, especially when their mothers did not take folic acid supplements (Pei et al., 2005). Other studies have failed to find an association between the *RFC-1 A80G* SNP and maternal NTD risk (Relton et al., 2004a, b); although an association between the *RFC-1 GG* genotype and low erythrocyte folate levels has demonstrated (Morin et al., 2003). *RFC-1 A80G* SNP may be a NTD risk factor, especially when maternal folate status is low, suggesting that sufficient folate can attenuate the effect of this polymorphism.

The objective of this study was to analyze the association of A80G polymorphism in the *RFC1* gene with the risk for having spina bifida affected-offspring and its interaction with C677T-*MTHFR* polymorphism in mothers and fathers from Southeast, Mexico. This design included only parents, supporting the hypothesis that mutation of *RFC1* gene on the parents side, mainly mother's might alter folate metabolism, since *RFC1* carrier is of particular importance during embryonic development for its role in transporting folate across the placenta. Moreover, metabolic changes, such as limiting the supply of folate to the embryo or facilitating the accumulation and increased transfer of homocysteine, could foster the formation of NTD.

## 2. Methods

### 2.1 Population

A case-control association study was performed, including as cases, 183 parents of children with open-dorsolumbar SB (119 mothers and 64 fathers). Case mothers and fathers were unrelated subjects belonging to 108 different families. The affected children were the first occurrence in the nuclear family and they were born consecutively between 1998 and 2004 at the General Hospital of the Secretary of Health of Yucatan, Mexico. Age of cases ranged from 15 to 57 years old and a mean age of 21.6 years. The control group was composed with 195 unrelated volunteer healthy parents (140 mothers and 55 fathers) who have demonstrated having healthy offspring in at least three consecutive children, not having SB or other type of NTD nor delivered an NTD-affected child. The control group was formed with volunteers who attended to Laboratorio de Genética at Universidad Autónoma de Yucatán for other diseases different to congenital malformations. Control subjects had a mean age of 35.3 years and range of 17–60 years. Folate dietary consumption based on a questionnaire of frequency of foods and folate erythrocyte concentrations were previously measured in case and control mothers, and no significant differences were found between them (Duarte-Pinzón et al., 2008). All selected subjects were born and had lived for at least three generations in Yucatan, Mexico. We also used anthropologic and demographic parameters such as language, birth place, surnames, genealogy, history of lifestyle; among others, to mach ethnically control with case subjects, belonging to the same ethnic group of Mestizos, defined as individuals born in the country having a Spanish-derived last name, with family antecedents of Mexican ancestors back at least to the third generation. In addition, we previously determined the absence of substructure or population stratification within the population of Yucatan by using 16 autosomal STR markers (González-Herrera et al., 2010), which may represent a confounder. Subjects with a chronic or degenerative disease, such as diabetes mellitus type 2, obesity or hypertension were not included. Informed consent was obtained from cases and controls according to the recommendations of Helsinki Declaration. This study was approved by the Bioethics Committee of Centro de Investigaciones Regionales, Universidad Autónoma de Yucatán, México. Confidentiality of participants was strictly maintained.

### 2.2 Genotyping

DNA was extracted from blood using standard techniques. Genotyping for A80G polymorphism in the *RFC1* gene was performed by polymerase chain reaction amplification and restriction fragment length polymorphism (PCR-RFLP). The SNP A80G was determined with PCR amplification using conditions and primers described by Chango et al., 2000: forward: 5′-AGT GTC ACC TTC GTC CCC TC-3′ and reverse 5′- CTC CCG CGT GAA GTT CTT-3′. PCR amplification produced a 230 bp DNA fragment, which was digested with HhaI restriction enzyme. Detection of the fragments was resolved on 4% agarose gel. After restriction enzyme digestion, analysis of *RFC-1* 230 bp fragments showed that the AA genotype had two fragments of 162 and 68 bp, the heterozygous AG genotype had four fragments of 162, 125, 68, and 37 bp, and the homozygous GG genotype had three fragments of 125, 68, and 37 bp. To ensure quality control of genotyping, 10% of samples were randomly selected and genotyped by a second investigator, resulting in 100% concordance. Samples that failed the amplification or digestion as well as doubtful results were repeated to ensure correct identification of variants.

### 2.3 Statistical analysis

Genotype and allele frequencies in cases and controls were determined by counting method and calculating proportions. The frequencies of genotypes and alleles were used to compare cases and controls by means of a standard $X^2$ analysis. Exact methods were considered preferable whenever expected values in any cell were < 5. The Hardy-Weinberg equilibrium analysis was calculated both in cases and controls, and was tested using $X^2$ statistics for goodness of fit (1 df). Association of *A80G-RFC1* genotypes with the risk of having a SB-affected child was estimated considering p values <0.05 as statistically significant and odds ratio (OR) with 95% confidence interval (CI) were calculated using STATA case-control odds ratio program with the Woolf method (STATA version 10.2). Frequencies of *A80G-RFC1* genotypes and alleles were also stratified by gender, in order to determine the maternal or paternal contribution to the risk for having a SB-affected child. Interaction of *A80G-RFC1* polymorphism with *C677T-MTHFR* was assessed using data previously reported (Gonzalez-Herrera et al., 2002).

## 3. Results

Genotype and allele frequencies for A80G polymorphism of *RFC1* gene for SB parents and their controls, Hardy-Weinberg expectations, as well as the comparison of frequencies between cases and controls on an association analysis are listed in Table 1. Genotype frequencies were distributed according to Hardy-Weinberg expectations (p>0.05) in cases and controls. The heterozygous AG genotype was as frequent as the homozygous GG genotype in cases, whereas heterozygous AG was the most frequent genotype in controls. Allele G showed a higher frequency than allele A in cases, whereas allele distribution was similar in controls. Comparison of A80G-RFC1 genotype frequency between parents having an SB-affected child and control parents did not show significant differences nor for the AG heterozygous genotype neither for GG genotype, except when compare the GG genotype versus AA+AG (p= 0.009). Distribution of frequency of allele G was also significantly higher in cases than controls (p= 0.04). These findings suggested that both allele G and GG genotype were associated with the parental risk of having an SB-affected child.

| Genotypes and alleles | SB Parents N= 183 | Control Parents N= 195 | Cases vs controls OR (95% CI) p |
|---|---|---|---|
| AA | 30 (0.164) | 35 (0.180) | Reference |
| AG | 77 (0.421) | 104 (0.533) | AA vs AG 0.863 (0.489 - 1.527) 0.662 |
| GG | 76 (0.415) | 56 (0.287) | AA vs GG 1.583 (0.871 - 2.878) 0.171 |
| Allele A | 137 (0.372) | 174 (0.446) | Reference |
| Allele G | 229 (0.628) | 216 (0.554 | A vs G 1.37 (1.01 - 1.801) 0.046** |
| | | | GG vs AA+AG 1.76 (1.15 - 2.703) 0.009** |
| HWE (p) | *(0.609)* | *(0.764)* | |

Table 1. Genotype and allele frequencies of *A80G- RFC1* polymorphism in parents of SB children and control parents from Southeast, Mexico. Counts (%). ** Significant

| Genotypes and alleles | SB Fathers N= 64 | Control Fathers N= 55 | SB Mothers N= 119 | Control Mothers N= 140 | SB fathers vs control fathers OR [95% CI] p | SB Mothers vs control mothers OR [95% CI] p |
|---|---|---|---|---|---|---|
| AA | 8 (0.125) | 10 (0.182) | 22 (0.185) | 25 (0.179) | Reference | Reference |
| AG | 26 (0.406) | 28 (0.509) | 51 (0.429) | 76 (0.543) | 1.161 [0.397 - 3.391] 0.500 | 0.763 [0.389 -1.496] 0.490 |
| GG | 30 (0.469) | 17 (0.309) | 46 (0.387) | 39 (0.279) | 2.206 [0.731 -6.652] 0.173 | 1.34 [0.656 - 2.738] 0.470 |
| | | | | | GG vs AG+AA 1.972 [0.928 -4.191] 0.056 | GG vs AG+AA 1.631 [0.968 - 2.751] 0.044** |
| Allele A | 42 (0.328) | 48 (0.436) | 95 (0.399) | 126 (0.450) | Reference | Reference |
| Allele G | 86 (0.672) | 64 (0.564) | 143 (0.601) | 154 (0.550) | 1.536 [0.908 - 2.597] 0.070 | 1.232 [868 - 1.748] 0.248 |
| HWE (p) | 0.937 | 0.999 | 0. 736 | 0.710 | | |

Table 2. Genotype and allele frequencies of *A80G- RFC1* polymorphism in parents of SB children and control parents from Southeast, Mexico stratified by gender. Counts (%). ** Significant.

Table 2 shows the genotype and allele frequencies for *A80G-RFC1* gene for SB parents and their controls stratified by gender in order to determine the maternal or paternal contribution to the risk for having a SB-affected child in the studied population. The heterozygous AG genotype was as frequent as the GG genotype in case fathers, whereas for case mothers as well as for control mothers and fathers, the heterozygous AG genotype was the most frequent. Stratification of the polymorphism *A80G-RFC1* frequency by gender did not show significant differences when comparing case fathers versus control fathers for any genotype or allele (p>0.05). Comparison of genotype and allele frequencies of polymorphism *A80G-RFC1* between case mothers versus control mothers, showed significant differences for the genotype GG when comparing against AA+AG genotypes, suggesting that the polymorphism *A80G-RFC1* is associated with the risk for having SB-affected offspring only in mothers (OR=1.63, IC 0.968-2.75, p= 0.04). These results demonstrate that the risk for having an SB-affected child is controlled maternally in the population of Southeast, Mexico.

| Genotype combinations RFC1/ MTHFR | SB Mothers N=119 | Control Mothers N=140 | SB mothers vs control mothers OR 95% CI p | SB Fathers N=64 | Control Fathers N= 55 | SB Fathers vs control Fathers OR 95% CI p |
|---|---|---|---|---|---|---|
| AA/CC | 4 (0.034) | 4 (0.036) | 1.18 [0.29 - 4.83] 0.546 | 0 (0.0) | 2 (0.036) | 0.00 [0.00-0.00] 0.211 |
| AG/CC | 12 (0.101) | 18 (0.129) | 0.76 [0.35 -1.65] 0.561 | 5 (0.078) | 10 (0.182) | 0.38 [0.12-1.19] 0.077 |
| GG/CC | 8 (0.067) | 9 (0.064) | 1.04 [0.39 - 2.81] 0.559 | 8 (0.125) | 2 (0.036) | 3.78 [0.76-18.64] 0.077 |
| AA/CT | 12 (0.101) | 13 (0.093) | 1.09 [0.47 - 2.50] 0.836 | 7 (0.109) | 4 (0.073) | 1.68 [0.46-6.09] 0.534 |
| AG/CT | 25 (0.210) | 44 (0.314) | 0.58 [0.32 - 1.02] 0.039** | 14 (0.219) | 11 (0.200) | 1.12 [0.46-2.72] 0.826 |
| GG/CT | 25 (0.210) | 17 (0.121) | 1.92 [0.98 - 3.76] 0.039** | 11 (0.172) | 12 (0.218) | 0.74 [0.29-1.85] 0.643 |
| AA/TT | 6 (0.050) | 7 (0.050) | 1.00 [0.32 - 3.08] 0.603 | 1 (0.016) | 4 (0.073) | 0.20 [0.02-1.86] 0.180 |
| AG/TT | 14 (0.118) | 14 (0.100) | 1.27 [0.54 – 2.63] 0.691 | 7 (0.109) | 7 (0.127) | 0.84 [0.27-2.57] 0.783 |
| GG/TT | 13 (0.109) | 13 (0.093) | 1.19 [0.53 – 2.69] 0.683 | 11 (0.172) | 3 (0.055) | 2.59 [0.94-13.63] 0.043** |

Table 3. Interaction of *A80G-RFC1 and C677T-MTHFR* polymorphisms in parents of SB children and control parents stratified by gender. Counts (%). ** Significant

Combined genotypes for both polymorphisms *A80G-RFC1* and *C677T-MTHFR* were determined in order to asses an interaction between these two genes since multiple SNPs have the potential to provide significantly more power for genetic analysis than individual SNPs for increasing the associated risk for having SB-affected offspring. The genotype combination with both heterozygous AG/CT was the most frequent in all studied groups, except for control fathers who showed the highest frequency for the genotype combination GG/CT. Comparison of genotype combination *RFC1/MTHFR* frequencies between SB parents and control parents did not show significant differences (p>0.05, data not shown). However, stratification by gender of *RFC1/MTHFR* interaction showed significant differences for the genotype combinations AG/CT and GG/CT in mothers (p=0.039), suggesting that AG/CT might be an interaction associated as a genetic protection factor and that the GG/CT genotype combination might represent a genetic risk factor having an SB-affected child for mothers. In fathers, the genotype combination with both mutants GG/TT was significantly associated with the risk for having SB-affected offspring (p=0.043). Frequencies of *A80G-RFC1/C677T-MTHFR* genotype combinations stratified by gender in the studied population, as well as the comparison of frequencies between cases and controls on an association analysis are listed in Table 3. Results of the interaction of *A80G-RFC1/C677T-MTHFR* suggest that for a genotype combination become a genetic risk factor for having SB-affected offspring in Southeast, Mexico; the homozygous genotype *GG-RFC1* should be present for both mothers and fathers.

## 4. Discussion

Variants of several folate-related genes have been found to be significantly associated with the risk of NTD, although, many genetic factors are also responsible for NTD due to the numerous candidates and population level differences. Previous investigations of the gene that are specifically involved in folate metabolism, such as 5,10-methylenetetrahydrofolate reductase gene (*MTHFR*) have shown that *MTHFR* is associated with an increased risk of NTD (Botto & Yang, 2000). There is a considerable body of data demonstrating that MTHFR gene 677TT homozygosity for the thermolability of the enzyme and *MTHFR A1298C* are genetic factors affecting the susceptibility of the NTD risk. However, in Yucatan, Mexico, no association between NTD and two common polymorphisms, C677T and A1298C of the methylentetrahydrofolate reductase (*MTHFR)* gene was found (Gonzalez-Herrera et al., 2002, 2007). Mutations in the *MTHFR* gene can only partially explain the protective effect of folate against NTD. In this study, we search for another genetic folate risk factor, which might explain the high prevalence of NTD, of SB type in Yucatan, Mexico. Therefore, other defects in folate metabolism, such as defective folate receptors and carriers, could also be causes of NTD. The carrier involved in cellular folate absorbed and transported, such as the reduced folate carrier (RFC), acts together with the folate receptor for folate internalization from tissue into the cytoplasm of the cells. Investigation of folate-related genes is necessary to reveal clues about metabolism underlying the potential embryonic protective effects of folic acid supplementation. Genes involved in the cellular folate transportation, such as *RFC1*, may be primary candidates for folate regulated NTDs (Shaw et al., 2003). Variance or abnormal expression of RFC1 can potentially have a major impact on folate metabolism and represents an excellent candidate for explaining susceptibility to folate-regulated NTDs (Shaw et al., 2002).

The A80G polymorphism has been demonstrated as a genetic risk factor for NTDs in both patients and their mothers (De Marco et al., 2003, Shang et al., 2008). These findings are agreed with our results obtained in the population of Yucatan, where we were able to demonstrate a significant association of both allele and GG genotype of A80G-*RFC1* polymorphism with the risk for having an SB-affected child. Previous familial based-association studies using transmission/disequilibrium test (TDT) have demonstrated the significant preference of the allele G to be transmitted to NTD-affected offspring in affected families compared with control families (Pei et al., 2005). In the population of Yucatan, the risk for having SB-affected offspring associated to A80G-*RFC1* polymorphism was mainly significant in mothers. Because the affected biological mechanism related to A80G-*RFC1* polymorphism is folate transport; additional folate supplementation is critical to maintain the optimal function of folate carriers and transporters, as well as folate adsorption, mainly in mothers. The folate transport occurs across the placenta in mothers , so maternal control of folate is determinant to maintain optimal folate serum and erythrocyte levels in order to assure an embryonic normal development. RFC-1 is a high-affinity transporter for the folate substrate 5-methyltetrahydrofolate. This carrier is of particular importance during embryonic development for its role in transporting folate across the placenta. The 80A>G mutation affects residue 27 of the protein in which the Arginine (or R; CGG codon) is changed into Histidine (or H; CAG codon). RFC-1 is a protein that requires a functional amino terminus for insertion into the cell membrane for folate transport. Mutation of RFC-1 80 AA to RFC-1 GG could impair folate transport from maternal blood to the fetus. Therefore, this homozygous genotype (GG) could be a biologically plausible risk of NTD (Shang et al., 2008).

As a maternal low folate/high homocysteine phenotype is associated with increased risk of NTD in offspring, women with the GG genotype may have an increased risk of having a child affected by an NTD relative to those with the GA and AA genotypes. In addition, GG homozygous women may be at increased risk of a range of other major pathologies, including cardiovascular disease, in which a low folate/high homocysteine phenotype is a predisposing feature (Stanisławska-Sachadyn, et al 2009). A previous report in California provided evidence for a gene-nutrient interaction between infant *RFC1* G80/G80 genotype and maternal periconceptional intake of vitamins containing folic acid on the risk of spina bifida (Shaw et al., 2002). Based on these studies, we hypothesized that infants with the *RFC1* (A80G) genotype would be at increased risk for NTD secondary to an impaired ability to transport folates to the cytoplasm of a critical cellular population. The metabolic changes, such as limiting the supply of folate to the embryo or facilitating the accumulation and increased transfer of homocysteine, could foster the formation of NTD, so it is the mutation of certain genes on the mother's side that would alter folate metabolism. Significant association between the *RFC-1* A80G polymorphism and NTD risk in Shanxi, China, especially for the occurrence of the upper type of NTD was observed (Shang et al., 2008).

The biologically plausible rationale for exploring genetic variation of RFC1 is based on the knowledge that RFC1 regulates the delivery of 5-methyltetrahydrofolate from the cell's endocytotic vesicle into the cytoplasm (Chango et al., 2000). 5- Methyltetrahydrofolate is required for the remethylation of homocysteine. RFC is also a protein that requires a functional amino terminus for insertion into the cell membrane for folate transport. Thus, increasing maternal serum folate from either supplements or diet could "correct" reduced kinetics of transport that result from a variant form of a folate membrane transport protein (Shaw et al., 2003). If a putative genetic defect was severe enough to eliminate RFC1- mediated folate transport through these systems, it is likely that it would be embryolethal. This has been substantiated by recent reports using knock-out mouse models for the folate receptor proteins, as well as for RFC1 (Gelineau-van et al., 2008). Mutation of *RFC1 80AA* to *RFC1 80GG* could impair folate transport from maternal blood to the fetus. Therefore, this homozygous genotype (GG) could be a biologically plausible risk of NTD (Pei et al., 2009)

There is evidence of an interaction between the methylenetetrahydrofolate reductase (*MTHFR*) 1298 A>C and the reduced folate carrier (*RFC1)* 80 G>A polymorphisms with the risk of birth defects in the Italian population (De Marco et al., 2003). Gene-gene interactions between *MTHFR* and *RFC1* gene polymorphisms and the risk of Down syndrome pregnancies in a group of young mothers showed a protective role for the *MTHFR* 1298AA/*RFC1* 80 GA or AA genotype, compared with the 1298AA/80 GG genotype, suggesting that interactions between *MTHFR* and *RFC1* gene polymorphisms could be relevant to the risk for Down syndrome (Coppede et al., 2006, 2007). These findings suggested that there is a significant interaction between maternal or offspring's GG genotype and the deficiency of maternal periconceptional folic acid. Otherwise, a modest gene-nutrient interaction between infant homozygosity for the *RFC1* GG genotype and maternal periconceptional intake of vitamins containing folic acid on the risk of spina bifida has been demonstrated: an increased risk for spina bifida among California newborns with the GG genotype whose mothers had not used vitamins with folic acid in the periconceptional period (Shaw et al., 2002).

Our study contributed with the identification of genotypes at risk for having SB-affected offspring in fathers and mothers from Yucatan, Mexico. Allele G as well as GG genotype of A80G-*RFC1* polymorphism are associated with the risk to have a child with SB, so this polymorphism might be recognized as a genetic marker for susceptibility to SB in the studied population. Results might impact the design of preventive programs in order to decrease the high prevalence of NTD in Yucatán, Mexico.

## 5. Conclusion

In conclusion, our findings suggest the association of allele G of A80G polymorphism in the RFC1 gene with the genetic risk for having a child affected of spina bifida, which might be controled maternally. Results also suggest that there might be an interaction between A80G-*RFC1* and C677T-*MTHFR,* since the genotype combinations GG/CT in mothers and GG/TT in fathers were associated with the higher risk to have a child with SB in Southeast, Mexico.

## 6. References

Au, SK., Ashley-koch, A., & Northrup, H. (2010). Epidemiologic and genetic aspects of spina bifida and other neural tube defects. *Developmental disabilities research reviews* Vol.16, pp 6–15, ISSN: 1940-5529.

Beaudin, A. & Stover, P. (2007). Folate-Mediated One-Carbon Metabolism and Neural Tube Defects: Balancing Genome Synthesis and Gene Expression. *Birth Defects Research* Vol.81, pp183–203, ISSN:1542-0752.

Botto, L.D., & Yang, Q. (2000). 5,10 Methylenetetrahydrofolate reductase gene variants and congenital anomalies: a Huge Review. *American Journal of Epidemiology* Vol.151 pp862–877, ISSN: 0002-9262.

Chen, C.P. (2008). Syndromes, disorders and maternal risk factors associated with neural tube defects (VI). *Taiwan Journal of Obstetrics and Gynecology* Vol.47, pp267–275, ISSN:1028-4559.

Chango, A., Emery-Fillon, N., de Courcy, G.P., Lambert, D., Pfister, M., Rosenblatt, D.S. & Nicolas, J.P. (2000) A polymorphism (80G>A) in the reduced folate carrier gene and its associations with folate status and homocysteinemia. *Molecular Genetics and Metabolism* Vol.70, pp310–315, ISSN: 1096-7192.

Coppede, F., Marini, G., Bargagna, S., & Stuppia, L. (2006). Folate gene polymorphisms and the risk of Down syndrome pregnancies in young Italian women. *American Journal of Medical Genetics A*. Vol*140*, pp1083-1091, ISSN: 1552-4825.

Coppede, F., Colognato, R., & Migliore, L. (2007). MTHFR and RFC-1 gene polymorphisms and the risk of Down syndrome in Italy. Author's response to the comments by Scala et al. [2007]. *American Journal of Medical Genetics* Vol.143A, pp1018–1019, ISSN: 1552-4825.

Czeizel, A.E., & Dudas, I. (1992). Prevention of the first occurrence of neural-tube defects by periconceptional vitamin supplementation. *New England Journal of Medicine* Vol, 327, pp1832–1835, ISSN: 0028-4793.

De Marco, P., Calevo, M.G., Moroni. A, Merello, E., Raso, A., Finnell, RH., Zhu, H., Andreussi, L., Cama, A. & Capra, V. (2003). Reduced folate carrier polymorphism (80A>G) and neural tube defects. *European Journal of Human Genetics* Vol.11 pp245–252, ISSN: 1018-48-13.

Duarte-Pinzón, V., López-Ávila, MT., González-Herrera, L., & Gamas-Trujillo, PA. (2008). Consumo habitual de alimentos con ácido fólico en madres de niños con defectos de cierre del tubo neural y en mujeres con descendencia sana. In: Ramírez-Sierra, M.J., Jímenez-Coello, M., Heredia-Navarrete, M. R., Moguel-Rodríguez, W.A. Investigación y Salud 3. Las ciencias de la Salud en el marco de los procesos de cambio y globalización. *Ediciones de la Universidad Autónoma de Yucatán*. Yucatán, México. pp253-273, ISBN: 978-607-7573-03-6.

Gelineau-van Waes, J., Heller, S., Bauer, LK., Wilberding, J., Maddox, JR., Aleman, F., Rosenquist, TH., Finnell, RH. (2008). Embryonic development in the reduced folate carrier knockout mouse is modulated by maternal folate supplementation. *Birth Defects Reseach* Vol.82, pp494-507, ISSN: 1542-0752.

González-Herrera, L., García-Escalante, G., Castillo-Zapata, I., Canto-Herrera, J., Ceballos-Quintal, J., Pinto-Escalante, D., Díaz-Rubio, F., Del Angel, RM., & Orozco-Orozco, L. (2002). Frequency of the thermolabile variant C677T in the *MTHFR* gene and lack of association with neural tube defects in the State of Yucatan, Mexico. *Clinical Genetics* Vol.62, pp394-398, ISSN: 0009-9163.

González-Herrera, L., Castillo-Zapata, I., Garcia-Escalante, G., & Pinto-Escalante, D. (2007). A1298C polymorphism of the *MTHFR* gene and neural tube defects in the State of Yucatan, Mexico. *Birth Defects Research* Vol.79, pp622-626, ISSN:1542-0752.

González-Herrera, L., Vega-Navarrete, L., Roche-Canto, C., Canto-Herrera, J., Virgen-Ponce, D., Moscoso-Caloca, G., Delgado-Nájar, E., Quintanilla-Vega, B., Cerda-Flores, RM. (2010). Forensic parameters and genetic variation of 15 autosomal STR Loci in

Mexican Mestizo populations from the States of Yucatan and Nayarit. *The Open Forensic Science Journal* Vol.3, pp57-63, ISSN: 1874-40-28.

Greene, N., & Copp, A. (2009). Development of the vertebrate central nervous system: formation of the neural tube. *Pregnatal Diagnosis* Vol.29, pp303–311, ISNN: 1097-0223.

Morin, I., Devlin, AM., Leclerc, D., Sabbaghian, N., Halsted, CH., Finnell, R. & Rozen, R. (2003). Evaluation of genetic variants in the reduced folate carrier and in glutamate carboxypeptidase II for spina bifida risk. *Molecular Genetics and Metabolism* Vol.79, pp197–200, ISSN: 1096-7192.

MRC Vitamin Study Research Group. (1991). Prevention of neural tube defects: results of the Medical Research Council Vitamin Study. *Lancet* Vol.338, pp131–137, ISSN: 0140-6736.

Pei, L., Zhu, H., Ren, A., Li, Z., Hao, L., Finnell, RH. & Li, Z. (2005) Reduced folate carrier gene is a risk factor for neural tube defects in a Chinese population. *Birth Defects Research* Vol.73A, pp430–433, ISSN:1542-0752..

Pei, L., Liu, J., Zhang, Y., Zhu, H., & Ren, A. (2009). Association of Reduced Folate Carrier Gene Polymorphism and Maternal Folic Acid Use With Neural Tube Defects. *American Journal of Medical Genetics* Vol.150B, pp874–878, ISSN: 1552-4825.

Ramirez-Espitia, J., Benavides, F., Lacasaña-Navarro, M., Martinez, J., García, A., & Benach, J. (2003). Mortality from neural tube defects in Mexico, 1980–1997. *Salud Publica de Mexico* Vol.45, pp356–364, ISNN: 0036-3634.

Relton, CL., Wilding, CS., Laffling, AJ., Jonas, PA., Burgess, T., Binks, K., Janet, TE. & Burn J. (2004a). Low erythrocyte folate status and polymorphic variation in folate-related genes are associated with risk of neural tube defect pregnancy. *Molecular Genetics and Metabolism* Vol.81, pp273–281, ISSN: 1096-7192.

Relton, CL., Wilding, CS., Pearce, MS., Laffling, AJ., Jonas, PA., Lynch, SA., Tawn, EJ. & Burn, J. (2004b). Gene-gene interaction in folate-related genes and risk of neural tube defects in a UK population. *Journal of Medical Genetics* Vol.41, pp256–260, ISSN: 1468-6244.

Shang, Y., Zhao, H., Niu, B., Li, W., Zhou, R., Zhang, T.,& Xie, J. (2008). Correlation of Polymorphism of MTHFR and RFC-1 Genes with Neural Tube Defects in China. *Birth Defects Research* Vol.82, pp3–7, ISSN: 1542-0752.

Shaw, GM., Lammer, EJ., Zhu, H., et al. (2002). Maternal periconceptional vitamin use, genetic variation of infant reduced folate carrier (A80G), and risk of spina bifida. *American Journal of Medical Genetics* Vol.108, pp1–6, ISSN: 1552-4825.

Shaw, G., Zhu, H., Lammer, E., Yang, W., & Finnell, R. (2003). Genetic Variation of Infant Reduced Folate Carrier (A80G) and Risk of Orofacial and Conotruncal Heart Defects. *American Journal of Epidemiology* Vol.158, pp747–752, ISSN: 0002-9262.

Stanisławska-Sachadyn, A., Mitchell, L., Woodside, J., Buckley, P., Kealey, C., Young, I., Scott, J., Murray, L., Boreham, C., McNulty, H., Strain, J., & Whitehead, A.(2009). The reduced folate carrier (SLC19A1) c.80G>A polymorphism is associated with red cell folate concentrations among women. Annals of Human Genetics Vol.73, pp:484-491, ISSN: 1469-1809.

van der Linden, I., Afman, L., Heil, S., & Blom, H. (2006). Genetic variation in genes of folate metabolism and neural-tube defect risk. *Proceedings of the Nutrition Society* Vol.65, pp204–21, ISSN: 0029-6651.

Whetstine, J., Gifford, A., Witt, T., Liu, X., Flatley, R., Norris, M., Haber, M., Taub, J., Ravindranath, Y., & Matherly, L (2001). Single Nucleotide Polymorphisms in the Human Reduced Folate Carrier: Characterization of a High-Frequency G/A Variant at Position 80 and Transport Properties of the His27 and Arg27 Carriers. *Clinical Cancer Research* Vol. 7, pp3416–3422, ISSN: 1078-0432.

# Part 3

## Surgical Treatment of Large Thoraco-Lumbar Neural Tube Defects

# 11

# Treatment of Large Thoraco-Lumbar Neural Tube Defects

Mehrdad Hosseinpour
*Pediatric Surgeon*
*Kashan University of Medical Sciences*
*Iran*

## 1. Introduction

Myelo-meningocele (MMC) is the most complex congenital malformation of the CNS that is compatible with life .Although the incidence of the MMC is decreasing, it remains one of the most common birth defect of the central nervous system, with an incidence of 0.5 to 1 per 1000 pregnancies in the USA and higher in some other part of the world, particularly developing countries.An MMC is typically closed within 24-48 hours after birth, and the goal of surgery is to close the neural placode in to a neural tube to establish a micro environment conductive to neural function.

Although MMC closure consist of the soft tissue and skin adjacent to be the defect, but repair of MMC larger than 5 cm in diameter is almost never easy. For this reason, increasing attention has been directed at soft tissue closure with multiple anatomic layers .

In 1956, Soderby and Sutton described the repair of MMC defect by plastic surgery. Desprez in 1971 reported the use of composite skin - muscle flaps for closure of large MMC. In 1977, Nelson described the use of delayed bipedicle flaps. In the same year, David and Adendorff used a large rotation flap raised across the midline MMC. In 1978, McGraw firstly described use of a posterior - advancement Lattissimus dorsi, myocutaneos flap to repair MMC.

In this chapter, we review the repair of large MMC defects by several methods described recently in literature.

## 2. Skin and fasiocutaneous flaps

### 2.1 Bilateral fasciocutaneous flap

The fasciacutaneous flap closure is supported by a rich vascular network with three main dominant vascular territories as bellow:

1. A prominent transverse segmental vascular pattern originating from the muscular perforator and lateral cutaneous branches of the lower intercostal arteries.
2. The parascapular and scapular fascial branches of the circumflex scapular artery.
3. Lateral extension of the superficial circumflex iliac arteries.

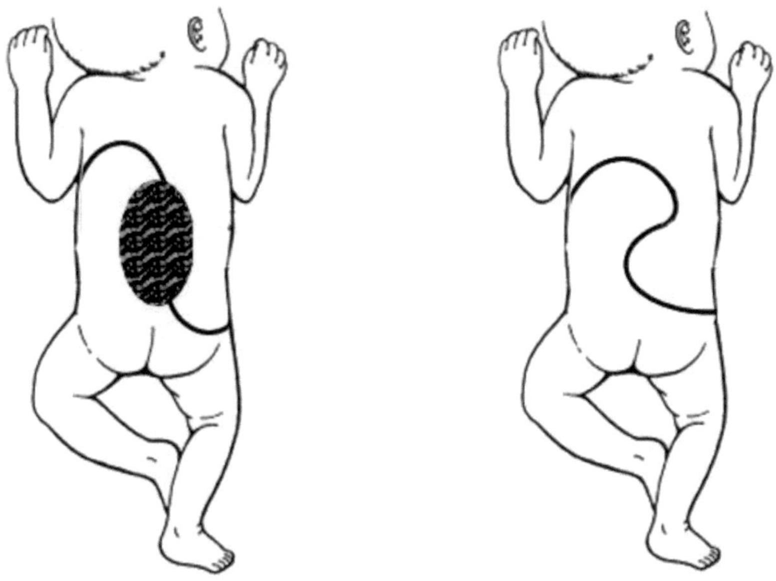

(a) (b)

Fig. 1. (a) (b)Bilateral Fascio Cutaneous Flap

In this technique, after the closure of neural defect by neurosurgery, two fasciocutaneous equilateral rotation flaps at both sides of defect are elevated. Elevation of the flaps is begun in superior -inferior direction, lifting the skin and the underlying fascia by sharp dissection. Once the flaps have been elevated, they are rotated and transposed across the midline to close the skin defect (figure 1a and b). The flaps are planned in such a way that the direction of rotation of one flap is against the other flap, and the design is oriented according to the skin reserve vector to accomplish closure with minimal tension. After elevating the flaps, they are sutured to each other. Skin and sub cutaneous tissue are closed by 5.o prolene and 4.0 PDS respectively. There is no need of drainage in most instances.

### 2.2 Delayed repair of large MMC

In this technique, the skin is incised in the midline proximal to the MMC. The incision is carried circumferentially around the neural placode and the overlying skin is saved as much as possible. About a 1cm width of dura mater beneath the skin is left to ease the subcutaneous suturing.

### 2.3 Limberg skin flap (1)

In this technique, a rhomboid defect is created around the MMC and a rhomboid flap is harvested cranially to the defect. After neural tube closure, a line perpendicular to the long axis of the defect is made (figure 2a and b).

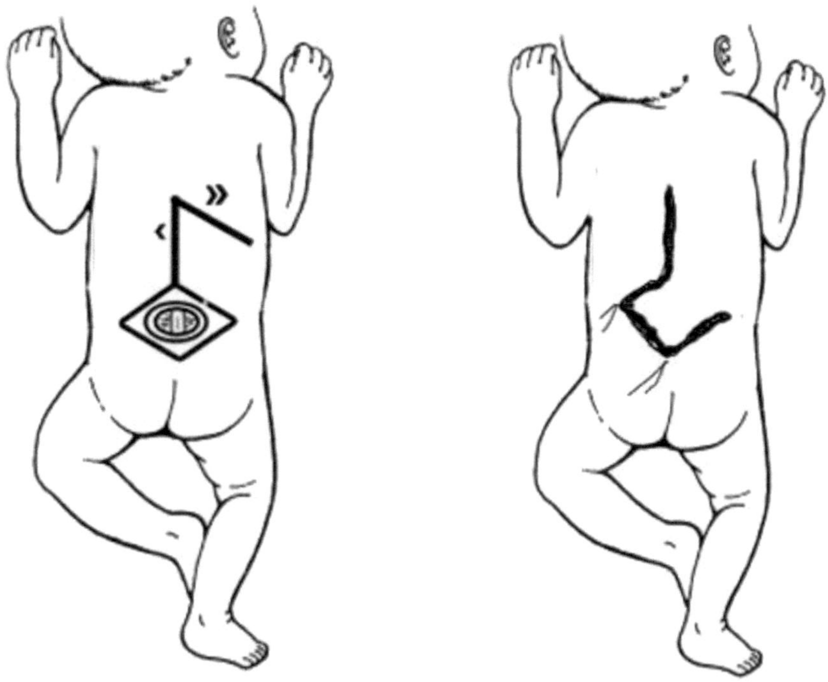

(a) (b)

Fig. 2. (a) (b) Limberg Skin Flap

The length of the line is equal to the length of one side of the rhombus. Subsequently , a second line at a 120 degree angle is drown ,making it parallel to a side of the rhomboid .The Limberg flap is then dissected at the level of the lumbar fascia. After flap dissected, the Limberg flap is rotated and adjusted to MMC defect and tension - free skin closure is performed.

### 2.4 Double 2-rhomboid technique

In this technique, after neurosurgical repair, the skin defect is surgically converted to the shape of the rhombus.

Equilateral 2-plasty flaps are elevated at the side of the rhombus and transposed across the defect.

### 2.5 Bilobed flap

The flap is based superiorly and laterally to the area to be covered. The first lobe crosses the midline above the defect, and the second lobe goes up the midline perpendicular to the first lobe (fig3a and b).

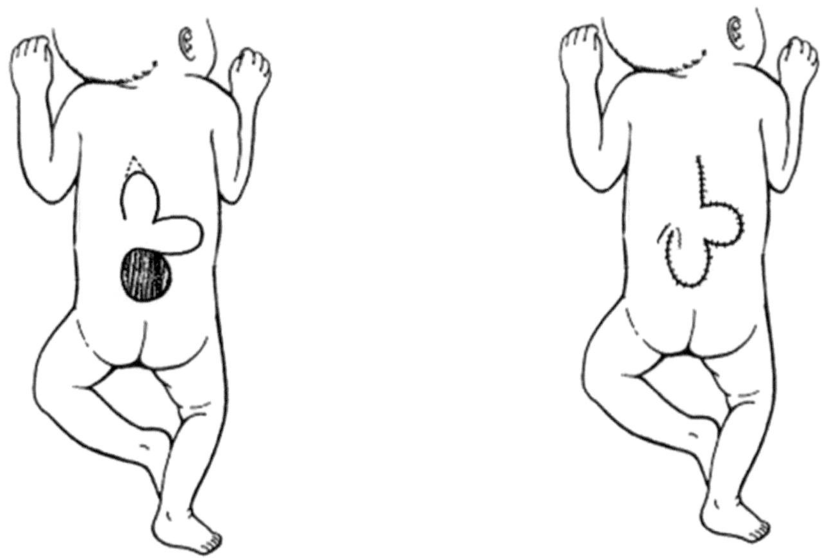

(a) (b)

Fig. 3. Bilobed flap

### 2.6 The repaired of MMC with tissue expanders (2-3)

The use of tissue expander in large MMC defect a relatively is new approach. In this technique, vertical incision is performed on the flanks. The expander pockets are dissected subcutaneously above the fascia parallel to MMC mass. The tissue expanders are inserted in to the pocket and suction drainage is established. The first saline injection is done on the 20th post operative day and this is continued on the outpatient basis at a rate of 15-25ml of saline weekly for six to eight weeks. When expansion is complete, the second stage operation is performed. Incisions, as long as the MMC defect and parallel to the margins are placed bilaterally over the expanded skin .The tissue expanders are removed and the capsule over the fascial portion is dissected suprafascially starting laterally and leaving a pedicle medially. Then neural tube is closed and the dissected capsule is turned over and sutured over the repaired dural defects. The expanded skin flaps are transferred to cover the defect using 2-plasty flaps.

### 2.7 Proximally based fasciocutaneous flank flap (4,7)

In this technique skin is closed by proximally based left side flank flap (figure 4). After measurement of defect dimensions, the flap length equal to 1.5 the width of the defect and flap width equal to the length of the defect. Drawing of the flap boundaries and dissection are started from distal to proximal under the thoracolumbar fascia. Flap is transposed to the defect with tension-free skin closure. Donor site is closed primarily or with split thickness skin graft from adjacent gluteal area.

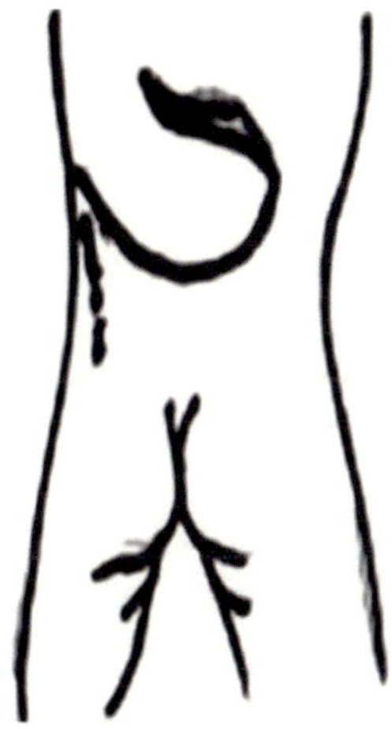

Fig. 4. Proximally based Fasciocutaneous Flank Flap

## 3. Muscle and musculocutaneous flaps

### 3.1 Bilateral Lattissimus dorsi Flap (5,9)

The lattissimuss dorsi(LD) muscle is the largest and one of the most versatile flaps, available for MMC closure.

The large size allows it be used to cover large MMC defects. The dominant vascular pedicle to the LD muscle from the subscapular -thoracodorsal vascular axis makes this muscle suitable for rotational and advancement flaps.

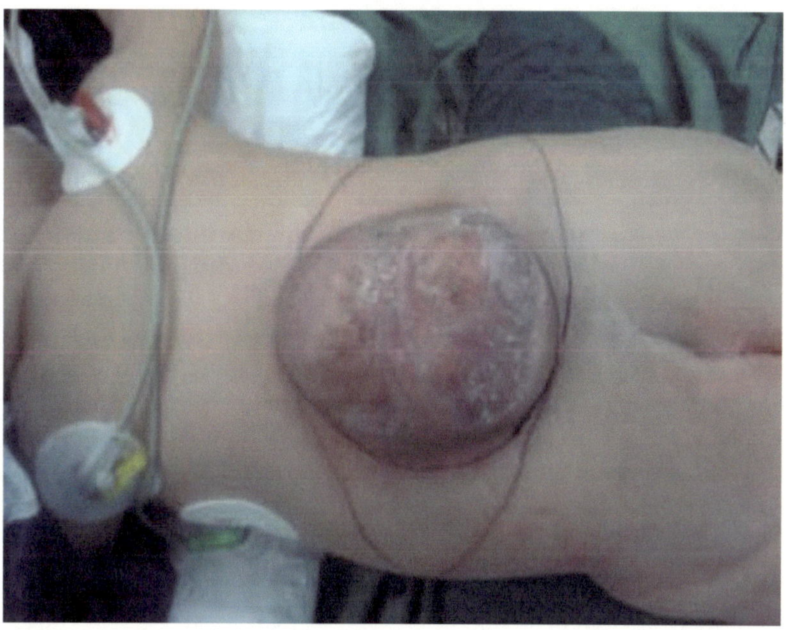

Fig. 5. Bilateral Lattissimus dorsi Flap(Design)

In this technique, patient is positioned prone and the designs of flaps are made (figure 5). Then, two triangular V-Y flaps are incised (figure 6) on each side of the defect. The tip of the triangle is extended to the posterior axillary line. The incision is started at the caudal line of the triangle and thoracolumbar fascia is freed from paraspinous muscles. The cranial border of the skin island is deepened to the muscle fascia and under the muscle, to create a proximally based muscle pedicle. The LD flaps, based on the thoracodorsal arteries are elevated bilaterally and advanced toward the midline with moderate tension (figure 7) and sutured together .The donor site are closed in a V-Y fashion.post operatively, patients are positioned prone for seven days.

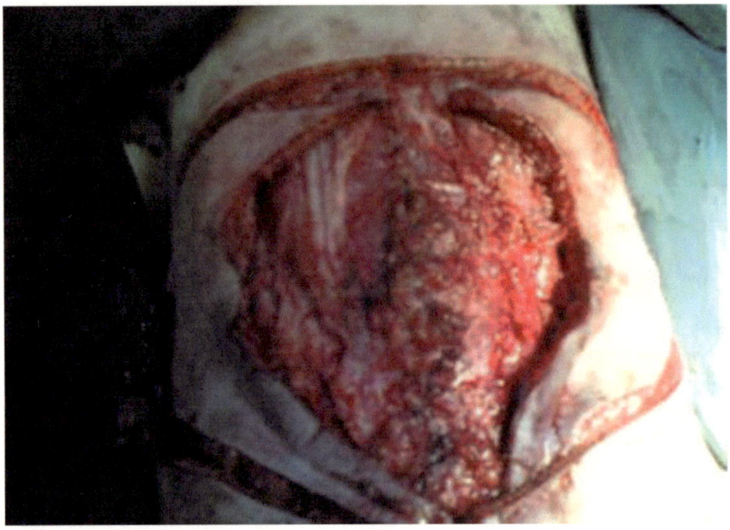

Fig. 6. Bilateral Lattissimus dorsi Flap (incisions)

### 3.2 LD + Gluteal myocutaneous flap (8)

In this technique during the neurosurgical closure of the dural defect, undermining of the skin is avoided. Following the tube closure, flap dissection is begun by incising the thoraco-lumbar fascia over the paraspinous muscles and carrying the dissection under the LD to its free border laterally. The perforating vessels are cauterized and divided for medical advancement. The LD is freed from its attachments to the external oblique and serratus posterior muscles by sharp dissection. Dissection is continued inferiorly deep to the lumbar fascia, including the fascia overlying the gluteus maximus muscles, but without raising the muscles. Dissection is carried out laterally and inferiorly as necessary to achieve tension free closure of the defect. After dissection, the reconstruction of the defect is achieved through enblock medial advancement of the bilateral interconnected LD myocutaneous, and gluteal region fasciocutaneous units.

### 3.3 Lower trapezius myocutaneous flap (6)

It is shown that there are two main patterns of vascular supply of the trapezius and that the muscle is principally supplied by three vascular sources.

1. The transverse cervical artery
2. The dorsal scapular artery
3. Posterior intercostal arterial branches

In this technique, the skin island is located at the inferior aspect on the trapezius muscle. It is designed between the vertebral column and the scapula with its vertical axis extending between the mid scapula and the inferior origin of the muscle.

The skin is incised to the posterior surface of the trapezius muscle. In elevating the skin paddle laterally, it is important to include the fascia overlying the LD muscle and then to dissect from lateral to medial under the fascia. This method automatically leads to the lateral border of trapezius.

The medial muscle fibers of origin are divided and the flap(s) is elevated toward the MMC defect. This flap can be elevated to the level of the base of the neck. Flap(s) is sutured on MMC defect with routine technique.

### 3.4 Reversed LD muscle flap (10)

The reversed LD muscle flap is based on perforators of the 9th, 10th and 11th posterior inter costal vessels.

They pierce the lumbar fascia and overlying sacrospinalis muscle to enter the LD muscle.

In this technique, incisions are extended obliquely from the axilla to the defect, then dissection continued and the muscle insertion is identified and divided. Then the deep lateral surface of the muscle is identified and dissections continued towards the posterior trunk midline, with preservation of the segmental pedicle from the posterior inter costal arteries. For adequate and tension -free turnover of muscle to the defect, superior muscle fibers of origin and the superior segmental pedicle are divided. Turning over is done along the oblique line connecting the segmental pedicle. Partial thickness skin graft is then harvested from the thigh and applied on the muscle.

## 4. References


[1] Campobasso P, Pesce C, Costa L, cimaglia ML. The use of the limberg skin flap for closure of large lumbosacral myeomeningoceles. Pediatr Surg Int 2004, 20: 144-147

[2] Arnell k. primary and secondary tissue expansion gives high quality skin and subcutaneous coverage in children with a large myelomeningocele and kyphosis. Acta Neurochir 2006, 148: 293- 297

[3] Celikoz B, Turegun M, Sengezer M. The repair of myelomeningcele with tissue expanders. Eur J Plast Surg 1996, 19: 297- 299

[4] Ozcelik D, Yildiz KH, Is M, Dosoglu M. Soft tissue closure and plastic surgical aspects of the large dorsal myelomeningocele defects (review of techniques). Neurosurg Rev 2005,28:218- 225

[5] Haktanir NH, Eser O, Demir Y, Aslan A, Koken R, Melek H. Repair of wide myelomeningocele defects with the bilateral fasciocutaneous flap method. Turkish Neurosurgery 2008, 18(3): 311- 315

[6] Atita AMR. The lower trapezious myocutaneous flap for reconstruction after surgery for head and neck cancer: NCI experiences.j Egypt Nat Cancer Inst 2002,14(3): 185-191
[7] Abdel-Razek E, Abuel-Ela A, Abdel-Razek A. Large Meningomyeloceles Closure with Proximally Based Fasciocutaneous Flank Flap. Egypt J Plast Reconstr. Surg 2006, 30(1): 1-5
[8] Ghozlan N, Eisa A. Reconstruction of Broad-Based Myelomeningocele Defects: A Modified Technique. Egypt J Plast Reconstr Surg 2007, 31 ( 2) : 213-219
[9] Hosseinpour M,forghani S. Primary closure of large thoracolumbar myelomeningocele with bilateral latissimus dorsi flaps. J Neurosurg Pediatrics 2009 3 : 331-333
[10] Nomori H, Hasegawa T, Kobayashi R.The "reversed" latissimus dorsi muscle flap with conditioning delay for closure of a lower thoracic tuberculous empyema. Thorac Cardiovasc Surg 1994;42(3):182-4